"Baldassar and Merla break new intellectual ground in this eminently readable and provocative book extending understanding of the nature of mobility and absence in contemporary family life. The essays ambitiously examine the intricate ways family members—including mothers and children, fathers and elders, those who move and those who stay—care for each other through processes of reciprocal exchange, across and despite distance. Theoretically brilliant and ethnographically rich, *Transnational Families, Migration and the Circulation of Care* is one of the most bold and exciting works to emerge in transnational studies in some years."

—Sarah Lamb, Brandeis University, author of *Aging and the Indian Diaspora: Cosmopolitan Families in India and Abroad*

"This is a wide-ranging and compelling study of migrant families coping with the practical and emotional difficulties of living and working across borders in communities which may be many thousands of miles apart. Modern ways of communicating (Skype, Facebook, YouTube and the like) may help, but of crucial importance are their social relationships, tried and tested in the past, but which now face the new challenges of caring transnationally."

—Ralph Grillo, University of Sussex

"This new book on care circulation and transnational family relationships expands the concept of family in contemporary societies. The stimulating selection of chapters combines a theorisation of transnational family practices with empirical studies, opening up new understandings of care, support, and socialisation over the life course across borders. The collection represents an important shift in focus from a Western notion of the nuclear family to a notion of social community involving kin and affinities within transnational settings—communities made possible through virtual technology on a global scale. The volume's central contribution will necessitate a widening of social and family policy taking into consideration consequences of global mobility."

—Ulla Björnberg, Gothenburg University

# Transnational Families, Migration and the Circulation of Care

Without denying the difficulties that confront migrants and their distant kin, this volume highlights the agency of family members in transnational processes of care, in an effort to acknowledge the transnational family as an increasingly common family form and to question the predominantly negative conceptualisations of this type of family. It re-conceptualises transnational care as a set of activities that circulates between home and host countries—across generations—and fluctuates over the life course, going beyond a focus on mother-child relationships to include multidirectional exchanges across generations and between genders. It highlights, in particular, how the sense of belonging in transnational families is sustained by the reciprocal, though uneven, exchange of caregiving, which binds members together in intergenerational networks of reciprocity and obligation, love and trust that are simultaneously fraught with tension, contest and relations of unequal power. The chapters that make up this volume cover a rich array of ethnographic case studies including analyses of transnational families who circulate care between developing nations in Africa, Latin America and Asia to wealthier nations in North America, Europe and Australia. There are also examples of intra- and extra- European, Australian and North American migration, which involve the mobility of both the unskilled and working class as well as the skilled middle and aspirational classes.

**Loretta Baldassar** is Professor in the Department of Anthropology and Sociology at the University of Western Australia and Adjunct Principal Research Fellow, School of Political and Social Inquiry, Monash University.

**Laura Merla** is a sociologist and Deputy Director of the Interdisciplinary Research Centre on Families and Sexualities (CIRFASE) at the Catholic University of Louvain (Belgium).

## Routledge Research in Transnationalism

1 **New Transnational Social Spaces**
International Migration and Transnational Companies in the Early 21st Century
*Edited by Ludger Pries*

2 **Transnational Muslim Politics**
Reimagining the Umma
*Peter G. Mandaville*

3 **New Approaches to Migration?**
Transnational Communities and the Transformation of Home
*Edited by Nadje Al-Ali and Khalid Koser*

4 **Work and Migration**
Life and Livelihoods in a Globalizing World
*Edited by Ninna Nyberg Sorensen and Karen Fog Olwig*

5 **Communities across Borders**
New Immigrants and Transnational Cultures
*Edited by Paul Kennedy and Victor Roudometof*

6 **Transnational Spaces**
*Edited by Peter Jackson, Phil Crang and Claire Dwyer*

7 **The Media of Diaspora**
*Edited by Karim H. Karim*

8 **Transnational Politics**
Turks and Kurds in Germany
*Eva Østergaard-Nielsen*

9 **Culture and Economy in the Indian Diaspora**
*Edited by Bhikhu Parekh, Gurharpal Singh and Steven Vertovec*

10 **International Migration and the Globalization of Domestic Politics**
*Edited by Rey Koslowski*

11 **Gender in Transnationalism**
Home, Longing and Belonging among Moroccan Migrant Women
*Ruba Salih*

12 **State/Nation/Transnation**
Perspectives on Transnationalism in the Asia-Pacific
*Edited by Brenda S. A. Yeoh and Katie Willis*

13 **Transnational Activism in Asia**
Problems of Power and Democracy
*Edited by Nicola Piper and Anders Uhlin*

14 **Diaspora, Identity and Religion**
New Directions in Theory and Research
*Edited by Waltraud Kokot, Khachig Tölölyan and Carolin Alfonso*

15 **Cross-Border Governance in the European Union**
*Edited by Olivier Thomas Kramsch and Barbara Hooper*

16 **Transnational Connections and the Arab Gulf**
*Edited by Madawi Al-Rasheed*

17 **Central Asia and the Caucasus**
Transnationalism and Diaspora
*Edited by Touraj Atabaki and Sanjyot Mehendale*

18 **International Migration and Security**
Opportunities and Challenges
*Edited by Elspeth Guild and Joanne van Selm*

19 **Transnational European Union**
Towards a Common Political Space
*Edited by Wolfram Kaiser with Peter Starie*

20 **Geopolitics of European Union Enlargement**
The Fortress Empire
*Edited by Warwick Armstrong and James Anderson*

21 **Rethinking Transnationalism**
The Meso-link of Organisations
*Edited by Ludger Pries*

22 **Theorising Transnational Migration**
The Status Paradox of Migration
*Boris Nieswand*

23 **Migration, Nation States, and International Cooperation**
*Edited by Randall Hansen, Jobst Koehler and Jeannette Money*

24 **Beyond Methodological Nationalism**
Research Methodologies for Cross-Border Studies
*Edited by Anna Amelina, Devrimsel D. Nergiz, Thomas Faist and Nina Glick Schiller*

25 **Transnationalism and Urbanism**
*Edited by Stefan Krätke, Kathrin Wildner, and Stephan Lanz*

26 **Transnational Marriage**
New Perspectives from Europe and Beyond
*Edited by Katharine Charsley*

27 **Transnational Politics and the State**
The External Voting Rights of Diasporas
*Jean-Michel Lafleur*

28 **Transbordering Latin Americas**
Liminal Places, Cultures, and Powers (T)Here
*Edited by Clara Irazábal*

29 **Transnational Families, Migration and the Circulation of Care**
Understanding Mobility and Absence in Family Life
*Edited by Loretta Baldassar and Laura Merla*

# Transnational Families, Migration and the Circulation of Care

## Understanding Mobility and Absence in Family Life

**Edited by Loretta Baldassar and Laura Merla**

Routledge
Taylor & Francis Group
NEW YORK LONDON

First published 2014
by Routledge
711 Third Avenue, New York, NY 10017

Simultaneously published in the UK
by Routledge
2 Park Square, Milton Park, Abingdon, Oxon OX14 4RN

*Routledge is an imprint of the Taylor & Francis Group, an informa business*



*Library of Congress Cataloging-in-Publication Data*

Transnational families, migration and the circulation of care : understanding mobility and absence in family life / edited by Loretta Baldassar and Laura Merla.
pages cm.—(Routledge research in transnationalism ; 29)
Includes bibliographical references and index.
1. Intercountry marriage. 2. Families. 3. Emigration and immigration. 4. Globalization—Social aspects. I. Baldassar, Loretta, 1965–editor of compilation. II. Merla, Laura.
HQ1032.T727 2013
306.85—dc23
2013008371

ISBN13: 978-0-415-62673-6 (hbk)
ISBN13: 978-0-203-07753-5 (ebk)

Typeset in Sabon
by IBT Global.



SUSTAINABLE FORESTRY INITIATIVE
Certified Sourcing
www.sfiprogram.org
SFI-01234
SFI label applies to the text stock

Printed and bound in the United States of America
by IBT Global.

# Contents

# Figures and Tables

## FIGURES



## TABLES

# Acknowledgments

This volume is the outcome of a productive collaboration that has benefitted from several discerning readers as well as the input of a number of seminar and conference audiences. For Baldassar, it builds on research begun with Cora Baldock and Raelene Wilding funded by the Australian Research Council. This initial project was extended and expanded to benefit enormously from the collaboration with Merla through the support of a European Union Marie Curie Outgoing International Fellowship. Merla has since continued to work on transnational families and caregiving with the financial support of the Belgian National Funds for Research (FNRS), the Belgian Federal Science Policy and a Marie Curie Career Integration Grant. Special thanks to our contributors who responded with enthusiasm, critical engagement and collegial spirits to our invitation to participate. All of the chapters benefitted from a workshop hosted by the Catholic University of Louvain with funding from the FNRS, the Institute for the Analysis of Change in Historical and Contemporary Societies (IACCHOS), the Leclerc Chair and the Special Funds for Research (FSR) Scheme.

A special and heartfelt thank you to Professor Ralph Grillo for his role as workshop discussant and, in particular, for his extraordinary generosity in reading and responding to various drafts in the course of producing this book. For constructive and incisive commentary on our work, we thank Marina Ariza, Christine Beasley, Ulla Björnberg, Paolo Boccagni, Giovanna Campani, Francesca Decimo, Florence Degavre, Gabi Dei Ottati, Angeles Escriva, Anca Gheaus, Graeme Hugo, Majella Kilkey, Sarah Lamb, Helma Lutz, Marinella Marmo, Suzan McDaniel, Stefania Giada Meda, Jane Millard, Rhacel Parreñas, Roberta Raffaetà, Wolfgang Schröer, Tiziana Torresi, Rosanna Trifiletti, Francesca Vianello, Karin Wall, Raelene Wilding, Caroline Wraith, Lana Yaroch and Minna Zechner. Special thanks to Asuncion Fresnoza-Flot for her assistance with the preparation of the bibliography and to Emanuela Sala for her work on the index.

Early drafts of the Introduction and Chapter 1 were presented at the following conferences, and the ensuing discussions with coordinators and audience participants were invaluable:

- ESF Exploratory Workshop on Rethinking Older Age: Transnational Migration, Home And Cultures Of Care, convened by Lena Näre and Katie Walsh at the Department of Social Research and Swedish School of Social Science, University of Helsinki, Finland, 23–24 August 2012.
- IMISCOE 2012 conference, 'Mobility as the New Paradigmatic Perspective in the Social Sciences', Amsterdam, 28–29 September 2012.
- International symposium, 'Transnational Aging: Current Insights and Future Challenges', Institute of Education, convened by Cornelia Schweppe and Vincent Horn, University of Mainz, Germany, 26–27 September 2012.
- ESA RN 13 Mid-term conference, 'Families, Care and Work Facing the Challenges of a Globalized World', Milano, 13–15 September 2012.
- ESA RN 35 Mid-term conference, 'Managing Migration in a World of Economic Crisis with New Profiles of Migrants', Paris, 3–5 September 2012.
- Department of Sociology Seminar Series, convened by Paolo Boccagni, University of Trento, 2 October 2012.
- Fay Gale Migration Roundtable Series, convened by Tiziana Torresi, University of Adelaide, 9 November 2012.

Thank you to our families, especially our partners and children, parents, siblings (including in-laws) and good friends, for their care and support.

# Part A

# Conceptualising Care Circulation

# Introduction

## Transnational Family Caregiving Through the Lens of Circulation

*Loretta Baldassar and Laura Merla*

> *'To investigate the different forms, orientations, and directions of care, one would need (. . .) to adopt an approach that follows longitudinally and spatially the migrant so as to capture care giving and receiving'.* (Kofman 2012, 153)

*In El Salvador, Yasmina, a lone mother of three children, struggled to provide for her family with a cleaning job. She both provided to, and received, financial and other forms of support from her mother Carlita and her brother Fausto, who also live in El Salvador. In addition, they all received regular remittances from Sara and Olga, Carlita's other children who live in the United States and Canada, respectively. In 2001, Yasmina accepted an invitation from her Belgium-based aunt (Carlita's sister) to migrate to Belgium, hoping to make a better living. Yasmina's son had recently migrated to Spain, and she left her two teenage daughters in the care of her mother. She travelled with a tourist visa and later became an undocumented migrant. The aunt financed her journey and provided her initial accommodation, but their relationship became difficult; Yasmina felt her aunt demanded too much in return, in the form of money and housework. When she found an undeclared job as a live-in domestic, Yasmina stayed at her aunt's only at weekends, where she also had to cook and clean, her aunt reminding her that this was the least she could do in repayment for her 'debt'. Living apart from her children was extremely painful. She remained in regular contact with her son and daughters and her mother, calling them as often as she could and exchanging practical and emotional support with them. She also sent them remittances, aimed at supporting both the children and their carer-grandmother. After two years, Yasmina was able to finance her daughters' move to Belgium. The girls travelled with Carlita, who had planned to spend three months in Belgium. The three women stayed at the aunt's house and were reunited with Yasmina on the weekends, but Carlita returned to El Salvador sooner than planned because her sister did not treat her well.*

*Over the next several years, Carlita regularly travelled between El Salvador and North America, dividing her time between Fausto, Olga and Sara's households, who took in turn the role of caring for their mother, taking her to the doctor and helping her in her daily activities while receiving her help in the form of babysitting, cooking and so on. Her four children supported her financially. The child with whom Carlita resided was also in charge of keeping the others informed of her health and personal situation. But now that she has become frail, at 84 years of age, Carlita spends most of her time in the United States, where she was recently granted permanent residency. Yasmina does not send her money anymore but is ready to step in if an emergency arises. She is in regular contact with her mother, whom she phones and messages on the Internet with the assistance of her daughters. Carlita is particularly keen to hear about her granddaughters, and floods Yasmina and the girls with advice. The granddaughters also send her money when an emergency arises. Yasmina deeply regrets not being able to visit her mother and siblings. Her undocumented status and the cost of flights make it impossible for her to travel outside Belgium. But she feels highly responsible for her mother's well-being, and she actively participates in the transnational family exchanges of caregiving that creates for them a network of solidarity.*

* * * *

*Viviana, a retired secretary who lives in Italy with her husband Natalio, a retired bank clerk, takes her duty as grandmother seriously, and often worries about how she can be a good grandmother even to her grandchildren who live in England, and especially to those who live furthest away in Australia. For her son and daughter, both professionals, who live close by, she helps out with regular weekly child minding after school and often prepares food for them to take home. This support is especially important to her son, whose work as a medical specialist involves spending three nights a week at a clinic a day's journey away by train. The whole family comes over for lunch every Sunday, and she has the grandchildren for extended stays during the long summer holidays. These 'local' or 'proximate' children and grandchildren assist Viviana and Natalio with all manner of practical tasks, such as the upkeep of their house and car, decisions about health care and the management of their finances, accompanying them to medical appointments and providing 'hands-on' care when they get sick, like the time they both had pneumonia and needed help with cooking and cleaning. It is important for Viviana to feel she is caring 'equally' for all her children and grandchildren, and she puts great effort into maintaining an up-to-date photo display of everyone, but especially those family members living abroad. Viviana takes the time to send special gifts to her grandchildren abroad, such as scarves she has hand-knitted, jewellery and other small trinkets.*

*Viviana describes the family as 'very close emotionally', and it has become a ritual to Skype call the Australia- and UK-based families after Sunday lunch, when all the Italy-based family members are together. She finds it difficult to Skype at other times because she prefers to have her son or grandson nearby to set up the computer and fix the connection, which is often faulty. Although both Viviana and Natalio hate flying, mainly because they do not speak much English, they make the effort to be present for the important occasions of their 'distant kin'. They attended the wedding of their daughter in Australia and the graduation of their grandson in the UK. They much prefer, however, to gift money towards the airfares of the far-away family members so they can visit them in Italy; 'that way everyone gets to see them and they get to see everyone', Viviana explains. She justifies the money spent on their visits by pointing out that she cannot provide them with the day-today care that she gives her nearby family, like child minding and cooking. For their part, the Australia- and UK-based daughters phone their mother in a weekly routine, on a different day each, but they also make additional calls whenever the urge takes them. The local children phone their parents daily. The siblings stay in regular and frequent contact with each other as well, by SMS texts and occasional phone and Skype calls, which increase around birthdays and anniversaries as well as before and after visits.*

*The UK family visits every year at Christmas, and the children in this family are old enough to visit on their own during the summer. The Australia-based family tries to visit every two or three years. All the siblings congregated together after Natalio suffered a serious stroke. The Australian daughter stayed for two weeks to help her mother care for him, and after she returned home, the UK daughter arrived to assist for a further two weeks. The Italy-based children have also visited their siblings abroad, and the Italy-based daughter made several trips to the UK to support her sister when she required short stays in hospital. The Italy-based family members have, on occasion, elected to send a family representative to Australia to attend a special event, including a first holy communion and a special birthday. All the Italy-based grandchildren are planning extended visits to their UK aunt to improve their English. They stay in touch with their cousins by regular Facebook posts and SMS text messages. They also Skype and phone each other to organise the details of their visits. Despite this constant and regular contact, Viviana feels the absence of her far-away daughters and their families deeply. She remembers them in her nightly prayers, and they are among her first thoughts when she wakes each morning.*

We chose to start this volume with two very different case studies.[1] Yasmina's family is in many ways exemplary of the situation of the female domestic migrants featured in the care chains literature, who are subject to discrimination and deprivation of basic rights in their society of destination,[2] and Viviana's family, whose middle-class members occupy a much more privileged position in both home and host settings. These case studies emphasise some of the key features, as well as some of the varieties and inequalities, of the transnational family forms presented in this edited collection. They highlight, in particular, the way family members from different socioeconomic and cultural backgrounds care for each other through a process of asymmetrical reciprocal exchange, across and despite the distance that separates them, and the way that care *circulates* between them. These cases also exemplify the three main propositions that shape this volume. The idea that care circulates within transnational family networks is central to this book, and this chapter examines the conceptual implications of its application to the analysis of transnational families. The care circulation framework that we are advancing helps to elucidate a further objective, which is to emphasise the importance of theorising mobility and absence as common features of family life. It also provides an analytical lens that allows us to examine the full range of family forms that have, to date, been compartmentalised in the existing literature between analyses of the south-north chains of domestic and care-sector workers and studies of a broader set of transnational family relations and migration types.

With increased mobility and improvements in both travel and communication technologies, more and more people are experiencing transnational family lives. Whether pushed or pulled out of homelands in search of safe asylum, better economic futures or improved lifestyles, increasing numbers of people are separated from their family by distance and national borders. Those family members who 'stay behind' or 'stay put' (as it were) in their place of birth or ancestral homeland also become part of social relationships stretched across time and place, even though they might never actually relocate or move at all. We propose that a focus on the disparate trajectories of care circulation helps us to better understand mobility and absence in family life, so that we might theorise transnational families as contemporary family forms in their own right. Absence, in this context, refers specifically to physical absence, and each of the chapters in this volume, like the case studies above, are examples of the various ways that a sense of 'co-presence' (Urry 2003) can be maintained despite separation. Indeed, we begin with the premise that, despite being separated by distance and over time, members of transnational families maintain a sense of 'family-hood' (Bryceson and Vuorela 2002a, 3), in that they continue to feel they 'belong' to a family even though they may not see each other or be physically co-present often or for extended periods of time. As Baldassar, Baldock and Wilding (2007, 13) write, 'the resulting idea of the "transnational family" is intended to capture the growing awareness that members of families retain their sense of collectivity and kinship in spite of being spread across multiple nations'.

We wish to highlight, in particular, how the sense of belonging in transnational families is sustained by the reciprocal, though uneven, exchange of caregiving, which we argue is a key feature of the practices and processes associated with 'doing family' (Morgan, 1996). Transnational caregiving, just like caregiving in all families (whether separated by migration or not),[3] binds members together in intergenerational networks of reciprocity and obligation, love and trust, that are simultaneously fraught with tension, contest and relations of unequal power.[4] We theorise the exchange of care in families (broadly defined) as inherently reciprocal and asymmetrical, governed by the 'norm of generalised reciprocity'—the *expectation* that the giving of care must ultimately be reciprocated, although it may not be realised. A pertinent example of this norm is what family and gerontology studies refer to as the generational contract, where parents care for their young, who in turn care for them when they age (Bengtson and Achenbaum 1993).[5] Anthropologists distinguish between various types of reciprocity, including the generalised form (Sahlins 1965; Lévi Strauss 1969), which refers to those exchanges that are not immediate and equivalent, in the sense that people give care without measuring exactly the amount they receive, but with the expectation and obligation that care will be returned to them. This said, as evident in the cases of both Yasmina and Viviana, family members often carefully monitor these exchanges, and they are governed by the multiple and constantly 'negotiated family commitments',[6] intimate and unequal power relations and private culture (Epstein 1978) that characterise family life. As this care is given and returned at different times and to varying degrees across the life course, the care could be described as *circulating* among family members over time as well as distance.

While the flow of care is by no means even and harmonious and is subject to constant negotiation by members, of factors both internal and external to the family, we see caregiving and its management as constitutive of transnational family life (Morgan 2011b). This does not mean that families are invariably a source of support and succour. While families are valued for providing security and fulfilment, they can also produce disappointment and even trauma. The feminist, family and gender studies literatures emphasise that an analysis of caregiving activity must be sensitive to the unevenness of reciprocal exchange, including the withholding and limiting of care (Kergoat 2000).[7] As in the case of proximate families, not all transnational family members give and receive care equally, and some—typically women—shoulder a far greater burden of care. While the circulation of care involves reciprocal exchanges between family members, both the transnational and local care burdens fall most heavily on women, who generally receive less than they give (Ryan 2007). In this context, care and the ability to exchange it can be considered a type of resource or form of social capital (Goulbourne et al 2010, Zontini & Reynolds 2007) that is unevenly distributed within families, subject to cultural notions of gender and identity roles relating to rights and obligations to care, which intersect with, and interrelate to, the historical care regimes of the various nation-states and communities in which families reside.[8] Here we draw on Wellman's (1988, 102) theory of network ties, which he defines as 'asymmetrically reciprocal, differing in content and intensity', including between close relationships characterised by strong ties. He warns against 'treating all units as if they had the same resources, all ties as if they were symmetrical, and the contents of all ties as if they were equivalent'(Wellman 1988, 20); only in this way can social structure be taken seriously into account, 'by studying directly how patterns of ties allocate resources in a social system' (Wellman 1988, 20).

Thus, we define care circulation as governed by 'generalised asymmetrical reciprocity' within transnational kinship networks. Far from being the private concern of family members, these caregiving exchanges are embedded in the broader political economy of migration and transnationalism. Indeed, the concept of care in feminist and gender studies is a highly politicised one, borne of the need to value the act of caring as unpaid *work* and to recognise caregiving as a fundamental, though generally invisible and unaccounted for feature of a nation's gross domestic product (GDP) (Leira and Saraceno 2006).[9] Similarly, the unpaid and more intimate dimensions of transnational lives, in particular of 'kin-work' (di Leonardo 1984) and caregiving, are often overlooked altogether, and their role in the more 'public' political economy of migration and diaspora is regularly undervalued (Gardner & Grillo 2002).[10] An analysis of transnational care circulation makes evident the links and intersections between kinship and economic and political motivations in migratory moves, highlighting the role of family and the domestic sphere in sustaining diaspora ties (Olwig 2002).[11] It also reveals the powerful non-economic factors that are highly influential in decision making about transnational movement and migration (e.g., Ackers & Dwyer 2002).[12] The various ethnographic case studies that comprise this volume highlight how it is primarily family relations as well as friendship networks and even the loose ties of associates—characterised by nonmarket-driven 'moral' and 'informal' economies—that represent a central motivation for migration and mobility and often comprise the infrastructures and structures (albeit informal) of transnational social fields.

Arguably, the most important literature to examine the negotiation of care within a global economic perspective, and in particular, its unequal distribution in transnational families, is the care chains literature (Hochschild 2000, 2005; Parreñas 2001b, 2005a, 2005b; Yeates 2009, 2012). This body of research specifically focuses on the commodification and political economy of care in 'south-north' female domestic labour flows, as exemplified by the case of Yasmina. Our focus in this volume is different, albeit complementary, with an emphasis on the asymmetrically reciprocal flows of caregiving located in kinship and moral economies of care. We offer a more detailed exploration of the intersections between the frameworks of care chains and care circulation in Chapter 1. Our main arguments are summarised here by way of introduction. The care chains literature tends to focus on care exchanges between two people who are linked together along a chain of 'dyads', with care flowing in one direction in exchange for financial returns that flow in the other. The care circulation lens broadens out the trajectories of these dyadic exchanges to consider the entire network of relationships around which care flows. This broader perspective avoids the risk inherent in a focus on one-to-one relationships, which tend to ignore the 'social structural context within which dyadic ties operate' (Wellman 1988, 36; Ryan 2007). There are important synergies here with Kofman's (2012) argument for a wider framework than is afforded by the focus on care that dominates the gendered migration literatures. She points out that care is but one element of a broader set of processes of social reproduction, namely, the 'different activities undertaken throughout the life cycle to sustain and maintain households, some of which are multi-sited and multi-national'. We agree that there is a need for analytical frameworks that can better capture the intersections between different types of migration, labour and family life that are more complex than the analyses of chains of care. Kofman recommends the notion of 'global householding' as a way of highlighting how 'economic and social resources are accumulated and deployed and how different types of migration enable such resources to be embedded and disembedded across space and time'. We return to this discussion in the next chapter. Suffice it here to say that we think a care circulation lens, with its focus on the practices and processes of the asymmetrically reciprocal exchanges of transnational caregiving, offers a productive way to trace and retrace the links and connections between members across distance and time, which constitute the workings of 'global households'.

In addition to a consideration of the wider network and processes of relationships and households, the care circulation framework enables us to expand the lens of analysis of migration and caregiving to include the full variety of family types and migrations. The asymmetrical character of care circulation not only concerns intrafamilial relationships, but also the transnational family forms that contain them. There is no such thing as 'the' transnational family, understood as a uniform family form defined by constant characteristics. Transnational families are as diverse as geographically proximate families, representing a wide variety of socioeconomic, educational, cultural, ethnic and religious backgrounds, and with extremely different levels of social, economic, cultural and symbolic capital (Bourdieu 1986), in both their home and host societies. The migration literature usually makes a distinction between them, based on class and migration status. On the one hand, there are the families of professional migrants and 'cosmopolitan' elites who 'seem to move more by choice and be in a better position to negotiate their connections, their nationalities, and benefits associated with their choice of a national residence. . . . The symbolic capital of education and language enable them to move freely, offering relatively easier access to border crossing and citizenship' (Bryceson and

Vuorela 2002a, 8).[13] On the other hand, there are the families of refugees and economic migrants like Yasmina, who, especially if they are poorly educated with limited language skills, tend to be 'pushed into transnational lifestyles by necessity because they cannot gain a secure economic foothold in their home country' or their host society (Levitt and Jaworsky 2007, 133). These labour migrants often lack 'the human and cultural capital to take advantage of opportunities in two settings' and are subject to discrimination in their access to employment and citizenship (ibid).

Between these two extremes are 'middle-class' migrants and their families, like Viviana's, who have access to enough economic, social and cultural capital within their extended networks to have a relative degree of control over their mobilities and transnational relationships. Despite their growing numbers, these families have been largely unexamined. Scott (2006), for example, argues that skilled international migration has 'become a "normal" middle-class activity rather than something exclusively confined to an economic elite', but that the resultant empirical and theoretical complexities have been overlooked.[14] Processes of deskilling and downward social mobility in host societies, further compounded by the current global economic crisis, make these class distinctions even more complex. These are related to the ethnostratification of labour markets, 'whereby immigrants are employed in the lowest positions, not because of a lack of qualifications but rather, among other reasons, due to the discriminatory practices of employers and the state itself' (Solé and Parella 2003, 124).[15]

These class and migration-type distinctions are also reflected to a large extent in the study of the mobilities of care, which to date has been divided between the more prominent global care chains research, which focuses on formal and informal migrant care workers (mainly female domestics) who leave their children behind (also referred to as the transnational mothering or parenting literatures), and the increasing research on transnational families, which examines care relations between a wider set of family members and extends the study of caregiving to all categories of migrants. To draw on Viviana's case once again, her family's mobilities represent what might be termed 'north-north' professional migration. These types of skilled migratory movements, including flows of students and graduates, have increased with globalisation in general and the current economic crisis in particular. Targeted migration, including preferences for business and professional entrants as well as labour and domestic workers, are facilitating the *mobility*, and more specifically the *circulation* (Agunias 2006), of individual workers rather than their settlement. These schemes are competing with family reunification as major sources of migrants in developed nations across the globe (Grillo 2008; Flavell et al. 2007; Hawthorne 2005), with a resulting increase in the dispersal of family members and the need for all types of families to exchange care across distance. The various types of transnational families are unequal in their access to the resources that support and sustain the transnational circulation of care, depending on their members' positioning vis-à-vis the migration, welfare, gendered care and working-time regimes in both home and host societies (Kilkey and Merla 2013), which are in turn influenced by a series of important interrelated factors, including class, gender and ethnicity (Lutz and Palenga-Möllenbeck 2011). The chapters that make up this volume offer a rich array of case studies, including analyses of the inequalities between transnational families who circulate care between developing nations in Africa, Latin America and Asia to wealthier nations in North America, Europe and Australia. There are also examples of intra- and extra-European, Australian and North American migration and care circulation, which involve the mobility of both the unskilled and working class as well as the skilled middle and aspirational classes.

We believe the exchange of care in transnational family settings takes on a special importance because of the lack of other ways to express family solidarity and belonging. Care circulation therefore provides an especially productive lens with which to examine transnational family practices and processes, and it has important analytical and methodological implications. By tracing the movement of care and monitoring the unevenness of its flows, including when it is lacking or abandoned, a focus on care circulation helps to identify all of the people who are involved in the social relationships that manage caring relationships. The resulting 'map' of caregiving actors and activity provides a detailed account of one of the central ways family relationships are constituted and maintained in transnational settings. It also brings to light the many ways family and caregiving activities intersect with the more commonly studied dimensions of migration, including economic, political, community and settlement. Mapping this caregiving activity requires an examination of the lives of family members in (and between) the various places they reside, and so begs a multi-sited methodology (Hage 2005; Falzon 2009), as well as posing the challenge of researching social and family life within the virtual world of new technologies (Miller and Slater 2000).[16] Equally importantly, a focus on the circulation of care helps to highlight the involvement not only of women, the traditional carers, but also of those actors who are less visible in traditional conceptualisations of care exchange, including men, children, extended family members, fictive kin and others. It also readjusts the focus from a preoccupation with the migrant as the provider of care to acknowledge how migrants are also the receivers of care. A major aim of this volume, then, is to examine the conceptualisation of care exchanges in transnational families in terms of the framework of circulation.

The lens of circulation not only helps to capture all the actors involved in family life but also the full extent of their care activity, including practical, emotional and symbolic, that defines their membership in a family. For this reason, we apply a broad definition of both family and caregiving. In line with recent social and cultural theory, we conceptualise family, household and home as processes (both ideational and structural) in which everyday practices of caregiving, 'emotion work' and intimacy are central (e.g., Duncombe and Marsden 1993).[17] Our definition of family includes both nuclear and extended types whose members are actively engaged in family survival and maintenance, ranging from those whose involvement is extensive and constant to those whose roles are more marginal. We recognise, too, that these roles and the extent of engagement can change over time and the life-course. For this reason, our definition of caregiving includes a wide variety of care exchanges, from the direct provision of support described as 'hands on' or 'caring for' that can only be delivered when people are physically co-present, to the more emotional support of 'caring about' (Fisher and Tronto, 1990) as well as the coordination of support provided by others (Kilkey and Merla 2013), both of which can take place through virtual forms of communication and co-presence (Madianou and Miller 2012; Baldassar 2008b). We draw on the classic work on (local) families by Finch (1989a), who identified five types of caregiving or 'mutual support' that are exchanged between family members, including: economic, accommodation, personal ('hands on'), practical and child care, and emotional and moral. All these types of care can be exchanged in transnational settings but to varying degrees and subject to a variety of factors, including gender, ethnic, class and power hierarchies as well as the cultural and structural histories of welfare regimes, all of which are examined in some detail in this volume.

In applying the lens of circulation to highlight how care circulates around a wide network of friends and family, crisscrossing both local and national settings, we are not suggesting that transnational caregiving is uncomplicated and easy, or even *as* 'easy' as in situations of propinquity. Rather, our aim is to better understand the practices and processes involved, and to acknowledge that virtual forms of care exchange play an important role in a growing number of families. In other words, of fundamental importance to our argument is the view that not all caregiving has to be embodied or proximate in order to qualify as care. This said, we are not suggesting that virtual forms of care are equivalent to embodied forms, but instead that it is the quality of the relationships, rather than the form or mode of caregiving, that is important. How individuals experience and understand this quality is greatly dependent on cultural and historical context. Yet the relevant literatures tend to adopt a Western normative ideal of physical proximity for healthy caregiving relationships, a point we discuss in some detail in the following chapter. In general, as is evident in the care chains literature described earlier, researchers have assumed that in order to care for each other effectively, family members must live in close proximity (e.g., Rossi & Rossi 1990).[18] Despite their growing numbers and diverse forms, transnational families tend to be stigmatised—by governments, public opinion (particularly in sending societies) as well as by some scholars—as somehow deficient or at risk, fragmented, broken and under strain (a point also made by Zentgraf and Chinchilla 2012). Nursing and gerontology studies in particular, but also studies of family and gender more broadly, have a relatively narrow definition of care as 'hands on' and therefore dependent on physical proximity (Leira and Saraceno 2006). In part, this focus on the embodied physicality of care was an important outcome of feminist approaches within these disciplines, which sought to recognise and appreciate the extensive skills and activities that make up caregiving as a significant type of *work* and contribution made primarily by women that, as noted above, is all too often ignored (Twigg 2000; Mol 2008). Feminist political theory has since broadened this debate to consider issues such as an ethics of care and embodied citizenship (see e.g., Beasley and Bacchi 2007; Engster 2004). However, these works tend to presume proximity is essential and generally do not consider broader notions of care in transnational contexts (but see Gheaus 2011).

This ideal of proximity leads to the consequent assumption that distance and absence automatically prohibit the exchange of caregiving. This volume seeks to interrogate this scepticism and the prevailing negative notions about migration and family life by bringing together leading authorities who have each conducted fine-grained research on this issue. We invited our collaborators to respond to the following questions: Is a care circulation framework an effective way to address the theoretical, methodological and policy implications of family mobilities in our contemporary world? In the vast array of family arrangements across the globe, is it possible to imagine the transnational family as an increasingly common and distinct mode of living? Does this very argument undermine the importance of highlighting the difficulties and discontinuities of transnational family lives?

## CHAPTER OVERVIEW

The ideas about circulation that we are presenting in this volume are the result of a fruitful and engaging dialogue with the various contributors to this book, who were all enthusiastic about applying the notion of care circulation to their own field of research and to examine the role of absence and separation in family life. Their reflections have contributed to the development of our initial thoughts into a fresh lens through which to analyse the mobilities of care. In the following chapter (**Chapter 1, by Baldassar and Merla**), we locate the care circulation framework within the broader literature on migration and families, highlighting the synergies with related concepts such as care chains, transnationalism and circulation in migration studies, as well as the conceptual implications of applying a care circulation lens to the mobilities of care. Part B of this book comprises four chapters that examine the 'care circulation' framework and further develop it conceptually, theoretically and empirically. This examination of the migration-family care nexus highlights the importance of taking into account the structurally diverse, asymmetrical, situated and gendered ways in which care may circulate within transnational family networks. The four chapters that make up Part C focus on the gendered experiences of absence and separation in transnational parenting and stress the importance of moving beyond the mother–child dyad as well as of challenging Western constructions of parent–child relations. Part D of this book comprises three chapters that each applies the framework of circulation to different types of migration flows and social strata, including students, the middle class and professionals. These contributions consider the impact of relative wealth and access to opportunities on the circulation of care in transnational families as well as their implications for migrant integration and settlement.

Part B begins with **Chapter 2, by Karin Wall and Claudio Bolzman**. The authors bring together the concepts of care circulation and family configuration (Widmer and Jallinoja 2008) and connect them by using the notion of *care configuration*, which they define as the family network of interdependent close persons as it relates to caregiving and support. Drawing on a wealth of ethnographic data from various migrant groups in Portugal and Switzerland, they chart the diversity of transnational families and the variety of actors involved in care circuits. Of central importance to their analysis is the application of a life-course perspective when analysing the mobilities of care, to show how actual practices, as well as the meanings and affects that are attached to them, vary to a great extent over time. The experience of physical separation and the feelings attached to having to deal with physical absence are not static, but change over time, depending not only on the objective situation of the migrant and his or her relatives, but also on subjective aspects including, among others, changes in migration and settlement projects, mutual expectations as well as the definition of self and of appropriate parenting at various stages.

**Chapter 3, by Paola Bonizzoni and Paolo Boccagni**, also identifies 'lifecycle' and 'time' as major variables for the study of care circulation. They provide an excellent overview of the current scholarship of transnational parenting with the aim of identifying the key themes and issues that are pertinent to the concepts of 'care' and circulation'. In doing so, the chapter identifies an important gap in the literature, namely, the experience of *caregivers* and the broader social context within which the caregiving, parenting and childhoods of transnational families take place. The authors employ the notion of care circulation to examine the ways in which the needs of children, parents and caregivers change over time in response to new circumstances, resources and opportunities, as well as constraints, giving much-needed attention, in particular, to the changing expectations, feelings and practices of children as they age.

Their contribution is followed by **Marina Ariza's Chapter 4** and her important analysis of the way diverse social spaces produce different conditions for the circulation of care. Based on a comparison of transnational mothering at various stages of the life course in Mexican and Dominican families living in the United States and Spain, this chapter highlights the way diverse migratory and security policies have a significant impact on the prospects for family reunion and how these in turn influence the social and affective experience of distance in transnational families. Contrasting Mexican and Dominican case studies is particularly interesting, as these groups differ in terms of family structures (highly stable, with predominantly male-headed households vs. highly unstable, with a predominance of female-headed households) and migratory patterns (male-headed and undocumented to the United States vs. female-headed and documented to Spain). Ariza's fine-grained comparative analysis makes a compelling case for the importance of taking into consideration the inequalities and asymmetries of care circulation in transnational contexts, in particular as they relate to migratory policies, gender, generation and ethnicity. Concluding Part B is **Laura Merla's Chapter 5**, which addresses the implications of mobilities and care circulation for social policy by 'situating' (Kilkey and Merla 2013) the circulation of care within institutional contexts. The author discusses the interrelations between institutional contexts and the capacity to circulate care, cultural constructions of appropriate care and the negotiation of family commitments. Drawing on the experiences of Latin American migrants in Belgium and Australia, as well as on the various contributions to this book, this chapter helps better understand inequalities in the capacity to circulate care that arise from institutional contexts while highlighting that the circulation of care itself can increase the agency of transnational family members by helping them overcome obstacles to their participation in family solidarity.

Taken together, the four chapters of Part B guard against the risk of presenting a uniform and static vision of care circulation in transnational families. They also highlight how transnational caregiving must be understood not as an activity of individuals or families alone but as a function of relationships between agents and social institutions within and across both home and host settings.[19] The case studies and literature review they present reveal how 'the processes of transnational caregiving are negotiated at the intersections of individual choice within what might be called micro patterns of kinship and obligation as well as within the more formal structures and infrastructures (or absence of them) of relevant services, technologies and resources at macro-state and meso-community levels' (Baldassar 2008a, 270). The macro factors that influence transnational caregiving include access to communication technologies, travel visas and health insurance, the social and migration policies governing settlement and immigrant integration including welfare services and employment and state provision of care services in both home and host countries. Meso factors include the community and voluntary associations that support (or impede) practices of transnational caregiving, the relevance of networks of co-nationals over time and the trajectories of 'community' settlement. Micro factors refer to family and personal histories and lifecycles, including the changing ways in which migration is understood. All these levels are informed by cultural and gendered notions of appropriate care, which influence kin relations as well as community and state provisions (and vice versa). Key questions to arise from this discussion include the interconnectedness of these 'levels', how much influence they exert on each other, how they are influenced by transnational family contexts and what particular mix of support they, in combination, provide. For instance, Merla highlights in her chapter the transformative potential of care circulation, which not only involves the mobility of people and caring but also of moral orders and gendered care cultures, which can enter into tension with local family regimes and lead to transformations both within transnational families as well as in the societies of destination and origin.

The notion of circulation captures both the way care is exchanged between family members—the manner and form of care exchanges—and the mobilities of people, goods, ideas and services in a globalised world. Part C revisits transnational parenting and labour migration flows, the traditional terrain of global care chains analysis, by challenging the dominant Western imaginary of mother–child proximity and analysing the mobilities of care beyond the mother–child dyad. The chapters in Part C underline the importance of taking into account local family structures, kinship systems and normative constructions of physical proximity. In **Chapter 6, Karen Fog Olwig** examines how family and kinship are constructed and reconstructed through the circulation of care in the context of Caribbean migration, and how this care circulation shapes, and is shaped by, notions of relatedness and the family networks associated with them. This chapter represents a vivid illustration of the lived experiences of migration and care and its evolution over the life course by giving voice to children, adults and elderly people. Through careful attention to historical and cultural contexts, the author explains how the migration of women from the lower classes is part of a system of circulation of care that is an integral and accepted aspect of family and kinship in Caribbean societies. Fog Olwig's detailed ethnographic account also reveals how the local population, through its participation in missionary religious churches and associations, is being exposed to dominant Western ideologies concerning the fundamental importance of the *proximate* nuclear family and the *intimate* mother–child tie. These ideas about appropriate family roles and relationships are changing the way educators, religious practitioners and welfare officials in the Caribbean evaluate transnational families. Left-behind children and stay-behind kin are being confronted with value judgments that challenge their notions about the appropriateness of migration and the absence of family members.

In **Chapter 7, Miranda Poeze and Valentina Mazzucato** present their study of Ghanaian transnational families, which foregrounds the children's experience of being geographically separated from their biological parents. They also highlight the importance of taking into account family norms from migrant-sending countries in order to understand how transnational parenting may affect children left behind. The authors show that the experience of separation is partly shaped by expectations regarding appropriate fathering and mothering in the homelands and can be facilitated by norms such as child fostering or social parenthood, which imply certain parenting ideals that are not accepted within the dominant Western family model. Children's feelings are also influenced by the *way* care is circulated and enacted, as well as by the history of relations with parents before migration. By focusing on children and their diverse experiences, the authors show that children, while going through a range of positive and negative feelings about their parents' migration, can be active agents in shaping this relationship.

These two chapters give voice to the usually invisible actors of care circuits, such as children and elderly people. As we argue in Part A of this volume, the application of a care circulation framework involves moving beyond Western-centred constructions of 'the family' as a nuclear household by taking into account wider sets of relationships as well as recognising the multiplicity of family forms. The chapters comprising Part C are particularly useful in shifting the focus from a concentration on parent–child and/or spousal relationships alone, to an analysis of extended family networks, which can include members related not only by blood ties but also by affinities. This is in line with the argument that researchers should not focus solely on specific dyadic relationships, but must always be aware of the ways in which these are embedded in larger networks of relationships (Widmer et al. 2008; Wellman 1988). A focus on the broader circulation of care between multiple family members helps to shift attention from women as the prime movers and victims in a transnational (market-defined) care system towards a broader view of gender relations and social reproduction within transnational family caring processes. It forces us to examine the dynamics of the dialectical relationship between structure and action in this particular set of relations, and it provides a useful frame through which to revisit key concepts in the study of family, mobility and care, such as care chains.

So far, men and fathers have largely been excluded from studies of parent–child relations in transnational settings, and the chapters by Fresnoza-Flot and by Kilkey directly address this gap. Drawing on the framework of circulation, in **Chapter 8, Asuncion Fresnoza-Flot** contributes to better understanding men's experience of mobility and separation by focusing on left-behind husbands and sons of Filipino migrant women in France. The author's ethnographic work in the Philippines reveals that these two generations of men are actively involved in the local and transnational circulation of material, symbolic and affective care, although their level of engagement does vary. Key elements influencing fathers' and sons' caring activities include the availability of women's care in the household, the age of the children and the level of female support to male carers. These findings nuance the idea that care labour is exclusively 'feminine' in Filipino transnational families while also confirming that men's caring is contingent on their wives, sisters and daughters. Concluding Part C is **Majella Kilkey's Chapter 9**, which seeks to foreground fatherly care in transnational families by examining the experiences of recent Polish migrant men in the UK through a fathering lens. The understanding and meaning of care and masculinity are transformed as care circulates between fathers and children. The data reveal the complex ways in which fathering norms around breadwinning and active/involved fathering are reworked in the context of father migration and transnational fathering, a process in many ways similar to women's redefinition of their mothering role in a migration context. This suggests that breadwinning or financial support should be acknowledged as an important dimension of care in (transnational) families. Kilkey also identifies what she calls 'counter-circulatory forces', which include the fathers' positioning as migrants in the UK labour market and their access to time and money, and more individualised factors such as the stage in the family lifecycle, the age of children and the quality of personal relationships.

As discussed earlier, one of the aims of adopting a care circulation perspective is to offer a framework that is pertinent to all types of transnational families and migrations, in order to bring together the current separation between those studies that mainly focus on domestic labour migration and transnational mothering and employ a care chains perspective, and those studies that look at wider sets of relationships and include not only economic but also skilled, professional and student migration. These particular migration flows are featured in Part D of this book. The experience of transnational family life is affecting a growing number as well as 'types' of families and north-north flows are increasingly relevant.[20] The current global economic crisis is likely to lead to a resurgence in emigration from European countries like Italy, Spain and Ireland, including young graduates and professionals (OECD 2012). Along with the significant migratory flows from 'south' to 'north', there are increasing 'north-north' and even 'north-south' flows (Solimano 2009). Thus, we argue that there is a growing need to better understand the transnational lives of these relative elites, some of whom are not particularly wealthy, (although they are likely to have families in the homeland who can support them), but are rich in the social and cultural capital that can enhance opportunities and life chances (Zontini 2010). Care flows concern economic migrants and refugees, as well as affluent, transnational elites, but the capacity of these various categories of migrants to circulate care across borders varies significantly. What we argue in this volume is that the asymmetrical reciprocal exchange of caregiving is a key element that constitutes family membership and facilitates a shared sense of family-hood despite absence and distance, whatever the social class or migration type involved. This does not mean that all transnational families and, within them, all family members, are equal in their capacity and level of involvement in caring circuits, even in relatively wealthy families. As noted earlier, care and the ability to exchange it is a resource and form of social capital that is unevenly distributed within and across families.

The distribution and circulation of care as a resource is a central theme in **Tracey Reynolds and Elisabetta Zontini's Chapter 10**, in which they investigate the interrelations between care circulation and social and cultural capital in Italian and Caribbean families based in the UK. They highlight how inequalities in terms of gender, ethnicity, language, generation, socio-economic and migration status can affect the levels and forms of social and cultural capital related to transnational care flows. Caribbean and Italian migrants experience inequality in their access to the resources necessary for receiving and providing formal and informal care, mainly because they lack insider knowledge of the caring sector and appropriate social connections. The authors identify the existence of 'key players', 'cultural mediators' and 'cultural gatekeepers' who occupy a privileged position within Caribbean and Italian community and family networks because their professional and educational backgrounds help them develop the cultural capital needed to facilitate their access to social care resources. They show that care circulated in transnational families can function as cultural and social resources that contribute to strengthening first- and second-generation migrants' sense of belonging to their local and transnational communities and maintain bridging and bonding networks (Putnam et al. 1993) across geographical as well as generational divides. For instance, second- and third-generation migrants who regularly use new communication technologies to keep in touch with distant relatives develop lateral kin relations that would otherwise have been lost. Their detailed case studies show that transnational kin and community networks can be mobilised to support a variety of initiatives including 'return' migration and visits to the homeland as well as to access the contacts needed to create small business and transnational business ties that lead to social mobility.

The quest for social mobility is a central motivation in the migration experiences of the Indian families in Australia discussed by **Supriya Singh and Anuja Cabraal in Chapter 11**. The authors draw on detailed ethnographic data on the circulation of remittances to compare and contrast the perception and experiences of Indian student migrants recently arrived in Melbourne and first- and second-generation economic Indian migrants already settled there. As in Reynolds and Zontini's chapter, the authors reflect on relations between the generations to show how family ties and connections are utilised as resources and capital that circulate between home and host settings, in this case with the aim of supporting young migrants to attain the middle-class life they are accustomed to, but find increasingly difficult to maintain, in India. A key conceptual contribution of this chapter is the argument that remittances must be seen as an important form of transnational care that flow in both directions. Their contribution highlights how transnational caring is influenced by a group's migration experience, life stage and generational changes. The Indian students, in particular, are providers but also mainly receivers of financial support—representing a two-way flow of money captured by the notion of 'boomerang' remittances, which challenges the prevailing view that remittances constitute a one-way flow from migrants to their home communities and families. The authors argue that an analysis of the circulation of care makes the two-way—circular—flows of remittances visible.

Interestingly, while the students and their families of origin are perhaps best defined as middle or upper middle class in India, their class position in Australia is more ambiguous because of their precarious student status, their tendency to be employed in working-class jobs in the taxi and service station industries and their difficulty in finding work in their chosen professions, even if they manage to successfully complete higher degrees. These aspirational students and their relatives use transnational mobility and the circulation of care as a resource for increasing economic, social and cultural capital that will benefit the whole family. It is expected that the student migrants will return the care they receive from their parents when they graduate, find suitable employment and become cosmopolitan elites. The authors underline how a focus on, and broader framing of, money circuits in transnational families highlight the intersections between the flow of 'the very personal money of family remittances, the community nature of diaspora philanthropy and the migrant dimensions of foreign direct investment'. This chapter offers a particularly pertinent example of the way the moral economy of care, in this case, through the flow of remittances, is linked to the broader political economy of migrant communities and the labour market (see also Zelizer 2005a, 2005b). It is also an example of the circulation of care in contexts quite distinct from, although comparable to, the classic global domestic care chains.

**Chapter 12 by Loretta Baldassar and Raelene Wilding** deals with the relatively more affluent transnational families of skilled and professional migrants in Australia, who have considerable access to financial, educational, health and employment resources but cannot afford to employ domestic workers, a practice that is not generally well regarded in Australia. These families participate in global care circuits that are quite different from those defined by the commodification of chains of care. Their caregiving concerns are largely focused on ageing parents and other extended kin connections in the homeland and are met through the circulation of informal, unpaid support between members, particularly women, within the family. Their relative access to the resources they need to exchange care makes the management of distance and absence easier than in less privileged families. But juggling the demands of local and transnational family, and meeting the time pressures and financial costs of both, present important tensions and difficulties that differ according to the gender, generation and cultural notions of appropriate family roles, as well as the levels and types of care available in the home and host countries. This contribution fills a gap in the literature by addressing the relative absence of analyses of middle-class and privileged families in transnational migration studies and by critiquing the often overly simplistic representation of women 'in the north'.

## CONCLUSION

There is an argument for considering transnational families as people practicing caregiving in deterritorialised contexts, and the framework of circulation might similarly invoke a sense of fluidity unencumbered by borders or boundaries. However, as the various chapters in this volume show, all migrants and their transnational family members are located in particular places at particular times, and their caregiving practices are variously affected by this 'territorialisation'.[21] As Yasmina and Viviana's stories show, transnational families must negotiate the expectations and regulations of (at least) two nation-states, often including the complicated 'borders' created by language and culture. In addition, as there are very few transnational structures, and even fewer that are designed specifically to facilitate transnational caregiving (e.g., reciprocal health care agreements and access to dual citizenship), these practices are organised by the, largely informal, structures of kinship and community, in particular the sense of obligation to engage in reciprocal care exchanges. Notions of obligation are debated within families as well as more broadly within communities, both local and national, and are influenced by and in turn influence existing and historical patterns of social structures and service provision in the countries of relevance (Grillo 2008).

Migration creates transnational families by putting distance between family members. This distance is thought to create broken and fragmented family ties. If, however, we were to concentrate on the transnational social fields and the virtual (and other forms of) co-presence created by the reciprocal exchange of communication and caregiving between transnational family members, we might be better able to examine these particular family forms more objectively. In order to begin to see transnational families as destigmatised family forms, in the sense that actors increasingly 'routinely' live their lives 'together across distance' and have developed practices to deal with the challenges this poses, we need to look beyond or transcend the conceptual (as well as the actual) road block presented by the separation inherent in the migration process. Partly, this is a question of challenging normative understandings of the delivery of care being dependent on physical proximity as well as rethinking our conceptualisation of caregiving and co-presence more broadly. In this volume, we suggest that one way to better account for the dominating role that notions of distance and absence have had on our understanding of transnational family life is to highlight the asymmetrical reciprocity and inherent circularity of both migration and transnational family processes. Transnational family exchanges, particularly those relating to caregiving, are defined by their (asymmetrical) reciprocal circularity. Further, the concept of circulation helps us to think of migration in terms of the family lifecycle as a dynamic set of processes across the life course, rather than a momentous event in time that damages family connectedness.

Care circulation can be defined as the reciprocal, multidirectional and asymmetrical exchange of care that fluctuates over the life course within transnational family networks subject to the political, economic, cultural and social contexts of both sending and receiving societies. The perspective of care circulation we are advancing is purposefully quite broad and 'flexible' and is meant to point to beliefs and practices about caring embedded in relationships wider than the nuclear family, which in turn are shaped and constrained by the broader (macro) socio-structural context in transnational settings. In recognising how families actively and effectively manage distance and separation, we are not suggesting that virtual forms of caregiving can easily be equated with proximate forms nor are we advocating that governments can abandon their responsibilities to support the reunification of migrant family members. Without a doubt, managing the exchange of care across distance is difficult, time consuming, challenging, exhausting, expensive and often painful and heart-rending. On the contrary, we wish to emphasise the many factors that limit and hinder the circulation of care across time and space and that create inequalities within and between transnational families, and we underline the importance of access to the technologies and resources that facilitate communication, travel and reunification, including, importantly, rights to citizenship and residency. Our objective in underscoring absence as a common feature of family forms is to encourage the development of national and transnational policies and services that facilitate family reunification and connectedness. The chapters that comprise this collection demonstrate that it is important to stretch our understanding of common family forms to include transnational families. This volume seeks to improve knowledge and understanding about the practices and processes people employ to maintain their caregiving relationships across distance so that we can be better equipped to support them.

## NOTES

1. In this chapter, we draw on data collected in several related research projects, including: (1) A comparative study of transnational care practices of Latin American migrants living in Australia and Europe, conducted by Laura Merla in 2007–2010 and financed by a Marie Curie Outgoing International Fellowship (MOIF-CT-2006–039076 transnational care). The study focused on migrants who occupy a low qualified and/or low remunerated position in Australia and Europe despite coming from a mix of working-class and professional backgrounds in their homeland. Data collection in Australia and Belgium comprised forty-four life-history interviews in the participants'

native language and participant observation with Salvadoran migrants living in Perth, Western Australia, and Brussels, Belgium (nineteen men and twenty-five women) (cf Merla Forthcoming, 2010, 2011, 2012a, 2012b) (2) Two ongoing research projects on transnational family networks of solidarity financed by the Belgian Federal Science Policy, the Belgian National Funds for Research and a Marie Curie Career Integration Grant conducted by Laura Merla, which analyse the processes by which family commitments are negotiated within transnational families by focusing on the experiences of Dominican and Brazilian migrants living in Belgium and their relatives living in the Dominican Republic and Brazil. This chapter reflects only the author's views. The European Community is not liable for any use that may be made of the information contained therein. (3) The *Transnational Families* Project conducted by Loretta Baldassar, Cora Baldock and Raelene Wilding and funded by the Australian Research Council (ARC) from 2000 to 2004. This study focused on transnational family and caregiving relationships and comprises more than 200 ethnographic interviews and participant observation with Australian migrants and their parents living in Ireland, Italy, the Netherlands, Singapore and New Zealand, as well as refugees from Iraq and Afghanistan and their kin living in transit in Iran (cf. Baldassar, Baldock and Wilding 2007). (4) The *Italian Lives* Project conducted from 2005 to 2009 and coordinated by Baldassar, also funded by the ARC, which involved the collection of approximately 170 life-history interviews and four group workshops (in which 115 individuals took part) with post-war migrants from across Western Australia (cf. Iuliano 2010). (5). The collaborative study *Australian Diasporas and Brain Gain*, funded by the ARC from 2009 to 2011, on which Baldassar was a chief investigator. This project examined diasporas in Australia and their transnational connections using a widely administered survey (total 2,355 responses), focus groups and interviews (cf. Baldassar & Pyke Forthcoming; Baldassar et al. 2012; Ben Mosche et al 2012).

2. See, for instance, Hochschild 2000, 2003, Parreñas 2001a, 2001b, 2005a, 2005b.
3. For geographically proximate kin networks, see, for instance, Attias-Donfut et al. 2002; Godbout and Charbonneau 1996; Finch 1989a; Bonvalet and Ortalda 2006, Coenen-Huter et al. 1994.
4. See, for example, Al-Ali 2002; Boccagni 2012a; Olwig 2002; Le Gall 2009; Zontini and Reynolds 2007.
5. See also Nydegger 1991; Finch and Mason 1991, 1993; Grundy 2005.
6. Baldassar, Baldock and Wilding (2007) developed this concept based on the notion of commitment in the work of Finch and Mason (1993).
7. See also Michel 1978; Cresson and Gadrey 2004; Lapeyre and Le Feuvre 2004; Damamme and Paperman 2009.
8. See also Kilkey and Merla, 2013; Baldassar, Wilding and Baldock 2007; Baldassar 2008a.
9. See also Waring 1999; Chadeau and Fouquet 1981.
10. See also Sharpe 2001; Baldassar and Gabaccia 2011.
11. See also Goulbourne et al. 2010; Shain 2007; Escriva and Skinner 2008.
12. Drawing on analyses of the Tongan diaspora, Cowling (1990), for example, discusses 'family networks', in which key family members facilitate movement of kin and remittance as 'custodians' and 'brokers',while Evans (1996: 119) refers to the 'dispersed household'. See also Lee 2003; Conway & Potter 2009; Baldassar 2007a; King and Williams 2000.
13. For a discussion of migrant elites, see Bullock and Paik 2009; Amit 2007; Coles and Fetcher 2008.
14. See also Conradson and Latham 2005; Abel 2013.

15. See also Constable et al. 2004; Martens and Verhoeven 2006.
16. Relevant here is the growing research on Human Computer Interaction; see, for example, Ames et al. 2010; Cao et al. 2010; Judge et al. 2010; Kirk et al. 2010.
17. See also Attias-Donfut et al. 2002; Cieraad 2006; Miller 2001; Maushart 2002; Walsh 2008; Goulbourne et al. 2010. This discussion is linked to the so-called 'emotional turn' in the social sciences and the growing literature on emotions and migration (Svašek and Skrbiš 2007b). Our own work on the topic (Merla and Baldassar 2010a; Baldassar 2007a, 2008b) explores the relationship between rational economic and emotional caregiving motivations for migration.
18. See also Lin and Rogerson 1995; Joseph and Hallman 1985; Bonvalet and Ogg 2006a.
19. See Baldassar 2007a; Kilkey and Merla 2013; Merla 2012a.
20. For example, regional flows within the recently expanded/enlarged European Union (Kilkey et al. 2013a; Williams 2007; Erel 2012). See also Khoo et al. 2011 for European migration to Australia.
21. Kilkey and Merla (2013) refer to this as 'situating transnational families care-arrangements'.

# 1 Locating Transnational Care Circulation in Migration and Family Studies

*Loretta Baldassar and Laura Merla*

'. . . we need more research on the portability of care as a concept.'
(Huang, Thang and Toyota 2012a, 131)

As stated in the Introduction to this volume, we define care circulation as the reciprocal, multidirectional and asymmetrical exchange of care that fluctuates over the life course within transnational family networks subject to the political, economic, cultural and social contexts of both sending and receiving societies. The framework of care circulation we are advancing draws on broad definitions of both family and care, including beliefs and practices about caring embedded in relationships wider than the nuclear family, which in turn are shaped by the broader socio-structural contexts in which families operate transnationally. In proposing a broad conceptualisation of care, it is not our intention to downplay the gendered and political aspects of the uneven nature of care exchanges. Some family members—especially women—carry a far greater care burden than others, and not everyone receives care equally. The lens of circulation allows us to acknowledge and examine the ways in which all family members, both migrants and 'non'-migrants, participate in a variety of caregiving activities and exchanges over time. This apparently private and domestic set of caregiving activities is a fundamental feature of transnational family life, intimately connected to those dimensions assumed to be more public and formal, including economic, political and social endeavours. The increasing mobility and profound impact of new communication technologies on our ability to care across distance and to manage absence in family life makes an analysis of 'the portability of care' a fundamental topic of our contemporary lives.

Building on the Introduction, this chapter serves to locate the framework of care circulation in the broader body of research on migration, transnationalism and the family. We begin with a discussion of the synergies and variances between the frameworks of care circulation and care chains in an effort to draw together and examine the full range of transnational families. To date, those families that are involved in global care chains, often referred to as transnational mothering or parenting, have been written about quite separately to those that are not, and vice versa. We argue that the lens of circulation is a useful framework for all types of transnational families. In section two, we examine the so-called 'mobility turn' in the social sciences and consider transnational approaches to migration in relation to families and the subsequent diversification of family forms. We argue that mobility has become an integral part of family life, and that this has both negative and positive consequences. In this context, we explore the somewhat controversial idea that the distance and absence that characterise transnational families should be conceptualised as regular features of contemporary family life. As already noted, it is not our intention to advocate transnational families as some kind of ideal form or to downplay the difficulties inherent in caring across distance. Rather, we wish to highlight the importance of understanding the impact of distance and absence on family life so that these family forms can be better supported. To provide a more detailed exploration of the framework, the third section of this chapter contextualises notions of 'circulation' in both migration and family studies research. We conclude with an overview of the practices and processes of 'transnational care' on which we draw and which we seek to expand through the lens of circulation. Throughout the chapter, we examine ways to define 'care circulation' and address the methodological and theoretical implications for further study.

## CARE CIRCULATION AND CARE CHAINS: CONCEPTUALISING CAREGIVING IN TRANSNATIONAL FAMILIES AND GLOBAL ECONOMIES

This volume is certainly not the first to consider the movement of care. Through the framework of global care chains and its elaboration, the delivery of care has been identified as an important, although still relatively underexamined, type of goods and service that circulates in 'global scapes' (Appadurai 1991). Hochschild's (2000, 2005) and Parreñas's (2001, 2005a, 2005b) classic work on care chains and its further elaboration by Yeates (2009, 2012) is especially pertinent to our discussion of migration, families and care.

In its classical, early version, the care chains literature tended to conceptualise the mobilities of care as one-way traffic, flowing from the 'global south' to the 'north' along a chain of women that usually included a carer in the south looking after a child whose mother migrated to the north to look after the child of a woman who works full time. The chapters in Parts B and C of this volume deal with this classic care chain scenario. Following this understanding of care flows, the migration of mothers who leave their children behind involves a care deficit for both migrants and their families back home (Pyle 2006). The framework of global care chains contributed to integrating research in the fields of globalisation, care and migration studies. Prior to this work, the literature on care had not taken internationalisation into consideration, and women from the south were largely excluded from the study of work-family balance issues (Leira and Saraceno 2006). The transnational mothering literature in particular provides an important contribution to our understanding of the global political economy by emphasising the commodification of care from a feminist, macro perspective. This literature is based on an analysis of the international transfer of 'motherly care' (understood as a linear process) performed by female domestic migrants from the global south, and it conceptualises transnational motherhood as an undesirable phenomenon that negatively affects parents, their children and the home community (Ehrenreich and Hochschild 2003a; Hochschild 2005; Parreñas 2001a, 2001b). This analysis has highlighted globally structured inequalities based on social divisions of class, race, ethnicity and gender. By showing the emotional costs of mother–child separation and the commodification of emotions (Hochschild 2000), the care chain literature has also brought emotional geographies into the realm of social inequalities (Yeates 2009).

This work has been critiqued for its focus on female domestic workers who were generally portrayed as helpless victims of the global economy (Ryan 2011). Studies of transnational mothering embedded in global care chains, in particular, tended to present a partial and static picture of transnational caregiving arrangements (Escriva and Skinner 2008). Little attention was paid to other types of migrants, such as the highly skilled, or to caring relations that involved other family members, such as the elderly or the extended family. Men and fathers were also generally excluded or portrayed as absent (Dreby 2006). The involvement of these various actors has been more commonly discussed in the broader transnational families literature, which extends the study of transnational families and caregiving to all categories of migrants and not just those who are working in the formal and informal care sectors.[1] Recent research in the care chains tradition has started to address these critiques (see for instance Huang et al. 2012b; Erel 2012). Several authors have shown, in particular, that mother–child separation often corresponds to a particular phase in the migration and family cycle, and that migrating with children, leaving them behind and reuniting in the home or host country are particular strategies that family units adopt based on institutional and personal opportunities, resources and constraints in both the home and host societies.[2] These examples highlight the agency of transnational family members.

The conceptualisation of care flows as unidirectional is informed by, and supports, the idea that migration automatically jeopardises family solidarity and that caregiving requires geographical proximity (Morgan 1975; Joseph and Hallman 1985), an issue we discuss further below. This is exemplified in Isaksen, Devi and Hochschild's (2008) analysis of the consequences of mothers' migration on the 'socio-emotional commons' of the south. These commons are characterised by 'a busy exchange of favors, large and small', which takes place in a community of kin, friends, neighbours and so on who exchange favours with one another (Isaksen et al. 2008, 414). Within transnational families, this translates as a brother looking after his parents, a migrant mother supporting the migration of her niece, grandparents taking care of the absent mother's children and so on. If we revisit these examples from a care circulation perspective, we might see that this brother, this migrant mother and these grandparents are actually participating in a circuit of mutual (though asymmetrical) support, in which care continues to flow and circulate within the family and in many directions. The authors argue instead that the migration of mothers over long periods of time 'attenuates, distorts, and sometimes ruptures the socio-emotional commons' (Isaksen et al. 2008, 418). This argument is based on the idea that physical co-presence in the form of daily face-to-face conversations, bodily contact, shared dinners and celebrations is essential for the maintenance of socio-emotional commons. Here co-presence is understood as strictly corporeal. The fact that migrants can, to various degrees, maintain a (sometimes daily) virtual presence in the life of their families via the use of communication technologies (e.g., Wilding 2006; Parreñas 2005b) is both underexplored and undervalued, as are the visits home to attend family events such as weddings (e.g., Fog Olwig 2002) or for caring purposes (e.g., Bacigalupe and Camara 2012). Although it is imperative to acknowledge how the practices and processes of transnational caregiving are embedded in the often unequal and unfavourable structures of opportunity that characterise migrant lives, this literature tends to portray virtual forms of connectedness as typically selective and fragmented and to assess them as invariably lacking and inadequate. Madianou and Miller's (2012) work offers a timely critique of this 'deficit model' of virtual communications through their detailed ethnographic account of effective virtual transnational exchanges. They argue that all relationships rely on mediated communication, reminding us that proximity does not necessarily ensure better quality family relationships.

The general lack of acknowledgement of both the extent and value of non-proximate forms of care in the care chains literature tends to reduce the mothers' participation in caring exchanges in the family to the sending of remittances, and to the view that informal family reciprocity 'comes closer to a market exchange' (Isaksen et al. 2008, 416). The conceptualisation of care flows between the north and the south as unidirectional is linked to the idea that migration involves the 'displacement' or 'diversion' (Parreñas 2003) of motherly love: Distance makes it impossible for migrant mothers to 'love' the children they left behind, and their love is diverted towards their affluent employers' children. This displacement of love leads Hochschild (2005, 35) to talk of a care drain, 'as women who normally care for the young, the old and the sick in their own poor countries move to care for the young, the old, and the sick in rich countries, whether as maids and nannies or as day-care and nursing-home aides'. But care drain may not necessarily occur in all transnational families (Sørensen and Guarnizo 2007) and risks presenting an overly simplistic assessment of the complex and extended care negotiations and relationships involved. Even though the maintenance of family solidarity in transnational settings is undoubtedly a difficult and painful process, just as it commonly is in proximate family contexts, the purpose of adopting a care circulation perspective is precisely to show that migrants and their relatives are both receivers and providers of care (Ryan 2007), and that care continues to circulate within family networks over the migration, family and lifecycle (Le Gall 2005).

The framework of circulation and the idea that caregiving is an 'entity' that circulates offers a different, but complementary, perspective to the care chains framework. As we have argued, the care chains literature is mainly based on the notion of the commodification of care—with the migrants selling their caregiving, which travels in one direction along a chain (usually from south to north) in exchange for money that travels in the other direction in the form of remittances.[3] Within this framework, care is conceived as embodied in the migrant domestic worker—the care cannot travel without the migrant, which makes sense in a labour market perspective. Domestic workers cannot look after the dependent family members of their employers without being physically present. In this perspective, two items travel along the chain in opposite directions: the migrant and his or her embodied care, and the money he or she receives and sends back home. In this context, the materiality and corporeality of care are foregrounded. If we move from a labour market focus to a focus on the moral economies of the family, we can see that not only do embodied and commodified forms of care travel along the chain, but also other 'virtual' forms of care travel in both directions (Madianou and Miller 2012).[4] In addition, care exchanges expand beyond the principle migration chain, foregrounded in the care chains perspective, and circulate between the various and extended members of the family. Thus, we argue that the idea of a 'chain' is not the most suitable way of portraying the mobilities of care from a family perspective. The 'chain' metaphor tends to limit these mobilities to back and forth movement between two nodes of a chain, where migrant and nonmigrant exchange various types of support, thus reinforcing the distinction between these two sets of actors, as well as putting the focus on dyadic relationships. Our fieldwork, as well as various valuable discussions with scholars from transnational and geographically proximate family studies (including the contributors to this book), suggest that the framework of 'circulation' is better able to highlight the fact that the mobilities of care are multidirectional, can take place simultaneously and diachronically and go beyond the migrant/nonmigrant chain of exchange.

In focusing on how care circulates throughout the extended network of family members, we are mindful that the notion of circulation may evoke the idea that care flows unencumbered and evenly between all family members in some kind of 'care-soaked' scenario, and this is certainly not the case. This interpretation of the 'circulation' lens would limit its analytical value by assuming all members of the network had the same access to resources, that all their relationships were equal and that they each exchanged equivalent levels and types of care.[5] As the case studies about Yasmina and Viviana presented in the Introduction to this book show, various types of care flow unevenly, both simultaneously and diachronically, between kin from various generations located in different places in the world. In order to highlight both the circulation of these care flows as well as their inherent inequalities, we define the caregiving exchanges between kin as 'asymmetrically reciprocal' drawing on Wellman's (1988, 102) theory of network ties, which he defines as 'differing in content and intensity'.

In addition, the care a person has given to a particular family member at a certain point in time may be returned to him or her by another family member. For example, Yasmina exchanges various forms of support with her mother Carlita, but this mobility of care—which might be conceptualised as a two-way flow between two nodes of a chain—is embedded in wider family relationships and circuits of care that involve her siblings, her children and her parsimonious aunt. It is these more extensive, although unequal and often fraught with tension family care exchanges, which become more visible through a 'care circulation' perspective. The 'circulation' of care does not mean that care automatically travels along a 'circle' that equally binds together all the members of a particular family network. The various circuits of care involving different family members may coexist within a particular family at certain points in time, and some relatives may never receive support from each other but may do so separately through the circulation of care in their broader family networks. For example, Viviana's Australia- and UK-based grandchildren may never exchange support with each other, although this potential lays dormant in the family network. However, they each exchange support with their common grandmother who is involved in circuits of care that include her children and siblings. The latter also provide and receive practical and emotional support from both sets of cousins. Here we again invoke network analysis and Wellman's argument that 'all social behaviour is best analyzed by looking first at the ways in which networks allocate flows of scarce resources to system members'. This allocation is rarely even, including in the case of caregiving; as a result, the care exchanges between family members are asymmetrical in both the amount and kinds of flows: 'Such asymmetric ties crucially connect network members to each other, and, through the other's additional ties, indirectly connect them to larger social networks' (Wellman 1988, 40).

A strength of the circulation lens is that it brings into view all of the actors and activities of caregiving, both actual and ideal, regardless of place or country of residence, migrant or nonmigrant status, gender, generation, age, etcetera, and so captures all of the care action (including its absence when expected or longed for) that comprises transnational family life. Therefore, it must be emphasised that the quality, quantity, direction, presence or absence of the circulation of care is highly variable, constantly negotiated and deeply influenced by factors both within and outside the family. While the care chains perspective tends to see the rich families of the north in care surplus and the poor families of the south in care deficit, setting up a dichotomy between caregiving and receiving (Kofman 2012), we apply the framework of care circulation to capture the asymmetries of care experienced by transnational families from various socioeconomic, educational, cultural, ethnic and religious backgrounds, and throughout each of these family networks, wherever members reside.

Comparing transnational caregiving in middle-class families with that of the care chains cases is treading on tricky conceptual ground. Several issues are pertinent here. The global care chains perspective tends to cast middle-class women of the north as subjugators of the care work of domestic migrant women workers, thus creating the care drain and deficit in the migrant women's families in the south. There is also a broader issue at play about the general resistance to analyses of the middle classes in the social sciences, given the taken-for-granted assumption of their relative significant wealth and access to resources (Miller 2010). The woman from the north and the woman from the south in the global care chain scenario are seen to represent completely different social positionalities. In terms of the experiences and practices of caregiving, they might be accorded comparable experiences at the emotional level, but not on many others. Without a doubt, there are important geopolitical and economic asymmetries in income and access to education, well-being and so on *between* these 'types' of women. There is also considerable diversity *within* these categories of women, in terms of power relations, ethnic hierarchies, citizenship and employment rights and so forth. Many women in the 'south' *as well as* in the 'north' carry significant care burdens that are not adequately met by either welfare provisions or paid help, or even a combination of the two, including for those women with significant purchasing power (Costa 2013; Saraceno 2010). It is important to also consider and compare the care circuits of these women from 'the north' if we are to more fully understand family care in a truly global context (see Chapter 12, this volume).[6]

Here we see useful synergies between the care circulation and the care chains approach in highlighting that care is a resource unevenly distributed and subject to a variety of inequalities, both within and between families. As the feminist literature has shown, families are hierarchical and asymmetrical social systems (Thorne and Yalom 1982), and the unequal, gendered division of labour is central to patriarchy (Delphy 1998; Connell 1987). The debate in the literature about the transformative potential of migration and transnational processes to reconfigure power relations, in particular of gender, is pertinent here.[7] If care is understood as a type of resource in families governed by unequal power relations, then an examination of care circulation can provide a window on the types of inequalities fostered within transnational family settings. Recognising that migrants continue to participate in family care circuits brings forward the need for policies that support this activity. As Merla and Degavre (2013) argue, European governments tend to consider migrants—and domestic workers in particular—as breadwinners discharged from family caring duties. Migrants who are employed in precarious and/or undeclared jobs in particular are excluded from de-familialisation policies, that is, policies aimed at helping adults 'uphold a socially acceptable standard of living, independently of family relationships, either through paid work or social security provisions' (Lister 1994, 32). These include measures designed to reduce the care burden of female citizens. However, these policies draw on a definition of 'family' as geographically proximate. Recognising migrants' transnational caring responsibilities calls for de-familialisation policies that are adapted to the specificities of balancing paid work in the 'north' with transnational family life. This also means 'facilitating access to the resources that determine family solidarity in situations of "non-proximate" care' (Merla and Degavre 2013, 113).

Framing the mobilities of care in terms of circulation addresses the need to bring to the fore some key differences between a family perspective and a political economy perspective, which are, we think, both relevant and complementary. The central notion of care in the care chains literature is commodification because of its treatment in the context of labour market exchange and the wider frame of political economy. In contrast, we are employing the notion of care as generalised, asymmetrical reciprocal exchange governed by the moral codes of family and kinship ties, that is, the moral economy. Clearly these are, on the one hand, quite different definitions of care, and, on the other hand, both types coexist. As Morgan (1996, 40) argues, 'households do not simply function on behalf of the wider economy and it is important to consider the ways in which the moral economy meets and interacts with the political economy in the business of family life located in and between households'. The interconnection between economic activities and intimate transactions are also highlighted in Zelizer's (2005b) notion of 'circuits of commerce', which include interpersonal care circuits and remittance circuits. These circuits are characterised by a distinctive set of social relations among specific individuals, which serve as a basis for shared economic activities, carry shared meanings and define a boundary between members and nonmembers of the circuit. This approach highlights that remittances not only serve the economic needs of transnational families, but they also establish specific connections between family members and convey powerful shared meanings, such as what it means to be a 'good' mother.

The case of migrant industrial districts and transnational family firms is another example of the links between migration, kinship and economic initiatives. In explaining the success of Chinese small businesses in Prato, Italy, despite significant tensions and hostilities from the local Italian community, Dei Ottati (Forthcoming, 11) refers to a 'localised thickening of economic and social relations' that 'facilitates the circulation of information among these immigrants and reduces to a minimum transactions costs within and between firms'. This is because the economic relations are largely embedded in the kinship and social ties of communities, 'which enforces a bond of solidarity enforced by the group' (Dei Ottati Forthcoming, 11). In other words, the asymmetrical reciprocal obligations, including of family caregiving, that characterise this group provide the opportunities, structures and infrastructures to support successful business and economic initiatives: 'a form of integration in which economic efficiency is reached mainly thanks to relationships of reciprocity rather than of authority' (Dei Ottati Forthcoming, 11). These types of ethnic entrepreneurship, community-based migratory moves and economic activities are not covered by the care chains perspective, and yet we would argue that the exchange of care that is constitutive of family life forms a fundamental foundation and motivation for this mobility and economic activity. Thus, we are certainly not advocating replacing the care chains literature with the framework of circulation and its more generalised reciprocal form of care. Rather, we are suggesting that the circulation lens allows us to examine family and care exchange more broadly in the various types of economic activities, mobility and migration, absence and separation that occurs across a range of families. In so doing, we wish to highlight how the care circulation framework can be employed to reveal the points of connection and disjunction between the labour market and the family.

Thinking of the mobilities of care in terms of circulation rather than a chain is not just motivated by a desire to make the multidirectional 'nature' of care flow more visible. It also contributes to a project that seeks to expand the scope of study. Here, family is taken in a wide sense, as going beyond nuclear households. Our volume sits firmly in the growing tradition of work on 'transnationalism from below', with a focus on the more private and quotidian constructions of transnational social fields at the level of families, households and the domestic sphere (Gardner and Grillo 2002).[8] This perspective highlights how family ties and obligations are integral to economic and political motivations in the decision-making process of both those who migrate and those who stay behind,[9] also evident in motivations for return (Conway and Potter 2009) and retirement (Williams et al. 2000; Ackers and Dwyer 2002). These processes are still largely ignored in official conceptions of the family and of migration, and they continue to be reflective of traditional static notions of families and households as well as implicitly unidirectional understandings of mobility (Kofman 2004). The circulation perspective that we are proposing helps to widen the analysis of the mobility of care beyond mother–child relationships. By taking a broad definition of care that includes both embodied and virtual 'love' and by tracing its movement, we bring more care actors into the frame and recognise the role played by wider family networks.

The conceptualisations of 'care chains' and of 'care circulation' are not mutually exclusive. As recent developments in the care chains literature have shown, the analysis of care flows as a chain is not incompatible with the interpretation of care flows in terms of circulation. As Yeates (2009, 46) notes, the chain 'conveys the networks of connection within and across borders, and the forward and backward linkages between different actors within the network'. In studies on transnational mothering and transnational families, the notion of circulation has been suggested and glimpsed for specific sets of relationships. For instance, Herrera (2010, 68) notes that the involvement of Ecuadorian grandmothers in the education of left-behind grandchildren 'sometimes blurs the dichotomy of caregiver and receiver and may be better understood as 'circulation of care' in which two or three sides are being cared for and taking care of each other'. Similarly, Hung Thai (2012) identified 'circuits of gratitude' involving emotional and material exchanges between Vietnamese transnational couples and the transpacific matchmakers who arranged their marriages. In their special issue on 'rethinking the transnational mobilities of care in Asia', Huang et al. (2012a, 2012b, 132) argue that the global care chains perspective, which they define as 'the predominant paradigm in the literature on transnational mobilities for care', needs to be expanded and complicated further to encompass

> more complex interactive relationship flows, where the boundary between the caregiver and the care receiver is more often blurred in a mutually dependent care relationship. Care does not only flow one way; the flows of care are bilateral and reciprocal. Despite this, what appears not to have changed is the strong feminisation of the care chain: caregivers still tend to be women.

The existence of forward and backward linkages along care chains has been highlighted in several studies of transnational mothering, and the broader transnational families literature also includes illustrations of multidirectional care flows, but so far none of them has explicitly conceptualised transnational caregiving in terms of circulation.[10] This chapter and this book aim to begin to shore up this gap.

As discussed in the Introduction, Kofman (2012), in particular, has noted the limitations of the care chain perspective in dealing with broader contexts of care. She advocates engaging with the concepts of social reproduction and 'global householding'[11] in order to 'place care work within a wider landscape of activities and sites and to connect supposedly disparate circuits of migration, in particular labor, family, and education, which are usually analyzed separately but which are in fact interconnected' (Kofman 2012, 144). While her definition of care is much narrower than ours, focusing on the support of people who are unable to care for themselves, her contextualisation of caregiving within the range of activities and institutions engaged in social reproduction makes her focus broader, though complementary. She sees the framework of global householding as a way of 'connecting the different processes and trajectories' of social reproduction, including care. Kofman (2012, 153) argues that a focus on global households—'an entity broader than the family and allowing for the formation of units not necessarily composed of relations through marriage or direct lineage'—would enable an analysis of 'the different forms, orientations, and directions of care' providing 'an approach that follows longitudinally and spatially the migrant so as to capture care giving and receiving . . . To this end, the use of the global householding framework, as the nexus of the life cycle and its diverse activities, including care, would be a concrete way of articulating the different circuits in the overall social reproduction of the household'. We believe a care circulation lens, with its focus on the practices and processes of the asymmetrically reciprocal exchanges of transnational caregiving, offers a productive way to map the actual and imagined connections between members of 'global households' across distance and time.

Another important aim of this book is to better understand distance and absence in family life. We propose that by applying a care circulation framework, we are better able to theorise absence and distance as common features of family life and so begin to see transnational families as family forms in their own right. This argument is the focus of the next section. At a time when mobility is intensifying and governments around the globe are increasingly targeting skilled migration in preference to family reunion (Hawthorne 2005), there is a growing need for social and migration policy as well as services and resources that facilitate reunion and connectedness. The transnational social sphere, while full of circulating people, ideas, goods and finances, remains relatively empty of transnational structures, infrastructures and support services to safeguard these people and their activities and relationships. Governments of developed economies are increasingly interested in facilitating knowledge transfer and trade links through their migrant diasporas (Williams 2007; Agunias 2006). What tends to be overlooked in the relevant policy deliberations is how transnational family and caregiving relationships often provide the basis and context from which economic links are developed and maintained.

## THE MOBILITY TURN: THEORISING DISTANCE AND ABSENCE AS PART OF FAMILY LIFE

Our discussion of care circulation is closely linked to developments in the conceptualisation and theorisation of migration and transnationalism.[12] The availability of increasingly affordable and safer modes of travel and communication across distance has fundamentally changed the process of migration. In contrast to the past, migratory moves today are more likely to be characterised by regular and frequent communication and linkages between sending and receiving areas.

To draw on our own research for relatively representative examples, the two major waves of Italian labour migration to Australia in the 1920s and 1950s were characterised by a family economic strategy devised to safeguard the livelihoods of left-behind kin. The migrants would remit as much of their earnings as they could in the hope that they would one day repatriate to a better life back home (Baldassar 2001; Baldassar and Pesman 2005). Technology being what it was, they commonly communicated with their loved ones through the exchange of regular letters, occasional phone calls and rare visits. These same migrants today, along with a growing 'new wave' of arrivals from Italy, enjoy significantly more active and complex patterns of communication with loved ones back home, including SMS texts several times a day; frequent e-mails, phone and Skype calls; as well as regular visits, often once a year.[13] Even far less wealthy migrants, including refugees, can reliably communicate with their distant kin weekly or monthly, although visits may be much rarer. Despite major obstacles to the maintenance of family solidarity across borders arising from a difficult insertion in the labour market, inadequate provision of leave options, restrictive visa regulations and inequalities in the access to, and use of, communication technologies, Salvadoran refugees who settled in Australia in the 1980s and early 1990s invest a lot of time, energy and money staying in touch with their ageing parents (mainly via telephone conversations) and fulfilling their filial duties notwithstanding the distance (Merla 2012a, 2012b; Merla 2011).

Put simply, in the past, migration was both conceived of, and experienced, as unidirectional—from home to host country—as well as finite or final, resulting in settlement and a new life in the host country. This view contributed to conceptualisations of the migrant's home and host societies as discrete, homogenous entities with little in common and few connections between them. Wimmer and Glick Schiller (2002) note how this seemingly unproblematic division of space tended to privilege the straight line theory of assimilation as the end result of migration and an either/or approach to home and host allegiances.[14] If migration, a process inherently involving movement, was conceptualised as finite and unidirectional, with an emphasis on settlement and assimilation, it is hardly surprising that the dominant notions about households—and the families they contain—are conceived of as rooted in or bound by static, geographical domains (Moore 1988; Stacey 1998). As Hardill (2004, 378, 386) points out, 'The term "household" is in fact usually associated with a locus of residence, but for the transnational households . . . members of one household can be simultaneously located in the sending *and* receiving country', arguing that 'because of the complexity of lives today we need to revisit these terms'. The concept of 'global householding', mentioned earlier, provides a pertinent example. The potency of assumptions about family and household occupying one locus of residence is perhaps most common in family and gerontology studies, which tend to define all manner of family function as dependent on geographical proximity, and this is perhaps most evident in the case of caring (Leira and Saraceno 2006). In general, as is evident in the care chains literature described earlier, researchers have assumed that in order to care for each other effectively, family members must live in close proximity.[15]

The notions of transnational migration and transnational families are attempts at better capturing the increased communication and closer linkages between the sending and receiving societies. 'Transnationalism' in this context is defined as 'a social process in which migrants establish social fields that cross geographic, cultural, and political borders' (Glick Schiller et al. 1992, ix). The conceptual shift to a 'transnational' framework exemplifies what is currently described as the 'mobility turn' in the social sciences (Urry 2000; Sheller and Urry 2006). Much of this thinking is an attempt to accommodate processes associated with globalisation, facilitate the integration of an increasingly diverse citizenry in the body politic of nation-states and eschew assimilationist and exclusionist rhetorics (like Fortress Europe) that have become all too common a feature of contemporary geopolitics (Furedi 2005). There is now a considerable body of research and theory that attempt to make sense of this increased mobility and connectedness,[16] including concepts such as diaspora (Cohen 1997), ethnoscapes (Appadurai 1990, 1996), network society (Castells 1996), networked family (Urry 2002), mediated relationships (Madianou and Miller 2012) and, of course, global care chains. Also relevant is the recent interest in notions of cosmopolitanism (Beck and Sznaider 2010), which reflect attempts at developing a social science more attuned to mobility, including its methodological implications (Beck et al. 2006). Far from denying the importance of physical proximity and corporeal senses, this literature examines how people compensate for and overcome distance and separation. Urry (2003, 163) highlights, in particular, the role of visits and intermittent co-presence as 'essential for developing those relations of trust that persist during often lengthy periods of distance and even solitude' .[17] A key point about the mobility turn in the social sciences is the attempt to highlight and examine how increased mobility and associated virtual forms of connectedness affect our lives, and not just the people who are actually mobile (Ostergaard-Nielsen 2003). The mobility turn is not just about those who move, but also about the connectedness despite mobility as well as the to and fro of that connectedness—its circularity.[18]

As we explain in the Introduction to this volume, the framework of circulation central to this book helps us to think of migration in terms of the family lifecycle as a dynamic set of processes across the life course, rather than a momentous event in time that damages family connectedness. While new technologies are effectively helping to shrink distance, we do not want to downplay the significant challenges and deeply heart-felt anxieties that characterise the realities of caring across distance. Without denying the often extreme emotional and practical hardships that members of geographically dispersed families confront, in this volume, we wish to highlight the agency of family members in transnational processes of care in an effort to acknowledge transnational families as increasingly common family forms and to further question negative conceptualisations of these types of families. In summary, we are suggesting that transnational families should be theorised as family forms that generate both positive and negative experiences, as geographically proximate family forms do, and that mobility and distance need to be seen as common features of contemporary family life. The framework of circulation is a productive way to achieve this aim by mapping the processes and practices of transnational caring.

The chapters in this volume all point to the general and robust scepticism (Zentgraf and Chinchilla 2012) about how effectively transnational families can discharge their caregiving obligations and how they can adequately care for and about each other, that is, how well they can actually 'do family', especially those families that are separated over long periods of time. Of particular concern is the potential for negative impact or harm that might be caused to family members by long periods of separation. Not surprisingly, the spotlight most often falls on those cases where mothers are separated from young children.[19] Transnational mothering challenges a central and deeply held dominant Western notion about the bond between mother and child being biological rather than cultural (Bowlby 1969) and the associated implications this has for mother and children to be both emotionally and physically close (Chavkin and Maher 2010; Banfi and Boccagni 2011; Lutz and Palenga-Möllenbeck 2012). All the chapters in this volume show how families and their members respond to and manage the considerable constraints they face in doing family, particularly parenting, transnationally. What they also emphasise and critique is the prevailing dominant Western notions about what constitutes 'normal' and 'healthy' family relationships (see in particular Chapters 3, 6 and 7, this volume). The notion of 'family' 'covers a multitude of senses of relatedness and connections' (Sørensen and Guarnizo 2007,161),[20] both within Western societies and across the globe. This richness is hidden from view in the dominant Western imaginary that identifies family with nuclear households bound up in notions of proximity and intimacy. As Sørensen and Guarnizo (2007) note, migration studies' tendency to identify the family with the domestic group has led researchers to assume that separation automatically leads to family disintegration, particularly when mothers leave husbands and children behind. The notions of transnationalism and transnational families have gone some way to highlight the existence of families maintained across distance. However, they are implicitly and overtly judged against the Western normative myth of proximate families. The ideal of proximity and intimacy for healthy parent–child relations leads to the consequent assumption that distance is a negative, major impediment to the delivery of caregiving.

This volume critically examines the implicit assumption that effective family caregiving requires intimacy and proximity. It is instructive to consider the argument about the relative absence of anxiety related to physical separation in the African compared with the Western case (Goody 1982). Levine (1976) argues that Westerners crave intimacy in social relations, and its absence generates anxiety. Elsewhere, Baldassar (2008a, 2008b) has discussed how older Italians desire a close relationship with their families, especially children and grandchildren, such that their perceptions about their health and well-being have been found to be associated with how close by their children are felt to be.[21] In contrast, Trajano (2009, 525) argues that because of the set of imperatives that define migration in Cape Verdean society, families experience separation as less painful and disruptive than in the West:

> These economic, political and cultural characteristics, which act as driving forces for emigration, represent the Cape Verdean expression of . . . the structural obstacles of the African cultural *ecumene*. Their regular and long-lasting existence in Cape Verdean society generates unbearable tensions that would tear the social fabric were it not for the ethos that emphasizes a lack of anxiety in regard to physical separation between those who stay and those who leave, and the maintenance of a strong feeling of relatedness, acting as a bridge for the physical distance, by means of continuity of material obligations.

Madianou and Miller (2012, 10) refer to 'anthropological accounts of many regions, such as the Caribbean, where the nuclear co-present family has never been the norm'. Fog Olwig's chapter on Caribbean transnational families (Chapter 6, this volume) shows that, 'From the perspective of people from the lower strata of Caribbean society, migration and care are . . . intimately linked and should be interpreted as a way of doing family relations in a mobile world of unequal social and economic opportunities'. Similarly, Agunias (2006, 17) describes the Caribbean as a pertinent example of 're-migration as a livelihood strategy to increase and diversify the income of the whole family . . . a complex, reciprocal flow rather than permanent one-way movements characterize Caribbean international migration'. He refers to Segal (1996, 25), who, like Fog Olwig, argues that Caribbean migration 'should be understood as a form of extended kinship over space and time with frequent rather than one-time movements' (Agunias 2006, 17).[22]

Thus, the way transnational family members experience absence from loved ones is much more dependent on the quality of their relationships, and the socially constructed meanings of mobility, than on the actual distance that separates them. Even the meaning of distance is specific to sociocultural contexts and influenced by the structural factors that frame mobility. For example, in the study by Baldassar et al. (2007), the New Zealanders did not define themselves as migrants, partly as a consequence of the unrestricted and relatively inexpensive border crossing to and from Australia. Most felt they were not living that far away from their homeland, despite the seven-hour flight and approximately five-hour time difference that actually separated them from loved ones back home. What these contributions show is that 'being together' may go well beyond daily proximity. Rather 'being together' as well as 'doing family' can be maintained by fulfilling a series of duties and mediations, even from afar. This points to the importance of including transnational families in our understanding of common family forms.

As we argue in the Introduction, members of transnational families increasingly and 'routinely' live their lives 'together across distance' and have developed practices to deal with the challenges posed by absence and separation. This means that we need to revisit normative understandings of migration and the conceptualisation of human mobility more broadly. In conceptualisations of caregiving, 'the' family and the nation-state tend to be defined within an interpretive frame that presumes sedentarism and physical co-presence as the norm and migration and mobility as, therefore, disruptive. As already noted, in gerontological studies, caregiving tends to be defined rigidly as personal or hands-on care delivered to dependent persons who cannot care for themselves (Ennuyer 2001), and thus cannot be provided except in contexts of physical proximity. The precondition of physical proximity for caregiving is inherently linked to the notion of 'the' family as a private geographic domain represented by a household. The standard, institutional model of the family, featuring a white, middle-class, heterosexual couple with two children, represents family members as bonded together by physical co-presence and bounded by the confines of the privately owned land and house that contains them (Morgan 2011b). In these conceptualisations, the structure of the family is viewed as a microcosm and primary reproducer of the patriarchal nation-state, a central concept in political science.

This approach to caregiving, families and states mirrors the way nations and communities were, until the advent of transnational migration studies, largely theorised as inherently connected to a geographical place. They are each defined and punctuated by various types of boundaries, including borders on maps, perimeters on plans and kinship groups on civil registry certificates. Within these fields, migration is primarily viewed as a process that literally and symbolically breaks away from the norm of sedentarism and therefore results in divided state loyalties, fractured families and an inability to fulfil obligations to care. The movement out of homeland states, and in particular the resulting distance between family members, is seen to rupture and inhibit continued connections to people and place. Not surprisingly, then, transnational family forms are by nature deeply suspicious and flawed. Ironically, many migratory moves are motivated by the need to provide for the family and care for its members. Over a century of migration studies reveals that these moves are also more likely to result in multiple identities and national belongings.[23] Further, recent research on transnational families shows that migration can result in expanded family networks of care as the use of new technologies gives rise to more frequent and complex, multidirectional communication flows between members, including across the generations (Madianou and Miller 2012; Nedelcu 2012). Perspectives of social life that are framed through a focus on social groups and processes, and therefore approach mobility as, potentially at least, a sociocultural norm,[24] lead to a methodological focus on the individual biography and life course of the people who move to consider how movement impacts on the static structures of the life world, rather than the reverse. In addition to work on transnational families, recent approaches in the sociology of the family, such as the 'family practices' approach (Morgan 2011a, 2011b) or the 'configurational approach' (Widmer and Jallinoja 2008) propose alternative frameworks that move beyond a focus on static, normative constructions of the nuclear family and stress the historical and spatial fluidity of kin relations.

While the families in this volume can all be defined as transnational, a growing number of related family forms approximate transnational families in the spatial and geographical spread and complexity of contemporary family living arrangements, regardless of their socioeconomic status. These families are affected by various forms of mobility, which, while not exactly migrations, result in the absences of family members (Hardill 2004). These family members are to a certain extent 'living apart together' (LAT), a term that applies to people who 'define themselves as a couple and (. . .) perceive that their close surrounding personal network does so as well' (Levin 2004, 226–227) but do not share a home, even if they work and live in the same town.[25] Short- and long-distance 'LATs' comprise a variety of couple relationships, including young couples who may study in different places and retired people who are emotionally attached to their house and do not want to leave it. According to Levin (2004), the decline in marriages; changes in labour markets, (which make it more difficult to find a job when relocating); search for gender equality in intimate relationships; and increased frequency of travel and accessibility of communication technologies all account for the increase and growing awareness of this type of living arrangement. Another example of this family formation (also discussed by Levin 2004) is evident in the so-called multi-local families that result from rising divorce rates and the recognition in many countries of shared custody as a reference model that result in growing numbers of recomposed families.[26] Members in these families, most particularly children, belong to more than one family household (Marquet 2009). Their various blended and/or stepfamilies live in separate households, which are often located at a distance, across a suburb, a town, a city or even countries. These children routinely spend time in 'separated, yet connected' (Smart and Neale 1999, 67) households depending on the particular custody arrangements, such as weekly or weekend exchange arrangements.

Another increasingly common multi-local family form found in many cities around the world today involves the commuter who travels to work and lives in one city during the week and returns to his or her home in another city on weekends. This experience is so common in Italy that these workers are referred to as *i pendolari* because, like a pendulum, they swing between cities on a weekly basis. In a growing literature on these 'commuter' families, members are also described as 'living apart together' (Hardill 2002; Smith 2001). We might also include fly-in, fly-out work arrangements, increasingly common in places where mining is a significant component of the economy (Taylor and Simmonds 2009). In Western Australia, for example, it is usual for mine employees to work and live on-site in a remote mining centre, flying back to their families in the capital city of Perth for one in every four weeks (Storey 2001). Comparable arrangements of this type include professionals and managers who might visit company offices and clients around the world, involving several extended work trips a year (Amit 2007). Doyle and Nathan (2001) argue that cross-border work is being similarly transformed to involve shorter stays, giving rise to new types of workers including international commuters, virtual expatriates, frequent flyers and short-term travellers who could also be considered transnational.

There is a corresponding increase in the diversity of transnational family forms. Perhaps most prominent in the migration literature are the seasonal or temporary workers who travel on short-term labour contracts of several months or illegally to fill labour shortages, like the thousands of Mexican and Caribbean seasonal farm workers who move each year to Canada during planting and harvesting seasons through the Canadian Seasonal Agricultural Worker Program (Basok 2000; Cohen 1987). Here, of course, the growing numbers of so-called domestic migrants who have dramatically and profoundly feminised the traditionally male south-north labour flows are centrally important and have given rise to the influential care chains thesis that we discuss in some detail above. Werbner (1999) describes these types of labour and domestic migrants as 'working-class cosmopolitans' to highlight their everyday lived engagement with cultural difference in ways that are often far more challenging than is experienced by the elites, who tend to share more class similarities than cultural differences with their colleagues.

The relatively much more affluent but equally highly mobile migrants include expatriate workers who might be based in an overseas office on a posting of several years during their career.[27] Shimoda (2012) argues that the host country nationals who work in these multinational and expatriate offices can be considered 'local' transnationals. While they do not cross geographical borders, they do cross cultural and organisational borders when they enter their foreign-owned and managed workplace. Ackers (2004) has shown that in the European context, this mainly male-led migration tends to place female spouses in 'a highly vulnerable and dependent position' due to their difficult access to employment and work-related social rights.[28] Finally, there are the largely long-term (or permanent) migrants who might live for decades in the host country only to return to their homeland on visits or for retirement. These include labour migrants and refugees as well as more wealthy professionals and elites. All socioeconomic classes of families are represented in this volume, and this diversity is particularly evident in the chapters in Part D, which present some of the variety of family forms and structures among the aspirational and middle classes. Hardill (2004, 376), for example, refers to transnational commuter-couples who live 'with one foot in two places—places that span national boundaries bringing two societies within one social field (Kivisto, 2001:566)'. What have been called Astronaut families with parachute children are a particular case of mobile families and refer to families where one or both parents live and work in one country and the children (and sometimes one parent) live in another country (Pe-Pua et al. 1998; Vertovec 1999; Waters 2002). These parachute children might grow up to join the growing ranks of international students who sojourn abroad to complete a university degree, yet another example of increasing mobility in our lives (Amit 2007) (see also Chapter 11, this volume).

While we do not deal with all of these family forms in this volume, we feel it is important to recognise their relevance to this discussion, to further emphasise the point that family life everywhere is increasingly affected by mobilities of varying types and degrees and the ever more common experience of caring across distance. It is also worth considering whether similar patterns of caregiving to transnational families are evident in families who live within the same country. This is particularly relevant to relatively large countries like Australia and the United States, where family members can be separated across even greater distances than families spread across different countries within Europe. But even in cases where families live relatively close by each other, the general time pressures of busy lives often mitigate against taking advantage of proximity, as do factors such as the inevitable tensions and frictions within family relationships. Baldassar et al. (2007), in their study of the Australian context, found that many people commented that they would probably *not* be in any greater contact with their family 'back home' even if they still lived there and that living so far away made 'being together' more special and meaningful than it appeared to be for their proximate kin.[29] Similarly, Madianou and Miller (2011, 148) acknowledge the potential 'benefits' of distance in helping to sustain healthy family relationships. Their careful and detailed analysis of transnational mothering by Filipina migrants is replete with 'examples of absence that exacerbates conflict with parents and equally rich with examples of absence that helps resolve conflicts with parents'. While it must be noted that they are dealing mostly with adolescent children, their critique is an important contribution to dominant ideas about this phenomenon. Arguably, then, in all families, including both proximate and distant forms, members must maintain a sense of family-hood despite absences (even across relatively short distances), and caregiving circulates over space and time.

## CIRCULATION IN MIGRATION AND FAMILY STUDIES

The framework of circulation is not new to migration studies, originally conceived to refer to seasonal labourers who moved between their homes in one country and their places of work in another country with such regularity that they were described as *circulating* between both places (Prothero and Chapman 1985). In the contemporary global context of significantly increased mobility, the notion of circulation is being revisited (Agunias 2006). Demographers such as Graeme Hugo (2005, 2009) point out that migration is rarely linear because most migrants eventually repatriate.

This careful attention to mobility has led to a reassessment of migrations of the past, which, while not characterised by the more regular to-and-fro mobility of today, show clear evidence of a degree of circularity (King and Christou 2012). In the case of the century of massive Italian emigration, what initially looked like a 'haemorrhage of humanity' with the apparent exodus between 1861 and 1965 of more than twenty-five million people (a number equivalent to almost half of the total population of contemporary Italy) has been reviewed in light of the significant rate of repatriations. Some twenty million people might have emigrated from Italy between 1861 and 1941, but the net loss of population over this period was only 7.7 million (approximately 39 percent) (Sori 1979, 19). The rate of repatriation was highest from the northern regions; for example, in the 1960s, almost eight and a half thousand men and women from the Veneto arrived in Australia, but in the same decade, just over six thousand (about 70 percent) were recorded as returning to Italy (Thompson 1980, 23; Baldassar and Pesman 2005). It is important to note that, until recently,[30] the collection of migration statistics was very much informed by a unilinear approach to mobility as returns and re-migrations went unidentified and return visits were completely overlooked (Baldassar 2001; Hugo 2012, Forthcoming). Price (1963, 10) notes that the official statistics for Australia 'simply record the total number of entries and exits, irrespective of whether the persons concerned are making their first or fifth entry or exit'. Di Leonardo (1984, 49) has shown the same is true for the United States; while the majority of Italian emigrants left intending to return, 'The evidence suggests that large numbers were counted as new emigrants and immigrants, by the Italian and American governments, as they left a second, third, or more times in their periodic returns and remigrations'.

Traditionally, the movement of migrants back to their homelands has been defined as return migration. Gmelch (1980) points out, 'As early as 1885, Ravenstein (1885, 64) noted the principle of return migration in his renowned list of migration laws: "Each main current of migration produces a compensating counter-current".' However, a focus on the physical migratory movement of the individual risks missing the complex and ongoing processes of connectedness over time, and Ravenstein's famous law could be interpreted as referring to more than just the flows of people. Hugo (2009) makes a similar point in his evaluation of this research. For him, return migration is an old phenomenon that is being transformed through globalisation. One of the 'new' elements Hugo refers to is 'a more extensive pattern of *circular* interaction' between home and host settings. This *circular interaction* is a reference to the significantly greater degrees of 'frequency and intimacy that [were] unthinkable until recently' (Hugo 2009, 213):

> In short, return migration needs to be considered as part of a wider process of transnationalism involving regular electronic interaction, frequent visiting and regular reinforcing of intentions to eventually return. (Hugo 2009, 214)

There is a degree of conceptual 'slippage' in the literature regarding exactly which movements the term circulation refers to. Most often, the notion of circulation is used to refer to the increased mobility of individuals.[31] However, as in the quote from Hugo cited above, circulation is also a useful term to refer to the 'patterns of circular interaction', which would include not just people but all the elements that create interaction and connectedness between people across distance. Caglar (2001, 607), for example, in discussing the conceptual value of a transnational approach, argues that it represents 'a new analytic optic which makes visible the increasing intensity and scope of *circular* flows of persons, goods, information and symbols triggered by international labour migration' (italics added).

An area of migration research in which the notion of circulation is increasingly debated is in relation to professional migration, and in particular concerns about 'brain drain' and the emigration of skilled young people (Harvey 2008; Tung 2008). This mobility of young graduates and other talent is not just affecting developing economies like those in India and Asia, but also developed ones experiencing economic crisis like Ireland, Italy and Spain. The mobility of highly skilled workers including doctors, nurses, engineers and IT specialists have been at the heart of this concern. Recent research is beginning to show, however, that these professionals often repatriate to their home countries after a period of time away (Conway and Potter 2009), and thus the notion of brain circulation has been advanced as a more appropriate term to describe this phenomenon (Saxenian 2005; Hugo 2009). Similar findings have been reported for *some* domestic and labour migrants who increase their skills and competencies during their time abroad, which they are able to capitalise on upon their return home (Agunias 2006).[32] Given the increased mobility that defines our contemporary lives, as well as the effective communication technologies that keep us connected, migration does not necessarily result in a loss of skills from the sending societies. Greater rates of repatriation and visits occur, during which 'feedback effects' may take place, in particular the so-called tacit knowledge of technology transfer, where migrants share information, know-how and instruction on the use of new technologies (Keller 2004). In addition, we might argue that these migrants can circulate their new-found knowledge and skills—their 'brain power'—through their personal, family and work networks and exchanges such that where they are located geographically is largely irrelevant.

To reiterate this point, circulation in the migration literature is most often a reference to the circular movement of people, 'a system of multiple, recurrent spatial movements of individuals, while the characteristic of multiplicity is as significant as the spatial movement and the system itself' (Illés and Kincses 2012, 198). But the people, while they circulate more often than ever before, actually move less often than their 'circulation activity' (what Hugo calls 'circular interaction'). In this way, 'brain circulation' might refer to the way knowledge can be transferred across distance between people regardless of where they reside. This idea of brain circulation led us to consider the notion of care circulation. Rather than focusing on the care workers, migrants or people who move, we asked, what would be the contribution to scholarship if we considered the circulation of care? The circulation of care, governed by cultural notions of obligation and generalised asymmetrical reciprocity, can occur in all families, wherever their members might reside, however distant or proximate, and whatever their socioeconomic class circumstances. The framework of circulation thus allows us to trace the care that circulates, such that the locus and mobility of the people involved, while equally important in terms of the multiple factors that influence care circulation, are not the primary focus of analysis. Of course, this is not to suggest that the circulation of care is similar in all the variety of family forms and social classes, nor that it is an easy and painless process.

The notion of circulation is also not new to family studies. We noted earlier how the circulation of care is often implied in research on care chains and transnational families but that it has not been formally examined. Similarly, the idea that care circulates within family networks is familiar to the socio-anthropology of proximate families and intergenerational solidarities, even if the term 'circulation' has been used largely descriptively and without being fully conceptualised. Key contributions in the field, including the classic work by Finch (1989b), have shown that caregiving in the form of goods and services flows—circulates—within family networks horizontally (between members of a similar generation) and vertically (across generations) both upwards and downwards over the family cycle.[33] Attias-Donfut (2000, 663, 664) talks of the 'circulation of exchanges' within family networks, as well as 'circular fluxes' of transfers between the generations.

The term 'circulation' in family studies has been particularly employed in relation to caregiving, or support, conceived as a form of gift-giving, following the seminal work of Mauss (1923) on the gift relationship, in which he argued that gift exchange is one of the bonds that cohere societies (see for instance, Bloch and Buisson 1994). According to Godbout and Charbonneau (1996, 61), the combination of the various forms of family support that circulate around children, homes, material support and money—as well as emotional and moral support—make the circulation of gifts complex and multiconnected and prevent individual members from closely tracking what is given and what is received in the long term. The authors see the circulation of gifts, which include care and support, as essential for the reproduction of kinship groups over the generations, and in particular for the intergenerational transmission of material and symbolic heritage (such as financial assets, family values and family principles). This focus on gift and 'generalised reciprocity' goes together with acknowledging the importance of reciprocal obligation and debt in family interactions. The anthropologist Levi Strauss (1969) developed ideas about gift exchange into a structural theory of group alliance, in which he argued that patterns of giving, receiving and repaying, as individuals and groups, reflect the deepest structures of societies. This is echoed in many case studies in this volume, which provide interesting data on the relationship between macro (state), meso (community) and micro (family and individual) factors and their impact on the circulation of care. This also involves understanding how particular mixes of private and public support arising from the articulation between families, states, markets and community organisations (conceptualised by some researchers as forming the points of a 'care diamond'; see Evers et al. 1994)[34] impact on transnational caregiving and receiving. Of particular interest here is the role of cultural notions of caregiving and obligation and how these are shaped by, as well as shape in turn, the policies, structures and infrastructures of family and support services.

Our book questions dominant constructions of 'families' and 'households' in research on transnational families by pointing to the diversity of family configurations and sense of connectedness. This is in line with Finch's (2007, 67) argument that:

> as a result of changed patterns of living there are now fewer and fewer people who can answer the question 'Who constitutes my family?' simply by pointing to a domestic group, or even by enumerating kin ties. Amongst those who cannot are people who live within 'chosen' families involving same sex partnerships and close friendships defined as family (Weeks et al., 2001); children and adults where there has been a divorce and where family membership has become multi-local, stretched across different households (Smart and Neale, 1999); and families where there has been a history of migration leading to transnational kin relationships, where families are stretched across continents, let alone across households.

While our analysis of care circulation features the social construction of 'the family' (albeit in its transnational form), we are also cognisant of the 'limits of the family construct' and how the notion of 'family' occupies an arguably privileged and hegemonic position within the sociology of relationships (Abel 2013). As mentioned earlier, it is imperative to take into account all of the important care-related social relationships in people's lives (Roseneil and Budgeon 2004). This involves debunking the notion of a single and uniform type of family form and structure (Bernardes 1986, 597). While the primacy of the kin network is clearly evident in the case studies in this volume, this is not to say that non-kin friendships and even the loose ties of associates (Amit 2007) do not play an important and integral role in social relationships and the exchange of care. As studies of British families show (Williams 2004), people work hard to sustain commitments to the persons (kin and non-kin) that matter to them. The notion of care circulation is based on the recognition of the diversity of 'families' within and across cultures, and thus invites us to move beyond heteronormative, static notions of the family to include all the actors of the care network—that is, kin and non-kin participants in transnational care flows.

In this volume, the framework of circulation is used to refer not only to the physical migratory movement of individuals between places, but to the other elements, in particular caregiving, that define their 'global' connectedness, including their links between family members in different places. People stay put for most of the time or for extended periods, but their labour and the fruits of their labour in the form of goods and services (money, gifts, letters, information), including caregiving, continue to 'move', and this circulation of elements that they propel defines, creates and sustains their transnational social spheres, transnational selves and transnational lives as well as their transnational family membership. The idea that caregiving involves the exchange of goods and services is central to the notion of 'transnational care' on which we build in order to propose a shift towards 'circulation'. Before concluding our discussion of this framework, we feel it is important to provide a brief overview of some of the ways people actually circulate care across distance and national borders; these activities comprise the practices and processes of transnational caregiving.

## THE CIRCULATION OF TRANSNATIONAL CARE

In this section, we draw on our own research to show how various types of care can be circulated in transnational settings to varying degrees and subject to a variety of factors. The notion of 'transnational care', as defined by Baldassar, Baldock and Wilding (2007), draws on Finch's (1989a) five-dimensional definition of care as economic, accommodation, personal, practical, emotional and moral. In transnational settings, personal (or 'hands-on') care can only be exchanged directly during visits, when people are physically co-present. Consequently, visits, and having the time, money and travel documents (including passports and visas) required to undertake them, are an important part of caring across distance. Financial support is arguably the oldest form of transnational care evident in the long history of remittances, which have traditionally been seen as the main motivation and justification for migration in the classical migration literature.[35] The exchange of financial support may take the form of cash remittances or other goods and services, including food and clothing, gifts and paying household and other bills. Practical care in transnational settings usually takes the form of exchanging advice and information, running errands and assisting with tasks, all of which may be provided both during visits as well as across distance, and these can involve extensive, regular and frequent communication, as in the case of transnational parenthood. Emotional and moral support is, arguably, the bedrock of all relationships and can be expressed in both proximate and distant contexts as well as through all other forms of care.[36]

The circulation of care across distance involves the social uses of communication technologies, including sending letters and messages by post, fax, e-mail and SMS texts; talking over the phone or the Internet (e.g., on Skype); and, more recently, staying in touch through social networking sites like Facebook and Twitter.[37] Access to technologies, including communication, travel, postal and international banking services, as well as their reliability and affordability and the knowledge and ability to use them, are becoming increasingly important factors in the practice of transnational caregiving. Here the importance of relations to the material world, of both technologies and 'non-human actors', is brought to the fore. Gille (2012) refers to this as 'methodological materialism', that is, the need to connect 'the social with the material'. Access to other types of resources is also essential, such as finances, time and social capital.[38] These factors account for and shape the asymmetries and inequalities, both within and between transnational families, in the capacity to circulate care. As Merla (2012a, 2) argues, 'access to, and use of, these capabilities is strongly influenced by both home- and host-country formal institutional and informal policies' and is shaped by gender, class and ethnic hierarchies (see also Chapter 5, this volume).

In their typology of the ways in which support is provided in transnational families, Kilkey and Merla (2013) include its direct provision in geographically proximate settings, the coordination of support and/or its direct provision through virtual communication from a distance as well as the delegation of the provision of support to others. They argue that it is important to acknowledge that a family member who delegates caregiving to a third person or institution does not automatically step out of circuits of care but may still be 'caring about' (Fisher and Tronto 1990) the person in need of support, stay informed of the level and quality of care provided and be ready to 'step in' when needed. In fact, caregiving in transnational contexts challenges the neat analytical distinction between 'caring for' (personal caregiving) and 'caring about' (emotional support), a distinction that is often difficult to sustain at the practical level (Leira and Saraceno 2006, 14).[39] For example, it is difficult to argue that emotional care is less necessary than personal care, and that it is not in itself a type of 'caring for', particularly in transnational contexts where there are limited opportunities for other forms of caregiving.

Transnational caregiving activity and its circulation waxes and wanes over the individual and family life course and migration process, and members may be 'inactive' in some periods and 'reactivated' in others (Grillo 2007). Bonvalet and Ogg (2006b, 51) see the reactivation of care exchanges in times of crisis as a sign that family solidarity is sometimes 'dormant'. There are also families in which care does not circulate, for example, when migrants purposely cease contact with kin to escape violence and abuse or to evade their caregiving obligations. This 'break' in family connectedness may be temporary and may change over the life course. Economically vulnerable family members in particular, including refugees, migrants without legal status and those with inadequate or unreliable incomes, might break ties when demands for transnational support are too onerous but reactivate them when they are better able to provide support.[40] Merla's (2011) study of Savaldoran refugees and economic migrants' transnational family networks shows that men and women's participation in the circulation of financial support varies over the life course depending on their legal status and position in the labour market. The inability to send remittances may lead them to invest in the circulation of other types of support, such as emotional and practical care.

The time and financial commitment involved in the exchange of transnational caregiving is an important consideration that influences not only the individual involved, but his or her local family as well. Putting time and money, particularly if these are scarce resources, into maintaining relationships with family overseas often means less time and money for local needs; therefore, having other household members willing to support transnational care is a significant variable (Wilding and Baldassar 2009). As Merla (2012a, 11) argues, 'Extended family networks . . . play a major role in helping migrants to overcome obstacles to transnational caregiving'. If, how and when support is exchanged is not a straightforward or simple process. Baldassar, Baldock and Wilding (2007) identify a dialectic at play that comprises capacity, obligation and negotiated commitments. Capacity to care is relevant in all settings, whether involving mobility or not, and refers to the physical (and mental) ability, opportunity and resources required to engage in caregiving. The notion of 'negotiated commitments' derives from Finch and Mason's (1991, 1993) classic work in which they discuss the notion of 'normative obligation'. Like the norm of reciprocity, normative obligation to give care is based on notions of duty and responsibility, supposedly at the core of family relations and frequently defined by policymakers as part of the moral fabric of society to which everyone should adhere. In practice, however, the actual support given to family members is not always the outcome of the 'proper thing to do' morally but of 'working it out' through the negotiation of commitments. These are the long histories of relationships and the circulation of care and support that cumulatively inform each decision to provide or withhold a certain form of care required by a particular person at a specific time—histories that are influenced by a series of factors, including power relations, gender inequalities, birth order and economic status.

Not surprisingly, much of the circulation of care activity in transnational families and the management of separation and absence of kin concern emotions and emotional lives.[41] There has been increasing interest in the social science of emotions, including in migration studies (Svašek 2008). Researching the emotional dimension of transnational relationships raises directly the issues discussed earlier about the cultural meanings and constructions of family roles and obligations in the contexts of distance and being apart (Merla 2010). Along with the reciprocal obligations to exchange care between family members, Baldassar (2008a) argues that the emotions of longing for and missing people and places appear to be an integral (though not an essential) feature of the kin work (di Leonardo 1984) and emotional labour (Duncombe and Marsden 1993) needed to maintain transnational relationships. She highlights how the activities of transnational communication and personal exchange are collectively described as 'keeping in touch' and 'staying in contact'. These phrases betray the central purpose of such practices as 'standing in for' physical presence, touch and contact. In addition to the labour and commitment involved in raising and saving money for remittances, the time and effort required to bridge the distance and create a sense of shared presence is not insignificant, as one research participant explained at length:

> I must tell you about distance . . . it's what I don't like about it . . . but distances estranges a little bit. Distance estranges . . . [you have to work at maintaining the relationship. . . . You have to listen to your feelings, you have to care, that is, you must care . . . You maintain the relationship by visiting, letters, phone calls, but first of all it is very important to keep them in your mind, caring for them all the time and not only when you phone or write to them. . . . This is made easier by having the photos around the house which help you to keep alive your memories.

A sense of shared 'presence' can be constructed in four main ways—virtually (through various communication technologies), by proxy (through objects and people whose physical presence embodies the spirit of the longed-for absent person or place), physically (during visits) and through imagined co-presence (Baldassar 2008a). The feelings of obligation, absence and loss, and the subsequent actions they motivate in people to try to create a sense of shared presence with their distant family members, comprise the activities and experiences that involve people imagining transnational family life into being. In this way, new communication technologies are pushing the limits of the lived experience of co-presence and have the potential to redefine our ideas about embodiment and the corporeal dimension of social relationships. While direct hands-on personal care, such as bathing and feeding, requires physical proximity, ongoing research is needed to better understand how technologies like Skype and the ability to be virtually co-present can compensate (or not) for corporeal absence. A key finding of our combined research in this regard is that the increased capacity to 'stay connected' offered by new communication technologies and/or relatively safe and affordable travel options actually increases the sense of obligation to engage in transnational communication and visits (Baldassar et al. 2007; Wilding 2007; Merla 2010). Far from replacing the need for physical co-presence, the exchange of virtual forms of communication may in fact increase it (Baldassar 2007a, 2007b).

Research on the communication practices of transnational families indicates that people will make use of whatever technologies are available to them to circulate care.[42] Our research suggests that, when available, new technologies are rapidly incorporated into family practices and a variety of modes of communication are used for different purposes. Baldassar et al. (2007) found, for example, that while everyday activities and concerns are regularly discussed in e-mails and phone calls, difficult and delicate news and information might be reserved for a written letter. Study areas such as Human Computer Interaction and ICT are developing a new lexicon to deal with the social impacts of the practices and processes of technology, including terms like 'scaffolding' (Ames et al. 2010), which refers to the support that one person gives to another to help make use of communication technology. We observed that children provide considerable assistance to their parents or grandparents in their use of new communication technologies such as Skype (Baldassar 2008a; Merla 2012b). Studies in 'media richness theory' describe how communication may escalate to a richer medium when the current one is not adequate. For example, family members may exchange an SMS to set up a Skype call, which may segue into a phone call and then be followed up with the sending of a gift. Similarly, Madianou and Miller (2012) show how polymedia—defined as a new communicative environment created by the emergence of Internet- and mobile phone-based platforms—have become an integral part of the way family relationships are experienced and enacted. For this reason, the social uses of technology have become a key feature of migration and family studies, and the chapters that comprise this volume offer a wealth of examples.

The intensity of care circulation varies over time. The Baldassar et al. (2007) study on transnational caregiving identified two main patterns of caregiving across distance—routine and crisis.[43] Crisis care involved responding to exceptional circumstances like the birth of a new baby, a serious and debilitating illness and death and dying. These lifecycle crises often involved a rapid reorganization of activities to permit an immediate and often extended visit to provide hands-on personal care as well as moral and emotional support. In moments of crisis, the importance of what people defined as simply 'being there' highlights the way physical co-presence is valued over other forms of 'staying in touch' through virtual technologies. In crisis situations, family members would rally together and increase all types of caregiving. In contrast, routine care defined the more regular exchange of care characterised by weekly phone or Skype calls and regular e-mails. These routine exchanges often developed into patterns of communication and included a mixed set of modes of communication—for example, daily SMS texts, phone or Skype calls every Sunday, long newsy e-mails periodically, and gifts for birthdays and special occasions. The particularities of age, gender and type of relationship impacted on these patterns as well as access to technology and the time and money to use them.

Our research findings suggest that the actual mechanical workings of these new technologies has increased the direct role and engagement of both men and younger generations in transnational family care exchanges because of their general tendency to be more familiar and proficient at using them. While the 'kin work' (Di Leonardo 1984) involved in keeping in touch with transnational family members was the preserve of women, particularly mothers and daughters, who wrote the letters and made the phone calls, we found in our samples that today it is not uncommon for fathers and sons, as well as grandchildren and cousins, to be directly involved in setting up the e-mail and Skype systems, coordinating and managing their use and maintaining their upkeep (Baldassar 2011; Merla 2012a, 2012b).[44] For example, Viviana, who we presented in the Introduction to this volume, asks her various local grandchildren to visit her so they can set up the Skype call to her daughters in the UK and Australia. Similarly, Viviana's distant grandchildren are regularly requested to assist with the technology of the call at the other end. In this way, the various cousins become involved in transnational communication exchanges that often lead to other forms and modes of contact, including exchanges on e-mail, Facebook and other social media sites. Here we see evidence of greatly expanded and intensified networks of communication and contact, including of the circulation of caregiving, than were possible before these technologies were widely available. This increased transnational family connectedness through the social use of new technologies belies the traditional association of migration with loss of ties and reduced capacities to exchange care.

## CONCLUSION

We have discussed how transnational families are in some ways similar to geographically proximate families, in that kin ties are constituted and maintained through the asymmetrical reciprocal exchange of caregiving. Yet transnational families are also impacted by distance and separation in specific ways. Distance makes the need to maintain family ties more pressing—and, therefore, more visible (Bryceson and Vuorela 2002a). The negotiation of transnational family togetherness in daily life requires particular skills and resources to transform physical absence into proximity through virtual communication. This is also true for multi-local families and not just transnational ones. What is particular about transnational families is that their members must deal with the opportunities and constraints of (at least) two national institutional settings, as well as transnational and international contexts. Highlighting the agency of transnational family members requires an analysis of the ways in which structural contexts frame the options and choices of migrants and their relatives, and how they 'respond to, resist, adapt to and/or bend the laws, rules and procedures emanating from specific policies' (Herrera 2010, 55) in order to keep their family ties alive.[45]

An elderly Irish woman from our study once commented that in the past when people migrated to Australia, family members would hold a wake; the departure was such a significant loss that it represented a kind of social death. Our research suggests that these days, migration is characterised by the increased use of new communication technologies that can help to ensure migrants remain very much a living part of family life. This anecdote is in many ways emblematic of the entire project of this volume; that the implications and impact of the act of migration—and mobility more generally—on family life has profoundly changed. The advent of new technologies means that care can be more readily exchanged across distance and continue to circulate through reciprocal (though asymmetrical) exchanges that consolidate and substantiate family and friendship ties. By concentrating on the transnational social fields and the various forms of co-presence created by the exchange of communication and caregiving between transnational family members, we are better able to examine these particular family forms more objectively.

In this volume, we suggest that one way to moderate the dominating role that notions of distance and separation have had on our understanding of transnational family life is to highlight the asymmetrical reciprocity and inherent circularity of both migration and transnational family processes. Transnational family exchanges, particularly those relating to caregiving, are defined by their flows back and forth and often in multiple directions. The chapters that follow trace the way care circulates around expanded transnational family networks to highlight the participation—and absence of participation—of various family members and not just those who have been traditionally more visible. While male migrants dominated the migration frame and women dominated the family studies framework, the involvement of extended family members, including the grandparent and younger generations, is highlighted through the care circulation lens. Furthermore, the lens of circulation is equally relevant to the poorer labour migrant families of the classical care chains literature as well as the relative elites of student, skilled and professional migration. While the scale, mode and degree may change, all transnational families are engaged in the reciprocal exchange of care that circulates among them. In the contributions that comprise Part B of this volume, the authors address the critical questions of gender, ethnic, generational and class differences and inequalities affecting the shape, intensity and quality of participation of all the actors involved in—or excluded from—care circuits.

For the purpose of this book, we limit our analysis to the family, but in order to be fully developed, the circulation framework will need to include other actors of global care circuits, such as wider communities in home and host societies. Research that examines the role of families and caregiving, broadly defined, in the processes of settlement and integration as well as the maintenance and development of homeland cultures and traditions offer productive sites of analysis. In line with Margaret Archer's (2000, 2006) compelling argument that 'we are what we care for',[46] we locate the 'portability of care' and its circulation in asymmetrical and reciprocal exchanges between people, wherever they live, at the centre of our research endeavour. The lens of circulation helps us to better understand the impact of distance and absence on our lived experiences and our conceptualisation of these. It also helps to highlight the arbitrariness of distinctions between what are often considered the more public and formal dimensions of culture and society, such as paid employment and civic life, and those defined as private and intimate, such as family caregiving.

## NOTES

1. See, for instance, Bryceson and Vuorela 2002b; Goulbourne et al. 2010; Olwig 2007; Zontini and Reynolds 2007; Baldassar et al. 2007; Bolzman et al. 2008; Le Gall 2009; Mazzucato and Schans 2011; Merla 2012a, 2012b; Razy and Baby-Collin 2011.
2. See, for instance, Andall 1999; Esparragoza 2003; Hondagneu-Sotelo and Avila 1997; Mazzucato and Schans, 2011.
3. Hochschild (2005) evocatively refers to this as the exchange of love for gold.
4. See also Merla 2011; Baldassar 2008b.
5. We also draw this critique from Wellman (1988, 20), who makes a similar point about the misinterpretation of network analysis: 'Many have limited the power of the [network analysis] approach by treating all units as if they had the same resources, all ties as if they were symmetrical, and the contents of all ties as if they were equivalent'.
6. For example, the representation of women in the north as gaining career and paid work advantage from the employment of domestics is arguably overly simplistic. Southern European women, in particular, are often blocked out of the labour market with limited prospects for career advancement that is not necessarily improved by the increasingly common presence of domestic women workers within their families (Campani 2012; Saraceno 2010). Furthermore, many domestic migrant women are from the middle classes in their countries of origin, and some of them, as argued by Morokvasic (2004), employ transnational mobility as a tool to maintain their middle-

class lifestyle through the improved pay they get from domestic work abroad compared with middle-class work at home. See also Flavell et al. (2007) for a discussion of the need for a more nuanced understanding of elites and migration.

7. See, for example, Abrego 2009; Dreby 2006; Parreñas 2005a, 2005b; Mahler and Pessar 2001; Pessar and Mahler 2003.
8. See also Fog Olwig 2002; Smith 2001; Baldassar and Gabaccia 2011. Along a similar thread and drawing on Werbner's notion of the diasporic public sphere, Baldassar and Gabaccia (2011) examine the idea of a diasporic domestic sphere.
9. As shown by Shain 2007; Goulbourne et al. 2010; Baldassar 2007a; Merla and Baldassar 2010a.
10. Relevant examples in studies of transnational mothering include Hondagneu-Sotelo and Avila 1997; Parreñas 2005[a], 2005b; Ryan 2011. For studies of transnational families, see, for instance, Hondagneu-Sotelo and Avila 1997; Parreñas 2005a, 2005b; Ryan 2011.
11. See Douglass 2006; Peterson 2010; Safri and Graham 2010.
12. See, for instance, Glick Schiller, Basch and Szanton-Blanc 1992; Vertovec 2001, 2009; Fog Olwig 2002, 2007; Bauböck and Faist 2010; Holmes 2006; Levitt and Glick Schiller 2007; Portes, Guarnizo and Landolt 1999; Abrego 2009; Parreñas 2001a, 2001b, 2005a, 2005b; Dreby 2006; Boccagni 2012b.
13. See Baldassar 2011; Baldassar et al. 2012.
14. See also Alba and Waters 2011.
15. See, for example, Rossi and Rossi 1990; Lin and Rogerson 1995; Joseph and Hallman 1985; Bonvalet and Ogg 2006a.
16. See, for example, Rouse 1991; Glick Schiller and Fouron 2001; Papastergiadis 2000; Boccagni 2012b.
17. See also Mason 2004; Baldassar 2001.
18. It is interesting to consider whether the notion of circularity offers something different than the notion of transnationalism, or at least it is important to reflect on the framework of circulation in the context of recent theorisation of transnationalism. The notion of circulation seems to have much the same meaning as transnationalism, insofar as both terms offer a more useful frame to complicate the notion of permanent unidirectional migration. It should be added that circulation and transnational processes in families are not new. Throughout history, there have been many and varied forms, including the medieval custom of apprenticeship, the longstanding practice in certain countries of sending young children to boarding school, the migration of wet nurses and artisans (Sarausa 2001), the separation from their families of members of religious orders (Yeates 2009) and so on. Rather, the scale of these processes has been radically transformed. Both terms clearly represent overlapping and complementary sets of processes. As already argued, circulation tends to refer to the movement of people. Circularity has been employed in the literature to define the migration type, as in the circular migration of relatively short annual or seasonal migratory moves, although now we better understand how even longer 'circuits' of migration spanning lifetimes also often end in return and are therefore also 'circular'. Transnationalism, as discussed in the literature, more specifically relates to the 'social field' in which the circulatory migrant moves, and refers in particular, to the way this social field is stretched across space and time, constructed and 'inhabited' by people who are separated by distance (Basch et al. 1994). The notion of circularity might be best understood as one dimension of transnationalism, referring more specifically to the people as well as the objects, ideas and

shared imaginings/meanings that move or flow across these transnational social fields, including of care. In addition, 'circulation' can occur within national borders and so encompasses local families as well, whereas transnational specifically refers to families separated by national borders. Hence, the analysis of care circulation can include both the proximate and transnational family relationships in which both migrants and nonmigrants participate.

19. See, for example, Carling et al. 2012; Hochschild 2005; Hondagneu-Sotelo and Avila 1997; Parreñas 2005; Hays 1998.
20. Sørensen and Guarnizo 2007; draw on Therborn 2004.
21. This link between physical presence and well-being is evident in the case of Italian migrants in Australia reported by MacKinnon and Nelli (1996, 74), who describe an obviously unwell elderly woman who was surrounded by her family when her doctor enquired after her health; she replied, 'Of course I am well, my whole family is here'.
22. See also Elizabeth Thomas-Hope 2002; Byron 1999.
23. See, for instance, Ahmed et al. 2003; Rutherford 1990; Lash and Friedman 1992; Lavie and Swedenburg 1996; Portes and Rumbaut 2001.
24. Relevant examples in the context of this discussion include research on nomadism and the practice of transhumance.
25. See also Caradec 1996; Trost 1998; Holmes 2004; Nowicka 2007.
26. It is important to acknowledge that in many countries, it is still difficult for men to get custody of their children.
27. See, for example, Kurotani 2007; Martin 2007; Walsh 2006, 2008; Coles 2008.
28. See also Boyle et al. 2003.
29. See, in particular, Chapter 6.
30. Since 1998, the Department of Immigration and Citizenship in Australia has given every person moving to and from the country a number, so it is possible to examine repeat movements of individuals.
31. For example, Hardill (2004, 378) refers to research that reports 'a rise in the circulatory movements of British citizens moving cross border on relatively short-term assignments before returning to the UK or transferring to another location'. See also Hardill and MacDonald (1998). Retirement migration (Williams et al. 2000) is another example, as are the growing numbers of so-called commuter families mentioned earlier.
32. However, this is certainly not the case for all domestic and labour migrants; see Kapur 2001 and Kapur, Devesh and McHale, 2005.
33. See also Attias-Donfut 2000; Attias-Donfut et al. 2002; Coenen-Huther et al. 1994; Finch and Mason 1993; Godbout and Charbonneau 1996.
34. See also Jenson 2003; Razavi 2007; Kofman and Raghuram 2009.
35. For one of the earliest studies of transnational family lives, see Thomas and Znaniecki 1974.
36. It is important to note that care can also be performed as an obligation or duty, both paid and unpaid, including between family members, without a sense of concern or emotional attachment. For an overview of this issue in the care literature, see Leira and Saraceno 2006.
37. There are also examples of distant kin 'babysitting' children by 'keeping an eye on them on Skype'.
38. Merla and Baldassar 2011; Merla 2012a; Kilkey and Merla 2013.
39. See also Baldassar et al. 2007.
40. See Baldassar et al. 2007; Baldassar 2008b, for a discussion of this dynamic in the case of Afghan refugees in Australia.
41. See, for instance, Merla and Baldassar 2010a.
42. Baldassar et al. 2007; Madianou and Miller 2012; Wilding 2006.

43. A point also made by studies of geographically proximate families such as Bonvalet and Ogg 2006b.
44. Although in the Salvadoran case, the use of new communication technologies was still limited (Merla 2012a, 2012b).
45. See also Baldassar and Merla 2011; Kilkey and Merla 2013; Merla 2012a, 2012b.
46. Reseach by Meda (2012), for example, uses a relational sociology (Donati 2012) framework to examine the intersections between what might be called different 'care projects' and their role in identity formation in transnational family and migration contexts, including care of origins (homeland) and differences (e.g., gender and generations) as well as care of distance (culture) and the care of the ties between them (transnational bonds). See also Rossi and Bramanti (2012) and Rossi et al (2010).

# Part B

# Care Circulation

## Theoretical and Empirical Considerations

# 2 Mapping the New Plurality of Transnational Families

## A Life Course Perspective

*Karin Wall and Claudio Bolzman*

## INTRODUCTION

Understanding how family relationships move beyond national borders and redefine themselves over space is the major challenge of research focusing on transnational family living. Migration literature has revealed the elusive and complex nature of family living across borders (Baldassar and Baldock 2000; Bryceson and Vuorela 2002b; Baldassar, Baldock and Wilding 2007) while also identifying *spatial dispersion* and *relational interdependency* as the two primary dimensions of transnational families (Vatz and Bolzman 2010). Dispersion refers to having members of the family spread out across several nation-states, whereas interdependency denotes maintaining a sense of bonding despite long distance.

Moving beyond this initial concept of transnational families, current literature stresses two important points. A first issue is the way transnationalism is disconnected from the conventional linkages between family and household (Parreñas 2001b, 2005a; Zontini 2007). The concept of *household* refers to a group of people who share the same residence and partake of daily life (Laslett 1965). It is a notion based on the concept of co-residence, in contrast to the concept of family, which is linked to the criteria of consanguinity and affinity. The family is nearly always included in a household, but not necessarily: Family relations go beyond the household, including a wide range of kin as well as other close ties, such as friends who may be perceived as family (Morgan 1996; Widmer 2010). In this respect, the framework of 'care circulation' (Part A, this volume) is crucial: By emphasising that care *circulates* across households and borders, it draws attention to exchanges that involve a large 'configuration' or network of close persons who are interdependent without living physically near each other. It conceptualises care as a multidirectional process, emphasising complex flows of support within the dispersed members of a family configuration, rather than a simple one- or two-way process.

A second issue in recent research is the need for a dynamic perspective, which captures the complexity and plurality of transnational families. A sense of family cohesion, underpinned by care and interdependency, and family practices have to be seen as processes that may change over time and also in relation to contextual factors such as life conditions, inequalities or migration policies (Wall and São José 2004; Clark et al. 2009; Baldassar 2008a; Kilkey and Merla 2013; Chapter 5, this volume). In particular, transnationalism needs to be understood as a set of practices fashioned throughout the life course, with key life stages shaping and driving a diversity of family obligations, support needs and exchanges of care. Those who migrate as single young adults, those in their middle years and the elderly are likely to be embedded in specific family configurations and develop different patterns of interdependency (Kobayashi and Preston 2007; Wall 2007).

These two questions underpin a third challenge, which is taken up in this chapter. How does migration experienced at different key points of the life course affect transnational family living? What is the influence of the family life stage on caregiving, and how does this interact with other important factors such as the family configuration and the migration project? Can we identify a plurality of transnational families or does geographical distance have such an overriding impact on family life that it systematically weakens the influence of the life course and leads to one predominant form (usually seen as negative, due to distance) of experiencing care and bonding across borders?

## MAIN FOCUS AND METHODOLOGY

Drawing on qualitative case studies carried out over the last ten years on migrant families living in different parts of Europe, in particular in Switzerland and Portugal, this chapter explores the new plurality of *transnational families* related to migration flows into and across Europe at the beginning of the twenty-first century. The in-depth interviews used in this chapter were collected in five cross-national studies on migrant families: the SOCCARE project (2001–2003), which included seventy-two interviews with migrant families living in Finland, France, Italy, Portugal and the UK; the RFA project on Family Reunification of the Elders from different countries (2006–2008), which included twenty-four interviews with elderly migrants and their families living in Switzerland; the Female Migration Vision Project (2005–2007), which included thirty-four interviews with Brazilian, Ukrainian and Cape Verdean migrant women with children living in Portugal; and the project on Latin-American Migrants in Switzerland (2007–2009), which included twenty interviews with migrant families. Interviews were analysed both vertically, to capture the stories of specific families, and horizontally, to grasp the recurrent patterns of transnational family living and how they relate to caregiving.

Our approach combines three theoretical underpinnings. First, the *life course* approach emphasises that family transitions (e.g., parenthood, divorce, repartnering) experienced by individuals over the life course are important factors in shaping close relationships (Bernardi 2011). Second, the framework of *care circulation,* as introduced by Baldassar and Merla (Chapter 1, this volume), focuses on the mobile nature of care practices, thereby drawing attention to care as a multidirectional process involving complex interdependencies between family members across borders. Thirdly, a *family configurational* approach stresses the wide range of carers involved in family structures and networks, thereby stretching our analytical outlook beyond the nuclear co-resident two-generational household. A configurational perspective posits that *family (or carer) networks* may include a variety of bonds (from close blood ties across several generations to ex-kin or friends) and involve exchanges of many different resources; it also draws attention to the *focal points* (e.g., significant events, activities, places) on which interdependencies in family networks are built (Widmer and Jallinoja 2008). For example, although transnational family members are separated, this does not mean that places and houses, through temporary co-residence or visits (Mason 2004), are not important 'focal points' of transnational living. Much as in postdivorce families, in which children live alternately in two or more households, migrant families may negotiate new boundaries of co-residency and physical proximity connected to one or more places of residence.

The notion of *care configuration* is adopted in this chapter to bridge and connect the concepts of care circulation and family configuration: It refers to the family network of interdependent close persons as it relates to caregiving and support. With the objective of identifying the plurality of transnational families from a life course perspective, our focus will be on three different life stages: adult life before parenthood (young couples), adult life with children (couples with children and lone mothers) and adult life in middle age (adults going through later life transitions such as grandparenthood, widowhood or retirement). The stories of migration are examined along three main analytical axes. First, it is important to identify the social and life course *position* of the main actor(s) in migration. Second, it is essential to understand his or her lived experience and subjective perspective on the situation: The *meanings* of transnational care and family life will depend to a great extent on the migration and family life projects of the person or couple who decides to migrate. Third, we look at the *care configuration* by examining family members' care responsibilities and practices, such as frequency and types of contact and support, as well as the type of family network and focal points that activate the exchange of care.

Our primary focus on these aspects does not mean that we ignore the profound influence of other contextual variables on migrant families over the life course. Migration policies, in particular family reunification policies in the receiving country, have a significant impact on transnational family living (Bolzman et al. 2008; see also Chapter 4, this volume). Other important factors may include labour markets and the experience of discrimination, as well as cultural and societal contexts such as gender cultural models or the push factors of migration (Baldassar 2007a). Gender and social inequalities, both in sending and receiving societies, are also crucial, especially in the context of growing female and illegal migration to many European countries (Ehrenreich and Hochschild 2003a). Finally, family variables such as the number of children born, the number of generations alive and changing family forms are all expected to influence the patterns of family networking and caregiving across borders. Although the main focus of analysis is on the impact of the life course, we will draw attention to these aspects as they emerge in many of the cases. This will help us explore the current complexity and diversification of transnational families.

## EXAMINING A PLURALITY OF TRANSNATIONAL FAMILIES

### Life Stage—Young Couples Before the Transition to Parenthood

This is a specific moment of the life course, one in which young couples who have recently entered into partnership are planning their future life together and seeking to set up a family. Although they decide to migrate in order to look for regular jobs for one or both members of the couple (Bolzman and Guissé 2010), the migration project is also embedded in a family and household formation project: The idea (sometimes referred to as 'the dream') is not only to improve employment and living conditions but also to save up money in order to set up a business and/or buy or build a house, thereby ensuring future family formation and parenthood (Bolzman, Carbajal and Mainardi 2007).

Gabi and Octavio, a young Brazilian couple in their 20s, are a typical example of these *young couples in the making*: They come from a small inland town where economic prospects were extremely poor in 2004; they have some qualifications (Gabi finished secondary school, and Octavio trained and worked as a computer programmer) but low paid job opportunities and no house of their own. Their migration project, well defined and discussed within the extended family before leaving, is to stay in Europe for five years in order to save up for a house of their own (close to their families) and for launching their careers. Gabi wants to set up as a hairdresser with the help of an aunt who is in the same line of business. Five years is also the ideal time span before entering parenthood. The couple will have been married for six years, and Gabi will be twenty-eight when they return, the ideal moment, they say, to make the transition to parenthood.

Family bonds spanning the two continents (Gabi has a younger brother working in the UK) are tightly knit and part of daily life and future plans: They talk to their close family members (parents and brother in particular) once a week on the Internet and share each other's life events and problems. Communicating, emotional support and future plans for returning are therefore the main forms of bonding. Gabi and Octavio's emotional well-being draws strongly on the concern expressed by their parents and extended kin. Other forms of care, such as financial support, are not only weak or totally absent but also not expected. Expectations are that the young couple will work hard and save up to have a house and a family of their own, and this implies putting close kin at home at some distance and not spending too much on visits: 'From the moment you get married, you have to think of your future, you have to let go of your parents just a little bit. . . . So, we came here, and we will have to work hard . . . but it's worthwhile'. (Gabi)

The care configuration of *young couples in the making* is anchored in the nuclear family but also branches out to other close kin, such as aunts and uncles and first cousins, siblings and their spouses and grandparents. It implies strong emotional interdependency as well as a sense of cohesion underpinned by projects of geographical proximity, house-building and parenthood in the near future.

What has been said for young couples on the basis of this case may, however, be examined in the context of other variables, such as the push factors of migration. Some couples migrate from countries that are going through major economic upheavals rather than just failing to provide good opportunities for young people. Political and economic upheavals in some Eastern European countries at the turn of the millennium, for example, make for slightly different projects and care responsibilities. First, the migration project is not as clearly delineated because future plans for return depend on developments in the home country and not only on the wishes of the young couple and their families. In fact, some young couples reckon they were forced to migrate due to unemployment. As a result, even if the project is perceived and couched in the same type of narrative—the couple's ideal is to improve their life and achieve sound economic basis for family formation—this kind of turbulent situation makes for greater fluidity in family bonding and caring across different countries. At least two important differences must be mentioned. First, commitment to future family life geographically close to the extended family in the home country cannot be as strong, thereby making for less cohesion on the basis of future proximity. In contrast, however, material care may, in these situations, be seen as more urgent. Those who stayed behind are seen to be in a precarious situation and need to rely on those who find themselves in more favourable economic circumstances. These *young couples in the making* who are still *on the move* may therefore be expected to contribute occasionally when close family members back home are in need, even if they are also expected to get on with their own lives. In some ways, then, in turbulent times, both migration and the need for transnational care may be seen as constraints on conjugal life in its early stages.

Ludmilla and Piotr, a young Ukrainian couple from Sevezskin in their late 20s, are an example of migration experienced as a constraint rather than an opportunity. The couple had been cohabiting for two years when things became very bad. Ludmilla was still a trainee (economist), and Piotr, a metallurgical engineer and the main breadwinner, was no longer receiving his salary. Two years after migration to Portugal, Piotr is working in his profession, whereas Ludmilla is working as a domestic employee; both are legal immigrants. They are in close contact with a first cousin living in Lisbon and also with their parents, siblings and aunts and uncles in Sevezsk. Work and family life have stabilised, and they are occasionally able to send money home to their parents. However, they have no plans to return or to save up money for a house in the Ukraine; for the moment, they are concentrating on their integration in the new country. Their parents also encourage them to invest in their working and family life; financial support is only requested when there are problems coping with debts or exceptional expenses.

In summary, in this life stage, young couples are expected to invest strongly in their jobs as well as set up a household and have children. In light of this major project, care responsibilities to other households in the home country, mostly of parents who are still working and middle age, are pushed into the background. Emotional bonds and support are strong, however, and this makes for strong 'potential' care, both economic and other, should the need arise either here or there.

## Life Stage: Adult Life with Children

In this life stage, we find many examples of transnational families in recent research on this issue, in particular the long-standing pattern of the breadwinner father who leaves his family behind. However, we also find other emerging patterns, such as couples who migrate together and leave their children behind; the lone mother (single or divorced) who leaves her children behind; and, more seldom, the breadwinner mother who leaves a husband and young children, or the breadwinner mother or father who travels with some of the children and leaves a spouse and/or an ex-partner and other children in the home country.

One of the predominant features of all the care configurations with children in this life stage is that the needs of young dependent children, independently of partnership, create strong care obligations and practices. Dependent children are a major focal point for care flows across borders, not only between parents and children left behind, but also from grandparents in the home country to families with young children in the receiving country. For example, couples that migrate with their children or give birth to a child abroad often ask for emotional support and practical counselling at a distance from their parents (Le Gall 2009). They contact them via Skype or by telephone to ask for information on bringing up babies and children. They also ask for advice when someone is ill and for parents' support in case of family problems, such as marital conflict or partnership breakup.

However, families with young children may include a wide range of family structures, revealing a trend towards diversification, which is linked not only to cultural differences across the globe but also to recent changes in family life as a result of increasing divorce rates, female participation in the labour market and more negotiation of conjugal roles in the context of gender equality, economic uncertainty and individualisation.

During most of the twentieth century, migration flows within and across countries and continents were linked to family migration, in which male providers were the first members of the family to emigrate, a pattern of migration that gradually led to reunification policies that allow dependent members of the nuclear family to follow in the footsteps of the husband/father as soon as he has a house and a regular job. This *caring long-distance father* type of transnational family follows a few typical pathways in terms of migration: The father emigrates alone soon after marriage and the birth of a first child; the father emigrates alone, leaving a wife and several children; after migrating alone before partnership and then coming back periodically to get partnered and start a family, the father moves to and fro, leaving his wife and children behind or 'sends for them' some time later. Labour migrant workers in postwar Europe often left their families behind on a permanent basis, coming back home for a few months every year and then leaving again. This was (and still is) frequently related to status as a 'seasonal' worker or as an illegal migrant worker not entitled to family reunification, but it can also be linked to labour migrants who have a specific intensive-saving project—to return at the end of a few years after saving up—and prefer not to move their families during this supposedly 'short' period. More rarely, it can also be linked to male providers who, in the face of economic difficulties in the receiving country and failure of the migration project to send money home or save up, became *absent long-distance fathers* who no longer contact or care for the families they left behind.

At the beginning of the twenty-first century, the *caring long-distance father* configuration still exists. António, a bricklayer, emigrated as a young man from the Cape Verde Islands in the late 1990s and met Dulce, his partner, when he went home on holiday. Dulce stayed on in Cape Verde for six years, where she lived with her parents and the two children she gave birth to during those years. António came home once a year, sent money regularly and would also speak once a month on the phone (they never had computers or access to the Internet). When she joined him in Lisbon, António had managed to move into a three-room (council) house, but Dulce decided all the same to leave the children with her parents: She wanted to work hard in order to improve family life and felt that the children were well cared for at home. The family reunited four years later. The couple sends remittances to Cape Verde regularly, both for her mother and to pay for the house they are renovating and hope to return to when they retire; they speak on and off on the phone and sometimes send parcels by post or through other migrants. Transnational family living, a common fate for the majority of Cape Verdeans, is neither questioned nor felt as a constraint, but rather it is viewed as a necessary part of life and an opportunity to be managed in the best possible way. Long-distance bonding, long-term separation sometimes involving abandonment, shared care for dependent persons across the extended family and living and dying far from home are closely embedded in this way of life and accepted as such. Societal context is therefore an important variable to be taken into account, as it may influence the greater acceptance or rejection of transnational family life.

The *caring father* pattern followed by step-by-step migration is no longer the main type of transnational family. Couples migrate jointly without their children, married women migrate before their husbands and children, lone mothers migrate alone or with their children and divorced men and women migrate with a second partner and leave children in the care of an ex-partner.

Couples with children who migrate together and leave their children behind (*caring long-distance parents*) usually wish to do so temporarily while they seek stable living conditions, legal status and jobs abroad (as above). This is often the case when family life is hit hard by economic problems, making it urgent for families to seek employment in another country. Angela (age thirty-nine) and her husband Nelson were highly indebted and in danger of losing their home in Brazil when in 2004 they decided to migrate together for a couple of years to pay off their debts. They left their sons, ages twenty and thirteen, at home, the younger in the care of the elder (and living close to other family members). But the younger son was unhappy away from his parents and asked repeatedly (on the phone) to join them. So plans were changed, and one year after leaving, when both had regular jobs (Nelson as a gardener and Angela as a daily), Angela went to Brazil to fetch him. The migration project, however, was not changed: The family only stayed for three years, working *from Sunday to Sunday* to pay off their debts; they went back to Brazil in 2007.

Older children left behind, of primary school age or adolescents, are expected to understand the need for temporary spatial dispersion of the family and to participate in the family migration project by caring for younger siblings. This is sometimes also expected of younger children, most of whom adapt well to staying in the care of grandparents. But separation is nearly always longer than expected, with economic and reunification problems as well as illegality and fear of not being able to re-enter the receiving country often making it impossible for parents to go back to visit their children. Prolonged separation may become difficult or unbearable, not only for young children but also for older children and their parents. Piatachoc and her husband left the Ukraine together in 2001 and had plans to fetch their nine-year-old daughter (in the care of her parents) as soon as possible, but it took them almost two years to find regular jobs, a house (shared with her brother and his partner) and legal permits. The years of separation seemed *never-ending*.

Another problem of care configurations in which dependent children are left behind is that long-distance communication, although regular (monthly, bimonthly or weekly depending on means, education and distance), is felt to be misleading, making it difficult for parents to assess whether the young children are well. Children and/or their carers will sometimes not mention problems, so as not to worry long-distance fathers and mothers. It is especially difficult if children fail to mention that they are being neglected or having conflicts with the adult carers to whom they have been entrusted. Helen, a divorced lone mother who migrated to Canada to try to make ends meet after a difficult divorce and left her three daughters in the care of her mother and stepfather, began to feel at a distance that something was not right. When she returned without warning, she found her children undernourished and neglected, but unable to communicate their troubles despite regular contact on the phone. From this point of view, transnational parenting is felt to be inadequate because face-to-face contact is felt to be necessary, at least occasionally, to make sure that children are being well cared for. Relational problems due to separation are also possible negative factors depending on how some children react to being left behind and waiting to be fetched. Calina's only son, age fourteen at the time of his parents' departure (both medical doctors who were unemployed in Moldavia), always expressed his hostility at being the only one of the nuclear family left behind (with his maternal grandmother), accusing his parents of *abandoning him*; he joined them two years later (before the reunification process was complete), but Calina is worried because parent–child relations and his integration in the receiving country remain strained:

> I left one son and found another one. (. . .) He didn't even want to speak to me on the phone. Because he started to think we had left him forever. (. . .) I can arrange everything in my life, but I can't arrange my son. I think that's the hardest thing I have had to go through with this immigration and I'm very sorry that he didn't come with me from the very first moment.

Another frequent type of family in this key life stage is related to migration pathways in which a young lone mother—separated/divorced or single—migrates, leaving children and other close family members behind. Women are usually confident about their capacity to earn well in the receiving country, in particular in the care and domestic work sector, and social networking creates opportunities for rapid integration in the labour market (Wall and Nunes 2010). The *caring long-distance lone mother* who leaves young children behind usually starts out with an intensive-saving project and hopes to return after a few years.

This is the case of Neuza, a twenty-three-year-old single mother who migrated alone, leaving a six-month-old child in Brazil in the care of her mother (a widow, who is also looking after an eight-year-old grandson left in her care by Neuza's elder sister, also a migrant single mother). Before migrating, Neuza lived with her mother and was unemployed, earning only a little money selling hand-made dolls. She decided to go to Portugal shortly after her child was born mainly because she needed money to bring up her daughter but also, if possible, to save up in order to renovate her mother's house. She arrived in Lisbon in 2005 and already had a job waiting for her (through a friend) as a *live-in* domestic employee for an upper class family, also caring for a ninety-three-year-old elderly person. With a salary of 500 Euros, she is paying off her debts in Brazil, sending money to her mother, and hoping to begin saving up for the house. If all goes well, she expects to stay in Portugal for only three years. She feels sad at missing the first years of her daughter's childhood, but at the same time she believes that coming to Portugal was the best decision, as she will be able *to provide a better life for her daughter.* She sees her sister (also in Lisbon working as a domestic employee) every week, and they are both in weekly contact with their mother and with their brother, who lives in the same town as their mother and keeps an eye on things at home.

Bonding and commitment in the context of caring lone parenthood is not always easy to build up across borders and several generations. The intensive-saving project is difficult to accomplish. Lone mothers may face other problems, such as having a second child out of wedlock in the receiving country or not being able to bring children from the home country because of economic or immigration restrictions. Managing alone in the receiving country is a major challenge and in some cases leads to poverty and difficulties in caring for children left behind. In light of these difficulties, the *caring long-distance lone mother* may turn into a care configuration of a *deprived long-distance lone mother*, as in the case of Julia. Julia was a three-year-old child when she was left with an aunt in Cape Verde. Her parents separated, and both emigrated abroad and remarried. Since then, she has only seen her mother once, when she was thirteen years old. It was against this background that Julia decided to migrate in the late 1990s, hoping to improve her life. She left on her own, leaving her one-year-old daughter with her aunt. Sometime later she had another child, also as a single mother. At the time of the interview, she was living in extreme poverty. She was working in a cleaning services company from 8 a.m. to 5 p.m., earning the national minimum wage (around 400 Euros). With this money and the child allowance from social security, she has to first pay the rent (around 100 Euros), then transport, food and clothes, and then still send money to Cape Verde. She has no financial support from the children's fathers and sometimes goes hungry to send money to Cape Verde. She hardly ever phones now and has never been to Cape Verde to see her daughter, now age seven. She feels lonely, ashamed and depressed about her daughters' future.

Deprivation, isolation and lack of future prospects can erode the pathways to transnational parental bonding in dramatic ways. But the nature of commitment may also change in a more positive direction in the context of other family transitions in the receiving country, such as stable repartnering. São is a forty-four-year-old *caring repartnered lone mother.* In Brazil she lived as a single mother in an extended family household with her retired parents and her brother's family, earning a low salary as a kitchen help. Migration to Europe in 2003 was seen as an opportunity to earn well in order to help educate her son, age fourteen at the time and a bad student, by putting him in a private school. São left him in the care of her brother and has been able to send money regularly to pay for his schooling and other needs, such as clothes and books. Two years after arriving, São met her new partner (divorced, one child), and they moved in together. Interviewed in 2007, she feels she wants to stay on in Portugal indefinitely, pleased with both her conjugal and economic life as well as with her son's progress (going to university to study engineering); she has planned to go with her partner to visit her son and family in Brazil.

In summary, in this life stage, parents living in different types of family forms (couples with children, lone parents, postdivorce families) are investing in their children's upbringing. Geographical mobility in this life stage puts the care needs of young children first in the migration project and seems to activate multidirectional care practices across countries and a variety of close kin relationships, with grandparents as well as aunts and uncles providing care for children left behind, and those in the receiving country sending money and support for three generations of relatives as well as asking for support. Intergenerational exchanges lead not only to care configurations focusing on children but also to emotional involvement and economic investment in the family homes where they live. However, in all the care configurations, the long wait for reunification is felt as a period that is too long for parent–child relationships.

## Life Stage: Middle-age Adults with Older/Adult Children

In this life stage, we find new types of transnational families. Middle-age male or female breadwinners frequently have to care simultaneously for adolescent children, adult children, grandchildren and needy elderly parents left behind. The financial burden on middle-age spouses or lone adults can be extremely heavy during this period of life: less focused on the problem of care for young dependent children, but instead spanning care responsibilities towards and across a wide range of close kin. In order to take on these new intergenerational responsibilities, they often modify migratory plans from intensive-saving into longer stay trajectories; they may go alone and return a few years later, postpone going home for many years or initiate migration and then encourage other family members to join them.

Antónia (age forty-seven, one year of schooling, domestic employee in three different houses) is a good example of a middle-age *caring long-distance mother-grandmother* who initiated migration as the main breadwinner of a three-generation family. As such, she was expected, just like the *caring fathers or mothers* described above, to start sending money home for daily expenses and to pay off debts. In fact, when she failed to send money during the first few months after her arrival in Portugal, her husband in Brazil asked her: 'What's happening, why aren't you sending any money?' Antónia and her husband (unemployed) accumulated huge debts while trying to help their adult daughter (age twenty-six) with a serious addiction problem. In 2002, Antónia migrated with her daughter to try to solve the family's financial problems and to give the daughter a fresh start, leaving her husband and a younger daughter (a twenty-year-old lone mother with one child) in Brazil; two years later, the house in Brazil was sold to pay for travel expenses, and they were all reunited; her elder daughter is working again and living with a new partner, her husband has found a job and the younger daughter is unemployed and living with her parents. Antónia is relieved: 'If I had to, I would do this all over again. It is not only money that counts, it's the will . . . to improve things, not only for me because I'm getting old, but for my daughters and my grandchild'.

In this period of life, other new and complex forms of mobility and transnational care relations can therefore emerge within the family.

Another example is that of the *gone-back-home father/spouse in later life*, a pattern observed among Italian, Spanish and Latin-American male migrants near official retirement age. These migrants can obtain an early retirement pension and want to go back to their home country while their partner wants to stay on to be close to their adult children and grandchildren. This is the case of Humberto, a former Chilean refugee who lived in Switzerland with his wife and two daughters for more than twenty-five years. At the age of sixty, he decided to go back to Chile, but his wife and adult daughters decided to stay in Switzerland where they have stable jobs and friends. Despite family opposition, Humberto travelled to Chile where he bought a piece of land and can also develop other intellectual and political activities: 'Life was meaningless for me in Switzerland. I had to come back to my roots, develop new projects to feel alive again'. Humberto communicates regularly with his family by e-mail or Skype.

At this life stage, we also find many cases of divorced or widowed middle-age women who migrate alone. However, the care configuration varies strongly according to the migration project and family structure. In some cases, a woman with adult independent children in the home country decides to emigrate to get married in a new country or to start afresh in a country with less social control and prejudices. In this case, she starts a more individualised 'new life' trajectory (Wall and Nunes 2010), nearly always finding and living with a new partner and keeping in contact with her adult children in the home country but assuming weak care responsibilities (gradually becoming a more distant caring mother-grandmother).

However, the transnational family is different when the middle-age mother-grandmother emigrates as the main breadwinner and continues to be the main manager of the family's problems (*widowed or divorced caring mother-grandmother)*. Natasha (age fifty-six, divorced for more than twenty years, working in the cleaning sector) is an example of a care configuration that spans four generations and includes friends as well as kin. When she was interviewed, she had been in Portugal for seven years (since the year 2000). Before migration, she worked as a ballet teacher in the Ukraine and was living with one of her married daughters and near her widowed mother (age seventy-three, retired, low pension). Natasha decided to emigrate in order to boost family income, at a time when her mother became ill and needed financial support and her daughter and son-in-law, both out of work, had a baby to raise. She was and continues to be an important provider for two households in the Ukraine: her own (where one of her daughters lives with a child) and her mother's. She thought she would return to the Ukraine after a few years, but family events (her daughter's husband died, her other daughter's husband had an accident and her mother needs expensive medicines) impelled her to stay on in order to provide for her family. In Lisbon, she works as a cleaner in a private school and does some extra hours as a daily. She rents a room in an apartment, which she shares with four other Ukrainian women, all divorced and over age fifty. She speaks to her family every week, oversees her mother's health at a distance (making sure that one of her daughters takes grandmother to her appointments) and goes home for a month once a year. She sends money every month (between 100 and 200 Euros), both to her mother and her daughter, but has to keep tight control of her budget to be able to do this. She doesn't know when she will return to the Ukraine. As she says,

> I have been here for so long now that I don't know anymore. I want to go back and I don't. I really like Portugal, I have friends, people are very generous here. . . I do miss my family, but I need to earn money for them. So for the moment I will stay on, while my health lasts.

This type of care configuration is possible when part of the 'beanpole' family lives near the needy elderly person. But caring for elderly parents when all adult children have migrated may give rise to other types of care configurations in which the dependent elderly person is brought to the receiving country to be cared for. This may be a major problem, however, because few receiving countries have reunification policies that include relatives in ascending line. As a result, the elderly person may do some "yo-yoing" for some time (going back and forth with tourist visas) or even circulate between different countries to be cared for by several adult children (*grandparents on the move between caring adult children).* Two cases illustrate this type of configuration and the problems with which they are associated. Mercedes is a Peruvian social worker. She married a Swiss engineer and came to live and work in Switzerland, where she had two children. The whole family later moved to Brazil in order to be closer to Mercedes's sister and mother. During her stay in Brazil, she visited her mother regularly in Peru. For financial reasons, however, the family decided to go back to Geneva. Nowadays, Mercedes keeps in contact with her elderly mother by using the Internet and pre-paid phone cards. She takes care of her mother at a distance and gives her advice on different health matters. She also managed to bring her mother to Switzerland for a six-month period. She stayed in Mercedes' three-room apartment but had to go back to Peru after the visa expired.

The second case is an example of elderly persons who move between different families and countries to be near their adult children and their grandchildren. Juana came to Switzerland with Fernando, her husband, and their two children during the early 1980s after the Chilean Military putsch. Juana and Fernando were in their early thirties then, and the family obtained refugee status. Juana's brother, Gonzalo, also came to Switzerland during the 1980s as an asylum seeker and obtained a residence permit after two years. Some time later, Virginia, the youngest sister, came to Europe and settled in Spain. Their parents, Roberto and Maria, stayed in Chile, where they had a grocery store. They were in contact with their children mainly by telephone. In the late 1990s, the parents, who were already over age sixty, decided to sell their grocery store and move to Europe to live closer to their children. Because they were not entitled to permanent resident status, the three children decided to set up a care arrangement by rotation: The parents spent the first three months with Virginia in Spain and were in contact with Juana and Gonzalo through Skype almost every day; then they went to Switzerland and stayed for three months with Juana, who had a bigger apartment than Gonzalo. Then they went back to Spain, to Virginia's home, and so on for four years. The rotational care arrangement was interrupted because Roberto developed cancer. Regular access to health services then became very important, and Juana applied successfully for family reunification. Roberto and Maria settled in Lausanne and stayed in contact with Virginia through virtual communication.

## CONCLUSIONS

The aim of this chapter was to explore the new plurality of transnational families by focusing on a diverse set of key life stages. We analysed the influence of the life stage on migration and family life projects, as well as its impact on the ways migrant families build up and safeguard specific 'care configurations'. Analysis reveals several important conclusions.

The three life stages are of particular significance for migrant families today and reveal that research must take into account an extended life course time frame that focuses not only on young adulthood but also on families in middle and later life. Different life stages position migrants (both female and male) in a variety of caregiving configurations: Today it is not only young adults and couples who migrate and take on care responsibilities, in particular for spouses and young children left behind, but also middle-age migrants who care for close kin belonging to three or even four generations or elderly persons who migrate to be nearer their adult children.

Contextualising transnational family life within the dynamics of the life course is crucial to understanding the linkages between the migration project and the exchange of care across borders.

Young couples without children are expected to build up family and professional life and have children, and the goals of migration are always incorporated into this 'early life' project: Financial obligations to other kin members are kept on hold during this life stage, while bonding and reciprocal emotional support are encouraged as well as family cohesion through future plans to build near to, keep up or renovate a family home. In this life stage, conjugal autonomy and individual occupational goals are also fostered by the key variable of individualisation.

In contrast, families with dependent children have major care responsibilities as parents who are bringing up and supporting children, with the latter becoming the major focal point of bonding and care across borders and the generations; the reciprocal exchange of care is especially intense when young children are left in the care of close family members.

Migrants in middle life, however, may also move into care configurations in which they occupy a key position as breadwinners and caregivers. Although caring obligations in this life stage focus strongly on needy elderly parents, in reality, many middle-age migrants take on significant care responsibilities for elderly relatives as well as adult children and grandchildren.

Drawing on life course and care configuration perspectives, we were able to identify a plurality of transnational families. Despite the growing diversification of transnational family living and the limited scope of this exploratory analysis (which only looks at three different life stages), it is possible to identify a first set of recurring or more predominant types.

In early adulthood (couples without children), we find one main type of transnational family: *young couples in the making*. In the life stage with young children, we find the well-known pattern of the *caring father* who migrated first, as well as the transnational families of *caring parents* and the *caring young lone mother*, who, within a short-stay and intensive-saving migration trajectory, leaves her young children with a close relative. In middle life, we find the *caring mother*, who migrates alone to save up or to provide for husband and older children in the home country and the *caring mother-grandmother*, who takes on care responsibilities across several generations. Examining the changes in female migration trajectories is therefore a key issue for understanding the emergence of new forms of transnational families. Women are migrating more often alone (as single or divorced women), with their partners or children or before them. This is greatly increasing the number of transnational family types.

As in nonmobile families, problems and constraints occasionally lead to some care configurations in which a gap exists between care obligations and practices. This is true for the *absent long-distance father* and the *deprived lone mother*. The latter are mothers who, in a situation of financial hardship in the host country, develop weak care commitments in relation to the children left behind.

Lastly, growing individualisation, also linked to increased life expectancy, is contributing to transnational family living in which middle-age/elderly persons also search for a 'new life' in another country while keeping up bonds but weak care commitments with close kin left behind (see e.g., the *gone-back-home father*).

The results of the analysis point to transnational family living as a dynamic form of creating bonds and care commitments. As such they are a significant source of social capital across the life course (see Chapter 10, this volume). Both for those who migrate and those who stay behind, transnational family living offers fertile ground for building a network of close relationships that underpins potential and active exchange of care and support. Like other families, transnational families include a wide range of close kin in their care configurations. The underlying principles of inclusion also follow trends observed in contemporary families: Partnership and blood ties based on bilateral filiation, in particular those related to the nuclear family across three generations (e.g., partners, parents, children, grandchildren, siblings, in-laws, aunts and uncles), occupy a central position in transnational family networks. But cultural diversity, migration and the changing nature of families also have an impact on the inclusion of other close persons: Matrilineal kin ties may emerge as more significant in some contexts (see Cape Verdean families above), partnership breakup and repartnering makes for inclusion of ex-kin and step-relatives and affinities built up through migration often encourage close relationships with friends or distant kin, such as cousins.

The care configurations at key life stages reveal that transnational families rely on similar aspects of bonding and care in close relationships as nonmobile families. Care and interdependency include communication and frequent contact, exchange of information and counselling, emotional and financial support, negotiation of gendered and generational divisions of care responsibilities and building up cohesion through a common pool of memories, activities and shared places of present or future co-residence. Over the last decade, the use of the Internet seems to be complementary to phoning and visiting, but many migrant families still had difficulties in accessing these forms of communication.

However, this is not to say that the care configurations of transnational families are not embedded in some specificity. Family and conjugal togetherness based on daily life (such as sharing meals, leisure activities, comforting and cuddling, sexuality, decorating and mending homes) have to be negotiated in time and space: regular visiting, spending some long periods together (a few weeks), checking up through others who are geographically closer, keeping up homes and a sense of common residence in one or several countries and inventing routines that impart a sense of anticipation and predictability of reciprocal exchange are all important for family bonds across borders. Sometimes they fail due to the constraints of migration (precariousness, high cost of travel); at other times, it is the lack of skills in changing physical absence into proximity through communication or family conflicts regarding the need for migration itself. Young children in particular are often unequal partners in the negotiation of migration projects and the routines of transnational family living. Care configurations in which reunification projects are frustrated or take two or more years, instead of one or two, sometimes lead to emotional problems that may be difficult to overcome. Children who lived in fusional and closed nuclear families before migration may be more likely to feel tension and strain than children who already lived in more open or extended families. However, the stories in this chapter clearly show that geographical distance and physical separation do not always have negative effects on family and child well-being. Like other families, transnational families are capable of redesigning and reinventing relationships and routines that respond to family members' needs for care and interdependency.

# 3 Care (and) Circulation Revisited

## A Conceptual Map of Diversity in Transnational Parenting

*Paola Bonizzoni and Paolo Boccagni*

### INTRODUCTION

This chapter provides a theoretical overview of the multifaceted processes of care negotiation and circulation that form the basis of transnational family life. Its central focus is on the changing relationships between emigrant parents and their kin—especially children—who are left behind. While considering a variety of case studies, we make special reference to the women-led labour migration flows that have increasingly headed for Western Europe in recent decades, with Eastern Europe, Latin America and the Philippines being the main areas of origin. Although transnational family life is by no means a prerogative of these particular flows, our choice reflects the growth of academic interest in the phenomenon, as well as our own research experience on it (e.g., Bonizzoni 2012; Boccagni 2012a).

It is our contention that a care circulation perspective (Part A, this volume) offers a promising way ahead in transnational family studies as it shares a fine resonance with the mobilities approach (e.g., Adey 2010). The same could be said of some new developments in the sociology of the family,[1] which highlight how social actors make sense of their family relationships and concretely, if variably, build up their affective and caring interlocutors. Once family practices are approached from an interactionist optic, rather than from a normative and institutional one, the dynamic evolution of family life in space and time can be better appreciated—on a local and even on a transnational basis. A pluralisation of family arrangements is thus brought to light, migration being a major, but far from unique, factor in accounting for them.

Building on these assumptions, we will argue for a more nuanced and multivocal understanding of transnational caregiving, particularly with regard to its structural reach and the social and cultural meanings underlying it. Overall, the chapter aims to provide a conceptual map of the burgeoning literature on the migration-care nexus, in the light of its impact on everyday family life and of the notions of *care* and *circulation*. Gender, lifecycle, culture and time are the main variables we will critically examine in this respect.

## TRANSNATIONAL PARENTING AS A GENDERED EXPERIENCE: PERSISTENCE AND CHANGE

Research on cross-border caregiving and transnational family life is often marked by a strong emphasis on the gender dimension. Transnational motherhood, in particular, has been at the forefront of a heated debate among scholars, in the general public and among other stakeholders—in the media, social and political spheres—in both home and host societies (Parreñas 2010).

This widespread concern has sometimes come close to moral panic about an issue that subverts gendered social expectations in the highly normative field of family life and relations. Female labour migration, in itself, challenges both the constructions of motherhood based on physical and emotional closeness and the constructions of fatherhood grounded only in (male) breadwinning (Parreñas 2005b). An open question is therefore whether, and under what circumstances, these tensions have durable effects on gender relationships, rather than inducing only temporary adjustments—in more or less conflictive, painful and affective terms.

Since the seminal contribution of Hondagneu-Sotelo and Ávila (1997) on Mexican migration, both commonalities and distinctive patterns have been highlighted in how transnational caregiving is performed by emigrant parents, as well as by their non-migrant children (and the latter's caregivers). Judging from the number of studies now available, transnational parenting experiences and care arrangements, while spanning the globe, are extremely diverse and variable (Carling et al. 2012; Dreby and Adkins 2010; Mazzucato and Schans 2011). A myriad of case studies has focused on both the systems of meanings and representations associated with parenting from afar and the ensuing social practices, thus uncovering the influence of migration on the ways care is valued, practiced and understood on a day-to-day basis (Baldassar et al. 2007). Such changes need to be read in the light of how culturally and locally specific gender relationships are challenged or reproduced in a transnational social space (Mahler and Pessar 2001; Pessar and Mahler 2003).

While fathers' migration is often understood as a natural expansion of their providing role (with no major effects of stigmatisation or social alarm),[2] mothers' migration is more frequently associated with new, and potentially conflicting, meanings and practices of care, as studies from several countries have shown.[3] Indeed, female labour migration entails a "stretching" of motherhood to include breadwinning (Asis et al. 2004), along with forms of care co-management that rely on non-migrants' active collaboration. Male labour migration, in turn, is more likely to be associated with a traditional division of family tasks as far as care and livelihood commitments are concerned.[4] In both cases, the transnationalisation of care obligations and practices may well pave the way for new social understandings of fatherhood—and, of course, of motherhood itself (Parreñas 2008).

Some authors have, however, shed light on the remarkable 'stickiness' (Asis et al. 2004) of traditional definitions of gender relationships in home societies (Dreby 2006). This contributes, in their argument, to several negative assessments of transnational mothering: the suffering[5] related to mother–child separation and the ongoing risk of stigmatisation and blaming, despite their intensive investment in long-distance mothering practices (i.e., remittances, phone calls, gifts, visits and so forth). A rigid definition of gender roles, whereby mothers are represented as the only possible nurturers, results in a pervasive social construction of the care provided by other kin as 'qualitatively inferior' and suspect, as studies in both the Philippines and Eastern Europe have shown.[6] It also provides some grounds for the charges of 'abandonment' their children may make,[7] as well as discouraging fathers from assuming a stronger caregiving role. Indeed, fathers may well be judged as 'naturally' incompetent by their female partners and the wider society (Parreñas 2010). All this being said, such accounts may well risk erring on the structural side, somewhat neglecting (or even demeaning) the very real suffering, and the broader range of emotions that are personally experienced—as much as socially constructed—by migrants and non-migrants alike (Horton 2009; Boccagni 2012a).

Coping with children's daily care arrangements after parental emigration depends on a 'caregiving triangle' (Suárez-Orozco et al. 2002; Åkesson et al. 2012), which connects migrant parents with their children and caregivers who are left behind and through which different forms of care are circulated. Both the composition and direction of the flow of care tends to vary with migrants' gender. Judging from the evidence available in several Asian countries, female emigration seldom induces a straightforward 'care transfer' to the fathers left behind (Parreñas 2010; Save the Children 2006; Scalabrini Migration Center 2004). It rather results in other women being involved, with most of them being part of the extended family (primarily grandmothers and aunts). Therefore, female migration typically entails more radical changes in the concrete practices of care and in its underlying meanings and expectations, thus reworking the ways in which family is actually 'done' (Cheal 2002; Morgan 1996). The reorganisation of care arrangements and the scope for involving kin as caregivers should also be read in the light of non-migrant fathers' reactions, which are, however, often missing from the picture (Carling et al. 2012).

In fact, the limited literature available on the role of fathers who are left behind provides a mixed picture (but see Chapters 8 and 9, this volume). Female migration may result in greater male involvement in caregiving tasks, at least compared with fathers belonging to non-migrant households (Gamburd 2000; Save the Children 2006). Still, such involvement may turn out to be limited, temporary[8] and constrained by the compensatory strategies men enact to reassert their masculinities.[9]

The ways in which women negotiate their increasing care responsibilities have been discussed at some length. Less attention has been dedicated to the ways in which men face the social devaluation and marginalisation they are exposed to—ironically, as both wage providers and family caregivers. As of now, however, empirical research has documented a great variety in the ways of experiencing and understanding transnational care practices. Gender ideologies, although relevant, are by no means the only factor that accounts for this (see e.g., Merla 2011).

## MAKING SENSE OF THE CHANGING CONFIGURATION AND OUTCOMES OF TRANSNATIONAL FAMILY LIFE

One of the reasons that female migration is depicted[10] as especially 'problematic'[11] lies in the transfer of care obligations to other caregivers. Substitute caregivers, as a widespread fear has it, may be unable to aptly replace biological mothers. This would result in poor support being provided for children in terms of affection, nutrition, medical care, schooling, disciplining and control (Bryant 2005; Cortés 2007; Scalabrini Migration Center 2004).

The quality of substitute care accessible to children left behind is strongly affected by the sociodemographic profile of the caregivers (i.e., age, education, employment, etc.)[12]; the stage in the family lifecycle and 'family type' (see Chapter 2, this volume); and the kind of relationship that connects them to the children and to emigrant parents—one more or less imbued with mutual acquaintance, trust and affection (Bonizzoni 2012; Bonizzoni and Leonini Forthcoming).[13] The quality of interpersonal relationships and the scope for mutual understanding and coordination within the 'care triangle' are critical to the efficacy of transnational caregiving (Åkesson et al. 2012; Suárez-Orozco et al. 2002). The diversity of experiences in family care shifting is also crucially affected by the composition of the household in which children are cared for, before and after parental migration. The caregiving triangle, in other words, is embedded in a set of wider social relationships, which may be more or less altered by migration, as new caregiving arrangements lead to reorganisation of family relationships, for the children, their caregivers and other relatives. This reorganisation will vary widely depending on the spatial reorganisation of households (with children and/or caregivers remaining in their home or moving to another household).

There are, however, at least two other factors that play a major role in accounting for such variations: timing and culture.

### Lifecycle, Time Management and Transnational Care Practices

Transnational family life and the attendant caring practices need to be better understood from a temporal perspective (Giralt and Bailey 2010; Glick 2010). This applies, first, to the differential impact of the age of non-migrant children on the 'disembedding' of care arrangements from parental proximity, and, second, to the intensity and distribution of their care practices over time (Baldassar et al. 2007).

The age of the children involved is critical for appreciating the contents and evolution of care arrangements (Carling et al. 2012; Suárez-Orozco et al. 2005). Children's scope for agency and the level of their cognitive development remarkably affect their role in transnational care relationships and their understanding of family migration (Bushin 2009). When in their infancy, children may not even realise the care fostering relationships they are involved in. At that age, they can develop an attachment to their main caregiver that equals, in all ways, a 'real' maternal relationship (Bonizzoni and Leonini Forthcoming). Children's limited ability to participate in transnational communication may also hinder migrant parents' capacity to develop significant intimacy and mutual acquaintance from afar. Under these circumstances, the risk of mutual alienation is arguably stronger, and dependency on caregivers for transnational communication is higher.

As children enter adolescence, separation from emigrant parents is likely to be more destabilising, thus enlarging the potential scope for tensions and conflicts (Scalabrini Migration Center 2004). Once they reach adolescence, children tend to be better able to express their own feelings and needs. They can also play a more active role in a variety of transactions from a distance, including remittances and the ways to spend them (Parreñas 2005b). Likewise, they may gain a deeper understanding of their social conditions (including the material improvements enabled by parental emigration) and of the rationale of their family migration projects overall. As these children grow up, their caregivers' role tends to become less pervasive—at least in terms of day-to-day social reproduction. Apart from becoming more autonomous, the children may be expected to take care of younger siblings (Parreñas 2005b, 2010). As they grow older, the risks they are exposed to tend also to change. During their infancy, critical issues typically have to do with health, nurturing or schooling (Save the Children 2006; Scalabrini Migration Center 2004). Entering adulthood, however, is a source of different concerns[14] and changed power relationships in the family. This may move families to rethink and renegotiate their spatial arrangements.

The continuity and frequency of transnational practices, in the second place, is critical to the efficacy and sustainability of caring from afar (Baldassar 2007a; Boccagni 2012a). This especially applies to remittances, home visits and phone calls—arguably the three most relevant indicators for operationalising migrant cross-border ties (cf. Soehl and Waldinger 2010). As shown by a plethora of studies (Baldassar 2001; Baldassar et al. 2007; Gardner and Grillo 2002; Mason 2004; Parreñas 2005b; Sutton 2004), long-distance family practices and rituals are permeated with a multiplicity of meanings and expectations, well beyond their most obvious function: ensuring children's social reproduction and, besides exerting control upon, potentially also re-creating intimacy with them. Such practices act as a public display (Finch 2007) of the ongoing significance of parent–child relationships, which is threatened by parental absence. They may also protect parents from allegations of 'abandonment'.

However, migrants' 'capability' to participate in these transnational transactions is highly differentiated (see also Chapter 5, this volume). This needs to be understood in light of the resources accessible to them (Baldassar et al. 2007; Merla and Baldassar 2011), as well as the geographical distances involved (Tymczuk and Leifsen2012), the role of care regimes and infrastructure (including information and communication technologies [ICTs]) (Madianou and Miller 2012), and, of course, their legal status (Fresnoza-Flot 2009b; Horton 2009; Raijman et al. 2003). This especially holds for home visits due to the geopolitical regulation of space mobility, but also to travel costs and to the labour market–related constraints (the latter being quite remarkable in domestic work, where transnational mothers are over-represented).

A strong case can be made for the mixed effects of transnational communication, once it is disembedded from face-to-face interactions (Carling et al. 2012). As migrant families find out, their cross-border transactions may create a sort of surreal 'timelessness' (Parreñas 2005b)—a bubble of 'virtual proximity'. This hinders their perceptions of the changes that involve their significant others and their life circumstances over time (Baldassar 2007b; Tolstokorova 2010). Physical reunions, given these premises, often result in a mixed emotional experience—both a desirable and destabilising one for the family members involved (Schmalzbauer 2004).

## Parenthood and Caregiving from a Cultural Perspective

Another major axis of variation in transnational caregiving lies in the social and cultural constructions of parenthood. Parenthood can be understood as a dynamic social institution, situationally affected by social factors that mirror predominant ideologies of gender (Arendell 2000). Put differently, both definitions and practices of motherhood and fatherhood are variable on historical and geographical bases. As shown by a number of sociological and anthropological studies, a huge variation in family life patterns exists before and, even more so, after migration. This applies to gender contracts in the family, relevance of extended families, cultural definitions of co-presence, care fostering, age-based family roles and household structures (Mazzucato and Schans 2011; Thompson and Bauer 2000). To better appreciate the effects of parent–child separation, therefore, the social and family context of preexisting emigration should be specifically analyzed.

As discussed by Baldassar and Merla in the Introduction to this volume, an important critique is pertinent to all those studies that tend to emphasise the negative effects of separation on intergenerational relationships (Åkesson et al. 2012; Coe 2008). As the objection has it, such studies tend to be conditioned by assumptions and theories[15] that ethnocentrically reflect the viewpoint of Western, white, middle-class families. As a result, undue emphasis is often put on parent (especially mother)–children ties, and early separation and child fostering would be constructed as a necessarily problematic issue.

As several studies have illustrated, practices of shared care and child fostering are relatively widespread and culturally legitimated in specific contexts of origin ranging from West Africa (Åkesson et al. 2012; Coe 2008) and Caribbean (Bauer and Thompson 2004; Foner 2001; Levitt 2001) to the Pacific (Lee 2003). This also has to do with mothers' active involvement in the labour market as main (and often single) breadwinners. In cultural contexts where children are expected to take a precocious productive role, their physical distance from parents is imbued with distinctive meanings and opportunities, compared with the cultural milieus where the transition to adulthood is relatively delayed (Luster et al. 2008).

In other words, research on transnational caregiving should systematically take into account the cultural construction of social roles based on age as well as on gender. This differentially affects the ways in which intergenerational separation is practiced and intimately experienced. In the local contexts where child fosterage has some currency, mothers are less likely to be heavily stigmatised (Åkesson et al. 2012; Coe 2008; Mazzucato and Schans 2011). Some even contend that transnational migration patterns would be particularly suitable to the typical arrangements of Caribbean families, resulting in extremely complex stepfamily structures, whereby fictive and chosen kinship ties may be no less relevant than the formally ascribed ones (Thompson and Bauer 2000). Such 'flexible' relationships would be especially suitable for the 'frontiering' and 'relativising' processes (Bryceson and Vuorela 2002b) entailed by transnational migration.

This said, cultural arrangements are far from immobile across time and space. Foster care, as a culturally defined social institution, can be experienced in completely different ways—depending on the kind of migration involved (i.e., internal vs. international). Furthermore, cultural definitions are prone to change over time, for a range of concurrent cultural influences[16]—including those derived from international migration.

## GENERATING, MAINTAINING (AND TRANSFORMING?) TRANSNATIONAL CARE ARRANGEMENTS

As the above remarks suggest, families' adaptations to the changing spatial configurations have been widely discussed. The same cannot be said of the temporal dimension of transnational family life—more specifically, the differential meanings and implications of transnationality across the life course, following the evolution of cross-border family ties (Evergeti and Ryan 2011; Giralt and Bailey 2010; Glick 2010; Ho and Bedford 2008). Yet a diachronic lens is fundamental to shed light on the constraints and motivations whereby families, indeed different family members with variable affective commitments and power resources, opt, or are forced, to maintain family dispersion across borders or, alternatively, how they overcome this arrangement.

Managing care relationships from a distance may be desirable, or at least acceptable, for a limited time-span or in certain phases of the life course (see Chapter 2, this volume). While transnational family life often leads to family reunification or return migration (at least concerning the migrant–minor child dyad), it may even reproduce itself across time under changed circumstances.[17] Migrant parents, along with their non-migrant counterparts, have to negotiate their caring arrangements against a changing and mixed background of constraints and resources, both in host and home societies (Bernhard et al. 2009; Coe 2008; Raijman et al. 2003; Whitehouse 2009; Boccagni 2011; Bonizzoni 2011). The evolving trajectory of their caregiving practices, however, is far from predetermined—in fact, it is a matter of incremental change as they cope with external circumstances that are often hard to predict.

The reasons that migrant families tend to maintain a 'dispersed' geographical arrangement, or instead pursue some 'return to proximity', are still underresearched. Both structural factors and grassroots family strategies, possibly resulting from extended intrafamily negotiations, are relevant here. While often a matter of sheer necessity, transnational caregiving arrangements can also be actively pursued (if not always deemed to be appropriate) by those involved, especially as far as migrant parents are concerned and also stay-behind parents eager to ensure their adult migrant children are coping well (see e.g., Chapter 11, this volume).

As several studies have shown, transnational parenthood mostly takes the contours of a forced transnationality, so to speak (Raijman et al. 2003; Bernhard et al. 2009; Horton 2009; Boccagni 2012a). Among the factors accounting for this, immigration policies in receiving countries are often stressed. Migrant settlement on a family basis can be complicated by the institutional regulation of immigrant legal status (Fresnoza-Flot 2009b), including the requirements associated with family reunion (Bonizzoni 2009; 2011). Indeed, the complex effects of immigration policies on family arrangements deserve further elaboration (Carling et al. 2012; Kraler and Kofman 2009; Mazzucato and Schans 2011; Bonizzoni 2011). Even within a generally restrictive framework, receiving country policies vary along several lines, including the fundamental rights that aliens are granted with regard to their opportunities for legal entry and regularisation (Baldwin-Edwards and Kraler 2009; Ambrosini 2011).

Constraints on family reunion are variable in turn. As far as European countries are concerned, moreover, factors such as the European Union (EU) enlargement and a common focus on highly skilled migration have contributed to an increasing pluralisation of legal statuses, and of the attendant rights, for migrant workers and their families (Morris 2002). Migrants' origin and qualifications, as a result, also affect the regime of rights accessible to them (Khoo2003).

Juridical regulation does not operate in a vacuum. It intersects, instead, with migrants' integration processes in the labour market, not to mention the pressures of a range of other relevant stakeholders (local authorities, trade unions, churches, non-governmental organisations [NGOs] and so forth). In the case of female labour migration, which often results in care or domestic work, low wages and intensive work schedules—often combined with undocumented status (Bonizzoni, 2013)–are equally important in accounting for their forced transnationality (Parreñas 2001a; Bernhard et al. 2009).

Altogether, the intersections of gender, social class and legal status significantly affect migrants' caring strategies at local and transnational levels. This should not lead us to neglect, however, migrants' personal agendas and perspectives. Some migrants, while still working abroad, can find several reasons to have their children—born abroad or in their homeland—raised in the countries of origin. This option may provide children with better education, health and housing (Parreñas 2005b), paving the way for 'remittance-driven upward mobility trajectories. Such a perspective, while hardly conceivable before parental emigration, seems far less viable in receiving countries, due to a range of negative factors—among them, labour market discrimination and ethnicisation, as well as the limited access to training and tertiary education. Moreover, this option enables children to be brought up in a social and cultural milieu that may be more consistent with their parents' values and lifestyles (Whitehouse 2009). At the same time, however, parents' own care resources risk being severely undermined by their difficult living conditions abroad—in terms of distressful work, poor networks of support and constant exposure to discrimination.

## TRANSNATIONAL FAMILY LIFE AND THE "STRATIFIED" CIRCULATION OF CARE: AN AGENDA FOR EMPIRICAL RESEARCH

Our analysis of the nexus between migration and family-based care practices would be incomplete without consideration of the cognate (and, to date, relatively understudied) notion of circulation. As two prominent theorisers of the "mobilities" approach recognise, while migration often results in extended physical separation between family members:

> The[ir] intimate networks of care, support and affection also stretch over large distances. Scholars of kinship and migration have long known that presence and absence do not necessarily conflict. Thus, "geographical proximity or distance do not correlate straightforwardly with how emotionally close relatives feel to one another, nor indeed how far relatives will provide support or care for each other" (Mason 2004). Indeed, intimacy and caring take place at-a-distance . . . so caring, obligations and indeed presence do not necessarily imply physical travel and face-to-face proximity. People can be near, in touch and together, even when great distances tear them physically apart. (Elliott and Urry 2010, 100)[18]

In principle, the notion of care circulation aptly stands for this mixture of distance and proximity; in other words, for all day-to-day attempts to socially and emotionally bridge the former and reestablish the latter. The notion of circulation, moreover, resonates with Appadurai's (1996) notion of 'translocality'" (McKay, 2006). This suggests migrants' potential to re-create their earlier life milieus from afar—to a variable extent and not without conflicts—even in the realm of family-bound, intimate relationships. At the minimum, however, practising care in a transnational setting is made more complex by 'the added layer of geography', which may exacerbate family members' 'differential access' to the resources necessary to their livelihood and communal life projects (Dreby and Adkins 2010, 684). It is critical, therefore, to appreciate the differential scope for care practices to bridge physical distance—in other words, for care to actually 'circulate' between migrants and those left behind. It is also important to consider gender roles and expectations and the cultural settings in which migrants and their stay-behind kin and quasi-kin are embedded.

Transnational caregiving inherently builds on forms of care circulation between people who are physically displaced from one another, with significant parental and/or affective ties, and whose 'desire' or need 'for closeness' (Adey 2010, 28) has been jeopardised by migration. If the essence of migrant transnationalism lies in the functional substitution of physical absence with social presence (Carling et al. 2012; Boccagni 2012b), cross-border caring is a good empirical terrain for testing such an assumption. Indeed, it can be understood as a diverse range of practices whereby the 'compulsion to proximity' (Boden and Molotch 1994) and 'longing for co-presence' (Baldassar 2008b) is displayed, if not realised fully.

As noted by the editors in Part A of this volume, it is imperative that the notion of care circulation should take into account the structurally diverse, asymmetric, situated and gendered ways in which care may flow over distance—depending on a range of factors that deserve careful elaboration. If the freedom to move is 'the main stratifying factor' of today's global society, as Bauman (1998, 2) famously argued, much the same goes with the *freedom to circulate care*, as far as transnational family life is concerned.

The development of the notion of care circulation needs to be understood in the light of the intersectionality of a number of factors that must be understood in context and with careful empirical analysis. It is our contention that six analytical dimensions should be specifically addressed as a way of mapping the transnational social fields created by what the editors to this volume refer to as the 'asymmetrically reciprocal' (but not necessarily consensual) efforts, interests and obligations to 'circulate' care. This involves, to begin with, the *kind of care resources* being circulated over distance. While hands-on care is still critically reliant on physical co-presence, all other forms of care could be helpfully distinguished based on the extent to which their enactment from afar can replace, by all measures, their enactment in proximity.

In the second place, the *channels and means* for care circulation also affect the performability of care practices, as well as their perceived efficacy and quality, from the viewpoint of both migrants and non-migrants. The degree of one's transnational engagement is still contingent on these structural factors, no less than on interpersonal wishes and expectations. This involves not only the reach of the technologies employed, but also the sociocultural relevance and persistence of the rituals through which caring obligations and attachments are displayed. The tricky and still relatively unstudied issue of care commodification is relevant to this point as well.

Third, the labels of care provider and recipient—apart from doing no justice to the mutuality inherent (if often asymmetrical) in care flows (what Baldassar and Merla [Chapter 1, this volume] refer to as the asymmetrical reciprocity of caregiving)—have to be deconstructed in the light of the *personal identities* and of the *key social and demographic attributes* of the subjects involved. Gender and generation differentially affect the perceived needs, obligations and commitments underlying transnational care exchanges. Less obviously, transnational migration often entails major changes in the family roles and reciprocal expectations and obligations. This makes any question of the 'who/whom' of care circulation—that is, the changing personal and social identities of the family members involved—all but rhetorical. The overall meaning of a family, no less than its borders, may change in more or less consensual ways, reflecting the migration-related changes in personal and collective biographies. Drawing on family studies (Finch and Mason 1993), Baldassar et al. (2007) refer to this set of issues as 'negotiated family commitments' to highlight how family members go through a process of 'working out' how care obligations will be distributed over time and among family members.

Fourth, as discussed above, the *temporal dimension* of cross-border care practices is largely underappreciated—due also to the significant investment in empirical research it requires, well beyond single case study designs (Mazzucato and Schans 2011). Factoring time into transnational family life involves a careful appreciation of timing and life stages, including the temporal extension, rhythm and frequency of the care practices stemming from family separation, as well as the cycle of care obligations and commitments across individual and family life courses, and with the key transitions that mark them. Even the 'temporal constructions' of family separation processes (e.g., an expectation of an 'imminent' reunification or a more extended detachment) have their stake, although they need not turn into real matters of fact.

Indeed—as a fifth point—the *geographical configuration* of transnational caregiving arrangements is far from irrelevant. Distance affects the costs and sustainability of care circulation in many ways, including the differential scope for matching it with periodical home visits, hence with hands-on care. This is also related to the political regulation of space; in other words, with the differential scope for mobility and circulation that stems from immigration policies, regimes of border control and the forms of legal categorisation of migrants.

Last but not least, the *reasons and motivations* underpinning the start and then maintenance of transnational family life are surprisingly understudied—indeed, they are basically understood as a matter of necessity and 'forced transnationality'. This, however, need not always be the case (see Chapters 11 and 12, this volume). The desire and need for proximity, among family members, may greatly vary across the life course. Different family members have different underlying assumptions of what a 'desired family geography' is or should be (Bonizzoni 2012). This affects, in turn, their perceived obligations and availability to care for each other. Once migrant families are understood as reactive social formations, in constant search for new adaptations to evolving life course needs and socioeconomic (as well as institutional) environments (Ho and Bedford 2008), the mutable geographic arrangements they assume can be better understood across their life course. One can then analyze how they concretely address the changing needs of their members, who experience a plurality of geographical configurations that are affected, in turn, by unstable economic and institutional environments.

Summing up, a heuristic typology can be built for exploring the scope, content and reach of the care circulation processes connecting migrants with their significant others left behind (see Table 3.1). Along each dimension, the development of transnational family life should be understood as a matter of kin-based cooperation, trust and reciprocity, but also—and often simultaneously—as a potential catalyst for conflicts and inequalities depending on sociocultural circumstances and the specific life trajectories of both migrants and non-migrants (Dreby and Adkins 2010).

*Table 3.1* Mapping Care Circulation in Transnational Family Life: Key Dimensions for Comparative Analysis

| *Dimension of Care Circulation* | *Definition* | *Key Questions for Empirical Research* |
|---|---|---|
| 1. Circulating—*What* | Kind of care resources being circulated on a translocal basis: material resources, time, affection, emotions, information | - What is the differential scope for circulating different care resources?<br>- How do reciprocal care obligations and commitments impact on the relevance of each resource (and on the perceptions, converging or not, of the actors involved)?<br>- How does the structure of opportunity in home/host societies interact with the actors' needs for (and interests in) care, in affecting cross-border care circulation? |
| 2. Circulating—*How* | Channels and means whereby care can be performed from a distance—phone calls, ICT communication, money transactions, mail, package circulation, intermittent visits | - What kinds of care can be circulated, with what frequency and intensity, depending on the channel/means for circulation?<br>- How is it that each channel/means shapes the caring process in distinctive ways?<br>- How is it that the accessibility and usability of different channels affect the caring process?<br>- In what respects, and under which circumstances, can ICT-based care replace proximity-based care practices? |
| 3. Circulating—*Who/Whom* | Actors involved on either side—demographic profile, gender and generational differences, family roles/responsibilities (and attendant sociocultural constructions) | - How does difference in gender and generations affect the expected forms of transnational care, as well as the negotiation processes underlying them, and their outcomes?<br>- How do social and cultural definitions of family membership shape the development of transnational care and affect its sustainability? |
| 4. Circulating—*When* | Timing of care practices along the migration and family life cycle, frequency and length of care practices, evolution of caring across time | - How are caring commitments embedded in migration and family life trajectories, as well as in those of individual care providers/recipients?<br>- What is the development of transnational caregiving across time—in the expectations of those involved and in matters of fact?<br>- How and why do different care practices vary in intensity and frequency? |

*(continued)*

*Table 3.1* (continued)

| *Dimension of Care Circulation* | *Definition* | *Key Questions for Empirical Research* |
|---|---|---|
| 5. Circulating—*Where* | Influence of geopolitical distance from homeland and borders on the scope and contents of transnational care (also in light of migrants' legal status), relevance (or not) of the 'desired geography of family life', care regimes and infrastructures | - How is it that geopolitical distance affects the viability, sustainability and social effects of different care channels and arrangements?<br>- In which respects and how does physical distance affect the prevalence and social relevance of different cross-border care practices?<br>- What accounts for the distance between the 'desired' and 'real' geography of family life in any given case? In what respects are care practices distinctive in the cases where extended physical separation looks more like a desire or anyway an ordinary fact than a migration-related constraint? |
| 6. Circulating—*Why* | Reasons, expectations, social and cultural factors accounting for migration, and then for caring commitments; relevance (or not) of family reunification, or of homecoming, as ultimate goal | - What family and personal factors account for the changing contents and shapes of transnational caregiving?<br>- What structural, historical and social factors shape the meanings and practices of care?<br>- What expectations and life projects are developed and negotiated in order to make sense of, or anyway accept, reciprocal (if possibly asymmetrical) care commitments and practices? |

## CONCLUSION

Against the literature reviewed in this chapter, a focus on care circulation enables greater elaboration of the dynamic and changing patterns of transnational family life, as well as the variety of care resources on which it hinges. That said, *which forms of care* actually circulate, and *how circulation affects* preexisting family arrangements, are questions that have no self-evident response, apart from being highly variable on a case-by-case basis. Hence, they should figure prominently in the future research agenda on the topic.

Approaching transnational family life through the lens of mobility, however, is not only a way to show the typically stratified and differentiated patterns of cross-border care circulation. Less obviously, such a lens can also shed light on the 'shifting geographies' of family life—that is, on the development of family relationships in terms of more or less stable geographical configurations, susceptible to change under internal and external conditions. Despite the plethora of case studies now available, comparative, cross-country research remains necessary.[19] In more substantive terms, the nexus between care obligations and transnational fatherhood is still relatively unexplored, hence the variable ways in which masculinity is challenged and/or reproduced in transnational migration (see Chapters 8 and 9, this volume); also unexplored are the distinctive experiences, views and expectations of non-migrant caregivers, along with their gendered roles vis-à-vis changing family and community arrangements.

Finally, as far as Europe as a receiving context is concerned, more attention should be given to transnational family life in the 'new' women-led flows from the Eastern part of the continent. Compared with the Filipino and Latin American flows that have been more extensively studied, Eastern European migration still deserves more thorough elaboration from the perspective of transnational care circulation.

## NOTES

1. Cheal 2002; Finch 2007; Gubrium and Holstein 1990; Morgan 1996; Silva and Smart 1999.
2. As new social definitions of fathering are gaining ground in home societies, transnational fatherhood may be equally constructed as a threat to the preexisting social order (Mummert 2005). What is in question, however, as for transnational fatherhood, is less the adequacy of the care accessible to their children left behind than the fathers' will and ability to contribute to the family life via remittances and other transactions.
3. See, for instance, on Latin America, Bernhard et al. 2009; Dreby 2006; Boccagni 2013; on the Philippines, Parreñas 2001a, 2008; on Sri Lanka, Gamburd 2000.
4. Male migration may well widen women's roles and responsibilities (cf. Cortés 2007). However, male migration does not seem to directly affect the daily organisation of children's care in terms of the kind and number of people involved.
5. Mothers, more than fathers, are expected to display (Finch 2007) their suffering as a confirmation of their love and commitment (Dreby 2006; Parreñas 2005a) towards children and other kin back home.
6. The social construction of so-called 'social orphans' is built on the idea of the 'inadequate care', which children are supposed to receive at home (CeSPI-FIERI 2007).
7. For how migrants strive to keep an active role in their family life from afar, it is mothers' physical absence—more than fathers'—that tends to be constructed as child abandonment. Indeed, while mothers 'stretch' their care duties to encompass livelihood provision, children do not necessarily accept this 'transubstantiation'" (Horton 2009), which challenges the tacit equivalence between love and co-presence.
8. Fathers may understand this transition as driven by temporary circumstances—hence, bound to be over as soon as mothers return (Save the Children 2006).
9. Non-migrant fathers may maintain a job that protects them from economically depending on their wives (Parreñas 2005a). They may also reassert their

masculinity through social practices (such as drinking or gambling) that are not easily compatible with a caregiving role (Gamburd 2000; Parreñas 2010; Save the Children 2006).

10. Broadly speaking, social researchers tend to underline the emotional suffering of children left behind (Parreñas 2001a; Thompson and Bauer 2000; Horton 2009; Coe 2008) and their poor educational achievement (Scalabrini Migration Center 2004; Save the Children 2006). Less obvious and more 'sensationalist' issues, such as children's deviance, drug abuse and even suicides, tend to be more often reported by NGOs, social workers and the media (Pribilsky 2001; Tolstokorova 2010).
11. The debate about social orphans is widespread in countries with higher rates of female emigration. It is almost non-existent, instead, in countries where men are more likely to leave their families behind (on southern America see, among others, Pribilsky 2001; Boccagni 2012a; on Eastern Europe, see CeSPI-FIERI 2007; on Asia, see Bryant 2005).
12. Grandparents' health conditions, for instance, may undermine their ability to care for children, while their educational level may prove inadequate to support them in schooling (Save the Children 2006). Elder brothers and sisters, in turn, may feel unease in exercising an almost parent-like role vis-à-vis younger siblings (Parreñas 2010). The legitimacy of caregivers in exercising a disciplining role, by the way, is often unclear or questionable. The same applies to the position of children in the new family arrangements. As shown by Olwig (1999), the legitimate presence of children in a 'new' household is accepted as the flow of remittance is sustained by migrant parents abroad; if this stops, it may well be questioned.
13. Judging from the studies that directly voiced children's life experience, the kind of tie they can develop with substitute caregivers is highly variable (Coe 2008; Dreby 2007; Olwig 1999; Orellana et al. 2001; Parreñas 2005a; Pottinger 2005). In fact, it ranges from 'parentification' processes, whereby grandparents or aunts are perceived as the main affective figures, to feelings of ambivalence, exclusion or rejection.
14. The fear of gangs and of violent and illicit behaviours, which may jeopardise the family's mobility strategy, has been traced to the root of transnational disciplining practices. This may lead families to raise children born in the host country at home (Orellana et al. 2001) or to rejoin children left behind (Bonizzoni 2012). This depends on the setting where the care resources and the social environment are perceived to be more favourable.
15. Among them, attachment theory, which has significantly affected sociological, but also socio-psychological studies on the topic (Suárez-Orozco et al. 2002).
16. Coe (2008) and Mummert (2005), for example, highlight the role played by some churches in changing normative definitions of parenthood in the contexts of origin (see also Chapter 6, this volume).
17. For instance, an emigrant parent can be followed (or replaced abroad) by the other parent, parents can experience separation or divorce while abroad, some children can be left home while others can be rejoined or born abroad and so forth.
18. Cf. also Baldassar 2008.
19. See, among the exceptions, Banfi and Boccagni 2011.

# 4 Care Circulation, Absence and Affect in Transnational Families

*Marina Ariza*

## INTRODUCTION

The aim of this chapter is twofold: to describe the dynamics of care circulation (Chapter 1, this volume) through the family cycle in two groups of Latin American immigrants interviewed in Madrid (Dominicans) and New York (Mexicans),[1] and assess the way in which various structural factors in the societies of origin and destination (migratory policies and family structure) condition the potential for care circulation in the transnational space.

Three questions guide the reflection: (1) To what extent does the stage in the family cycle affect the patterns of care circulation in transnational spaces? (2) What are the similarities and differences in care provision between these two groups of transnational families (Dominicans in Madrid and Mexicans in New York)? (3) How do migratory policies (in sending countries) and family structure (in societies of origin) influence care circulation? The analysis is based on twenty-four interviews conducted between 2006 and 2007 in the four locations involved in these two migratory flows: Spain and the Dominican Republic and New York and Mexico.

The work is divided into three sections: The first part explains the analytical framework within which the empirical examination of data takes place, the second part presents this empirical examination, and the third part includes a discussion of the findings. The conclusions summarise the most important findings.

## THE CONTOURS OF TRANSNATIONAL FAMILY LIFE: ANALYTICAL BASES

Unlike the relative spatial delocalisation of global economic transactions, transnational family life takes place in the gaps between two or more nation-states, which it transcends yet by which it is also constrained (Kearney 1995; Levitt 2001, 14). The growth of transnational communities parallels the political limits established by nations and attempts to take advantage of the spaces opened up by the inequalities existing between societies of origin and destination (Portes 1996). Transnational family members use all available resources (whether human or technological) to reduce the physical distances separating them (Baldassar 2007a). The different conditions in which family exchange takes place denote some of the marked social asymmetries characterising today's global world, in which freedom to move has become, according to Bauman (1998), the main stratifying factor.

Several of the concepts developed in this field of research describe the complexity of long-distance family interaction. Two widely accepted notions, transnational motherhood and global care chains (Hondagneu-Sotelo and Avila 1997; Hondagneau-Sotelo 2001; Hochschild 2000),[2] refer as much to the expansion of affective links in sending and receiving societies as to the efforts to ensure care provision for relatives remaining in the localities of origin. Both concepts were developed by observing the experience of international immigrants incorporated into the low manual sectors of the labour market where most were domestic workers. The family undertaking is largely possible because of the density of networks of social relations that transcend the countries involved in the transnational space. Bryceson and Vuorela (2002b, 11, 25) propose the notions of 'frontiering' and 'relativising' to name the practices of creating connections and materialising the family as an imagined community implemented by migrants. These notions refer partly to the creativity shown by the members of these families in—through the selective expansion of their relations and bonds of loyalty—preserving the sense of belonging that gives them continuity in the enormous hiatus created by absence. The reflection of these authors is born of their observation of transnational European families.

In keeping with the original proposal of Finch (1989a), Baldassar et al. (2007), drew up an analytical framework to understand the factors on which care exchange and moral support between migrant parents and children depends. For the authors, this is the function of the dialectic relationship between the capacity (ability) to produce it, the obligation (in terms of the cultural norms that prescribe it) and the negotiation of family commitments. These conditions vary as a result of family relations, specific migratory histories and the moment in the family and individual cycle (Baldassar et al. 2007; Baldassar 2007b). They have made an effort to systematise the factors that permit care exchange on the basis of the experience of immigrants from Europe (Ireland, Italy, Holland), Oceania (New Zealand) and Asia (Singapore, Iraq, Afghanistan)[3] living in Australia.

The analytical efforts mentioned—which do not exhaust the existing conceptual proposals—illustrate the complexity of the analysis of transnational families. The heterogeneity of situations is such that one or more concepts are unlikely to be able to comprehensively cover them. The specific analytical scheme used in my data analysis is described below. I begin with the assumption that the two transnational social spaces in which these transnational families participate are based on normatively established relations of reciprocity (Faist 2000, 203; see Chapter 1, this volume).

Taking up Bryceson and Vuorela's proposal (2002b, 8) regarding the need to differentiate between the social levels that intervene in transnational family life in contexts of globalisation, I distinguished four analytical levels (Figure 4.1).[4] First, a macro level, provided by the strength of political borders in establishing criteria for the inclusion or exclusion of family members into a national (or supranational territory, such as the EU); second, a medium socioeconomic level represented by the conditions of transnational economic reproduction of these families by virtue of the insertion of some of their members into the labour markets of two or more nations; third, a second, medium level, resulting from the way in which local contexts and cultures of societies of origin and destination condition the social reproduction of these families; and, last, a micro-social level comprising the different care and attention needs determined by the moment of migration, the stage in the family cycle and the position occupied by the migrant within the family.

By delineating these levels in the case of the two groups of immigrants (Dominicans and Mexicans) and the countries I am comparing (Spain/Madrid, United States/New York), I found that the two transnational spaces produced by the combination of these levels create different conditions for the circulation of care. The description of these differential conditions guards against the risk of disregarding the asymmetrical ways in which care flows. The macro level, of the migratory policies of Spain and the United States as receiving countries, has a decisive, structural effect on the possibilities of exchange (Cohen 2000; Fresnoza-Flot 2009b). The greater relative flexibility of Spanish migratory policy, the existence of more forms of legal access for unskilled labour immigration and the relatively swift transition towards the naturalisation of Latin American nationals in that country (Calavita 1989, 2006; Colectivo IOE 2002) mean that a substantial part of the Dominican immigrant population in Spain, as opposed to the vast majority of the Mexican population in the United States, comprise legal residents who can travel freely between the points on the *continuum* of transnationality.[5]

Whereas in this comparative exercise, migratory policies as opportunity structures (Castles 2004) constitute a factor of differentiation between Dominican and Mexican transnational families, economic insertion is an element of homogeneity since the overwhelming majority of immigrants interviewed in Madrid and New York (with the exception of one) were domestic workers.[6] This aspect places objective limits on the resources that can be mobilised within the transnational sphere, and therefore on the quality of care provision. It should be pointed out that socioeconomic homogeneity is relatively greater among Mexican immigrants in the United

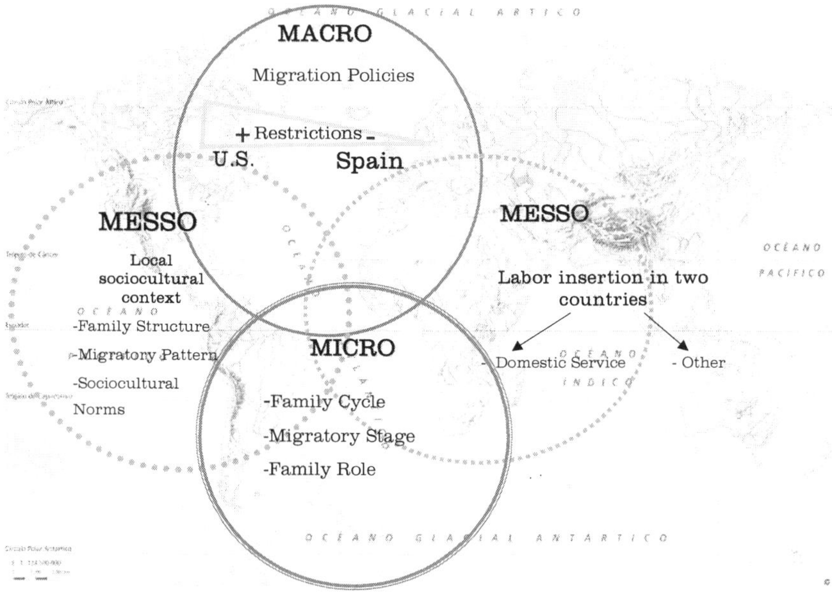


*Figure 4.1* Transnational social space boundaries.

States than among Dominicans in Madrid. The fact that domestic service in Spain is one of the legal channels for the admission of extra-communitarian immigration makes it one of the favorite gateways into the labour market for women with a wide range of sociodemographic profiles. In my data, three out of eleven of the Dominican immigrants held undergraduate degrees and belonged to lower middle-class social sectors.

At the other meso analytical level, that of the sociocultural conditions of local contexts, I highlight the family structure and migratory patterns of the societies of origin, which are also factors of differentiation between the transnational families compared. Within the context of Latin American countries, the Mexican family structure is distinguished by its high stability, the predominance of legal marriages over consensual unions, the high percentage of nuclear households and the low, albeit growing, presence of households with female headship (24.5 percent in 2010) (Instituto Nacional de Estadística y Geografía INEGI, 2011). Conversely, the Dominican Republic, in keeping with the so-called Caribbean pattern of family formation, is characterised by a high degree of marital dissolution, a predominance of consensual over legal unions, a lower relative importance of nuclear households compared with extended households and a higher percentage of female-headed households (35.2 percent in 2007) (ENDESA 2008; Ariza et al. 1994; Ariza and Oliveira 1999, 2001, 2007; Chapter 6, this volume). These aspects account for the greater presence of female heads of household in the universe of Dominican immigrants.[7]

As part of the contextual factors of the medium level, the differences in migratory patterns are one of the most striking aspects and can be summarised as follows: the clearly female selectivity of Dominican migration to Spain compared with the predominantly male profile of Mexican migration to the United States,[8] the virtually one-directional destination of Mexican international migration versus the greater diversification of Dominican emigration[9] and the higher percentage of households with international migrants in the Dominican Republic (9.6 percent in 2002)[10] in relation to Mexico (4.4 percent between 2004 and 2009) (INEGI 2009). The last two aspects denote the higher degree of transnationality of Dominican society as a whole, despite the extraordinary volume of Mexican international migration.

Last, at the micro-social level, the women interviewed occupy one of three positions in these transnational families: They are mothers (the majority), grandmothers or daughters, and they are distributed among three stages of the family cycle: the early stage, the stage of consolidation and the advanced stage.[11] These two aspects shape many of the needs and obligations regarding the reciprocity of persons linked by family bonds.

## Data and Method

The analysis is based on eighteen in-depth interviews with female immigrant workers from Mexico and the Dominican Republic carried out in the cities of New York (for Mexicans) and Madrid (for Dominicans) between May 2006 and April 2007 (eleven Dominicans and nine Mexicans), plus six interviews with the immigrants' relatives in the places of origin or destination (three from the Dominican Republic and three from Mexico), comprising a total of twenty-four.[12] For the purposes of this chapter, a subset of interviews was selected, namely, those that met the condition of belonging to divided families—in other words, families that had not achieved full reunification of their members at the time they were interviewed. The methodological strategy followed two complementary paths: (1) an exhaustive examination in the destination cities of the workers' pre- and postmigratory trajectory, a detailed description of the labour sequence before and after migration (paying particular attention to domestic service) and a compilation of the changes that had occurred in family structure and family interaction as a result of the displacement and the transnational networks and links if any; and (2) ethnographic tours in the places of origin and selected interviews with some of the women's families in the sending communities of both countries (Mexico and the Dominican Republic) as a means of triangulating the information. The cases were selected through a snowball procedure.

The period of reference was the same for the two groups of immigrants: that they should have arrived in the city between 1986 and 2005–2006. This criterion is linked to the start of the past wave of Latin American immigration to Spain and the moment New York emerged as a key destination for Mexican immigration. The selection of countries and cities was based on the fact that

Spain and the United States constituted the main international destinations for Latin American emigration until Spain's current economic crisis. Further, due to their migratory policies and another series of aspects (geopolitical location, migratory systems), they constitute different contexts of reception. During the period of observation, 1986–2006/2007, both countries implemented border control policies aimed directly at containing the flow of immigration from Third World societies, which were particularly reinforced during the 1990s, with a peak from 2001 onwards in the United States. In Spain, the most important outcome of these policies was the establishment in 1993 of the requirement of a visa for a set of Latin American countries including the Dominican Republic, plus five processes of regularisation between 1991 and 2005. With regard to the United States, the groundbreaking measure was the 1987 Immigration Reform and Control Act that legalised approximately three million immigrants. The lack of a regularisation process since 1987 confines most unqualified immigration—particularly Mexican immigrants—to a nearly permanent state of illegality.

## THE DYNAMICS OF CARE CIRCULATION AND ITS DIFFERENT SOCIAL CONSTRAINTS

### Care Circulation Through the Family Life Cycle

Three analytical axes are used in the following analysis of family interaction: (1) the stage of the family cycle and the role women play (daughter, mother, grandmother or both) (see also Chapter 2, this volume); (2) a list of the different forms of care[13]; and (3) a description of the affective aspects involved in long-distance interaction, if they existed. I began with the assumption that care circulation in the transnational space happens through three dimensions of mobility in the global sphere (Svašek and Skrbiš 2007a): mobility of persons, ideas and practices and of objects and images. Thus, whereas shifting between one country and another forms part of a person's mobility, remittances (both monetary and non-monetary)[14] constitute the objects that shift while looking after the welfare of children and other relatives (parents) is located within the sphere of practices and ideas.[15] This distinction follows only analytical purposes since they are often combined. Thus, when a person travels, she may take money, goods and ideas. Nevertheless, transnational social spaces as described above may deter their simultaneous occurrence. In transnational families, this mobility is structured around reciprocal relations based on affective bonds.

#### *Early Family Cycle: Migrating to Help the Family Progress*

Of the six immigrants located at this stage of the family life cycle, two were daughters and single (with parents living in the place of origin) whereas four were mothers (with children in the country of origin). They were all between ages twenty-two and twenty-nine and had spent less than five years separated from their loved ones[16]; three were from Mexico and three from the Dominican Republic. The only one with regular migratory status was Dominican.

The two young women who were daughters (one from each country) had never had children and had lived with their families before they left their countries of origin. In both cases, the migratory project reflects individual reasons linked to the need to lend direction to their own lives[17] (Ariza 2005). From the outset, this aspect involved fewer obligations in terms of reciprocal relations and care in the transnational sphere. During the short time they had been outside their country, interaction had mainly taken place through the irregular sending of monetary remittances and continuous telephone communication; neither of them had, at that point, been able to return to her country of birth.

Although strictly speaking, these migrants did not acquire the explicit commitment to leave their countries to improve the well-being of their relatives in their place of origin, it continued to be part of their objectives due to the normative expectations of the family role of migrant daughters in these social sectors.[18] The persons towards whom care is predominantly oriented are parents and sisters. Thus, although Marisol, a Dominican immigrant who had spent a year in Madrid, did not initially set out to provide financial assistance for her sisters, she felt happy to be able to assign some of her income to them as often as she could. This support was partly an act of voluntary reciprocity for the support she was given when the time came to migrate. Conversely, Gertrudis sent her mother more sporadic remittances, after building her own house in Mexico, as protection from the misfortune of having a 'bad husband'.

As one would expect, motherhood places its own particular stamp on the dynamics of long-distance interaction. This notion is reflected in the accounts of the four young women who, at this stage of the family life cycle, were mothers (two Dominicans and two Mexicans) with children under the age of ten. Three of the four women are separated from their partners, while the fourth (a Mexican) was married. They had all left their children in the care of their maternal families. Although the *leitmotiv* of the migratory project is essentially to achieve a better future for their children, this sometimes extends to other close relatives (parents and siblings). Monetary remittances are sent regularly (either monthly or fortnightly) and account for a high proportion of the income they earn (between 50 and 80 percent). Non-monetary remittances (clothes, books, toys) are more sporadic.

In addition to remittances, a palpable expression of the migrant's affective presence in the family home (Sørensen 2004b; Singh 2006), shared socialisation and raising of the children also occupy an important place. Children's academic performance and discipline are a constant source of concern for mothers. Within this sphere, collective care management is no easy task. This is partly due to the fact that the axis from which authority emanates is not always clear (Bernhard et al. 2008). Whereas the absent mother is assumed to have the last word and is occasionally consulted, the fact of not being physically present reduces her authority (Chapter 3, this volume). The tentatively 'temporary' nature of family arrangements means that grandmothers feel that certain issues are not entirely their responsibility, giving rise to a degree of laxity that deeply affects the migrants. Some grandmothers have been forced to accept the responsibility of looking after their grandchildren at a stage in their lives when they were beginning to enjoy a certain amount of independence, as shown in the account given by Ines's mother, interviewed in a rural community in Hidalgo, Mexico:

> I was used to not having children or anyone and going out whenever I wanted . . . so I said to her, how can you leave them with me? I have to go to meetings, to school and everything . . . because I had to help her out.

On the subject of the behavioural problems of her oldest grandson, who is nearly ten, she said:

> He doesn't obey me . . . it is a good thing his mother's here now to raise him . . . .

In this scenario, school performance often becomes the most objective indicator used by mothers to gauge their children's situation and attempt to correct their behaviour. Grade sheets often become the currency for mother–child interactions. It is common practice for mothers to use the promise of future material goods to justify their departure and shape their children's behaviour. This practice reflects the well-known aspects of manipulation and blackmail that occur when remittances become the main factor structuring long-distance family interaction among immigrants of low socioeconomic strata (Parreñas 2003, 2005a; Sánchez-Carretero 2005; Dreby 2006).

In keeping with the greater degree of transnationality in Dominican society, for two of the six immigrants at this stage of the family life cycle, collective care management included the circulation of resources and frequent communication betweem New York, Madrid and Santo Domingo (Figure 4.2).[19] Thus, whereas Marisol, a twenty-eight-year-old woman, tried to get ahead in Madrid where she had recently arrived, her mother, a legal resident in the United States, was on one of her intermittent work stays in New York employed as a domestic worker for an American family. Thus, Marisol's transnational household, comprising herself, her twin sister (a marketing employee) and her father (retired), supported themselves on the basis of the material and affective resources that circulated between these three points on the transnational *continuum*.

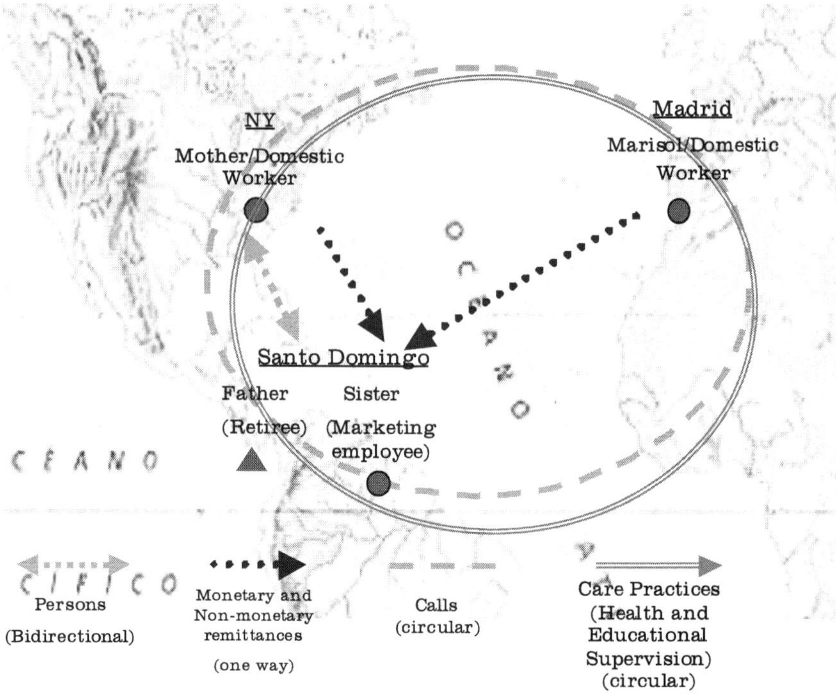


*Figure 4.2* Care circulation in Marisol's transnational family (early family stage).

Two features should be highlighted in the sphere of affectivity: the changes perceived in the mother–child interaction and the tangible marks of migratory grief caused by the separation. With the exception of one young migrant, all the mothers detected changes in the affective interaction with their offspring as a result of migration. Sometimes children avoid speaking to their mothers by phone, or, apparently upset and uncommunicative, they quickly hand the phone over to other adults standing nearby. This behaviour forms part of the pattern of 'feigned indifference', mentioned by Dreby (2007), as a common reaction among pre-teenage children in migrant families.

There is often a certain amount of confusion about the mother figure, with children calling their grandmothers 'Mummy', which migrant women find deeply distressing: 'I am afraid my children will adapt more to my parents than to me' (Inés, Mexican) (Cohen 2000; Dreby 2007).

The accounts of these women, who had only emigrated a few years before, revealed obvious signs of the process of grief entailed in separation, as well as marked feelings of sorrow and guilt, which they relieved by imagining that they would return in the near future. They often mentioned feelings of depression (sadness, grief, weeping, lack of appetite, weight loss). The most difficult aspect to handle was their separation from their children, which they could not help regarding as abandonment. But grief not only affects migrant mothers and their children experience; it also affects grandmothers and other relatives. The mother-grandmothers interviewed recalled their separation from their daughters with great sorrow.

### *Consolidation Phase: The Struggle to Stay Close and Progress*

The four immigrants (two from Mexico and two from Dominican Republic) in the consolidation phase of the family life cycle were between ages thirty-one and forty-eight and had children ages thirteen to eighteen.[20] With the exception of one who had only arrived in Madrid a year before, they had all spent between six and nine years in the receiving country. Two women (Dominicans) were separated and the heads of households in their places of origin; the two remaining Mexicans lived with their partners. The children lived within a variety of family arrangements.[21] Three of the immigrants had an irregular migratory status, and only one, a Dominican, had legal status (naturalised).

Once again, remittances (whether monetary or non-monetary) and regular telephone calls were the most frequent forms of interaction between the mothers and the children they had left behind. In the case of the Dominicans, family households depended entirely on the money they sent, which explains the high percentage of income they sent (more than 50 percent). In the case of one Dominican immigrant, care circulation included—as in the previous stage—resources that moved between New York, Madrid and Santo Domingo, locations among which members of their family household were scattered.

Collective management practices for child care show common patterns. Supervision is delegated to immediate relatives or other members of the same household (parents and in-laws in Mexican households; mother, sisters, brothers-in-law and domestic workers in Dominican households), but it remained a difficult, potentially conflictive process in several respects. The children were in the midst of adolescence, an age of affirmation and rebellion. Problems of authority, lack of discipline, disobedience and poor academic performance or apathy were widespread, according to the immigrants' accounts. In the words of some of them, their children had 'tantrums' and had to be spoken to 'firmly'. At other times, they understood that their behaviour was the result of the grandchildren being spoiled by the grandparents, which was often mentioned in the immigrants' accounts. Since I did not have interviews with non-migrant mothers with children of similar ages as a means of control, it is impossible to tell whether this behaviour is the result of maternal absence or simply of adolescence. A plausible hypothesis is that it is the result of the interaction of both processes, exacerbated by the atmosphere of relative laxness attributed to the grandparents' child-raising techniques.

Sometimes these collective management practices can be extremely close. Juana, one of the Dominican mothers who had barely spent a year in Madrid, supervised her children's welfare on a daily basis: She checked whether they had had their bath at the right time, monitored their homework, and reminded the father (and ex-husband) of the dates of doctors' appointments, what school supplies to buy and to buy bread on the way home. This zealous supervision even extended to household maintenance (bill paying, cleaning the drains etc.). For this mother, it was particularly important to attempt to provide her children with a similar level of well-being to that of Spanish children, in a sort of compensation and social equality mechanism. In addition to punctually sending monetary remittances, she sent a box with the food in a typical Spanish child's diet to Santo Domingo every month.

> My older son likes cars and sophisticated toys, robots and so on, so I send him all that. . . . Everything Spanish kids eat, from sweets to tuna, arrives at my house every month in a box, with clothes and toys, and everything I find I can send them.

But some mothers realise that they can do very little and resign themselves to the fact that effective supervision is in the hands of the relatives who stayed behind. Anastasia (Figure 4.3), who had been living in New York for nine years, had never been back to Mexico and therefore had not seen her two eldest children, who stayed in Mexico, since she left. Anastasia claimed: 'My mother-in-law is there to keep an eye on them'. Concern over their children's welfare is a central feature of the women's discourse. Some complained that their children are not looked after as they would like them to be or expressed their chagrin at finding out how neglected their children had been in their absence. In the words of Mónica, a Dominican who had lived in Madrid for six months: 'I didn't feel comfortable with my family because they did not treat my children well'. These risks led some of them to openly use the sending of remittances and gifts to the relatives in charge of their offspring as an overt means of blackmail to guarantee that their children were treated well. As one of them openly admitted, 'I buy them'. Sometimes these children become the hostages of these relatives since they guarantee that the money will arrive.[22] In other cases, they are subjected to situations of abuse in which they are not told that the money has arrived or else it is funneled off and used for other purposes by the caretaker responsible for them.[23]

As in the case of migrant mothers at the early stage, and with the sole exception of one Mexican woman, they also mentioned the results of separation on affective relations. The main one is the sorrow at not being able to

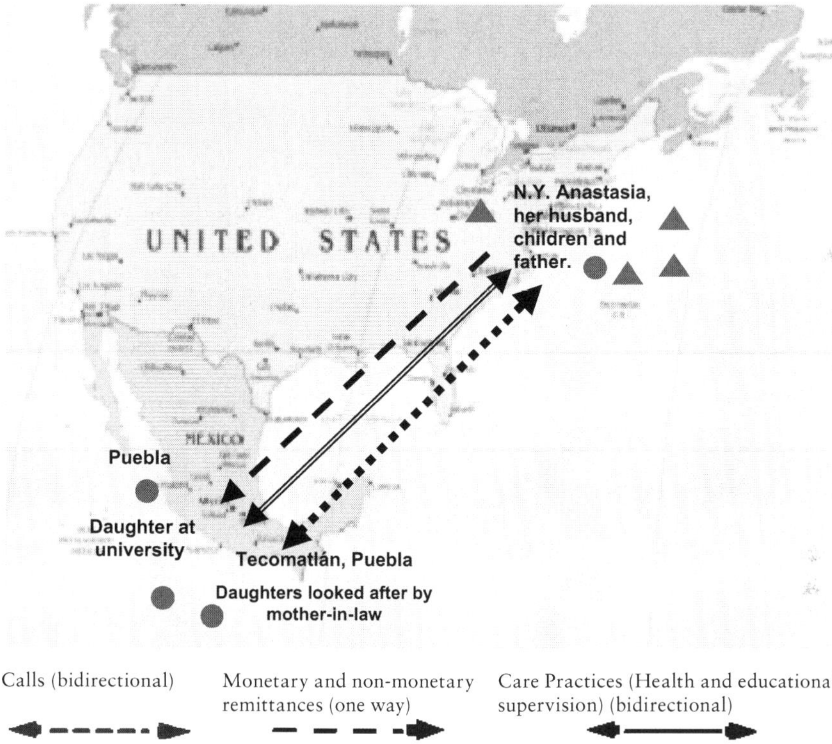


*Figure 4.3* Care circulation in Anastasia's transnational family (middle family stage).

be physically with their children and the overt or veiled guilt over what they regarded as neglecting their maternal duties. However, they took comfort in and were proud of the fact that the material well-being they had provided for their children was much greater than what they would have had if they had stayed in their countries of origin.

However, although remittances, telephone communication and other collective care management practices were fairly similar features of care circulation in the Dominican and Mexican transnational families, a substantial difference emerged with regard to the mobility of persons. This difference emerged when one contrasts the accounts of two immigrants who had been away from their homes for the same length of time (six years) yet in different places of residence: Mónica, who was living in Madrid and had became a naturalised citizen after just two years; and Hortensia, who was living in New York and was undocumented. Mónica had not only visited the Dominican Republic several times during this period but, supported by family reunification laws, managed to bring over two of her daughters and used other means to obtain a work contract for her older son, who had already been in Madrid for two years. Conversely, Hortensia had not been back to Mexico once, even though the oldest of her four children had just been to New York after crossing the border illegally.

### *Advanced Family Cycle: Time to Hand Over*

There were eight women at this stage of the family cycle (six Dominicans and two Mexicans) ranging in age from forty-eight to fifty-nine. Although two of them were childless (both Dominicans), most were mothers (six) and/or grandmothers (four). All the children were age nineteen or older. As a group, they had spent an average of ten years living in Madrid or New York, with a range of two to fifteen years. Regarding migratory status, most of them were legal, although two of the immigrants were illegal (one from each country). Several of the legal residents had begun the process of family reunification, with some of their children living with them and others not.

As in the previous stages, frequent telephone calls were the most common form of communication, although there were different patterns regarding the sending of remittances. Among the women who were unmarried daughters, there was a pattern of maximising savings in order to build their own houses. This pattern was combined with punctual financial assistance for needy relatives. Elderly parents and nieces and nephews or siblings were the recipients of long-distance care.

Conversely, half of the women who were mothers and/or grandmothers had stopped sending regular remittances and, at the time of the interviews, did so in response to specific requests or on the occasion of specific family rites (birthdays, Christmas celebrations). In most cases, these women's children had formed their own families, and the immigrant women were no longer primarily responsible for the reproduction of households in their countries of origin. There was, however, a subset of Dominican heads of household who had not handed over the responsibility of domestic reproduction and continued to be the main providers not only of the second but also of the third generations of their offspring.[24] Thus, Beatriz, a Dominican woman who had spent twelve years living in Madrid, exclaimed proudly at the age of fifty-nine: 'I will die working for them, I still work . . . [ ] . . . I still work for them'.[25] Although she had covered most of her eight children's needs throughout her long migratory career, and had half of them living with her in Madrid, Beatriz still covered the expenses of several of her grandchildren in the Dominican Republic due to the fact that their mother, who was unemployed at the time and living in Spain, was also the head of her own family. This pattern of behaviour, based not on economic rationality (Baldassar 2007b) but in ideals of reciprocity and the continuous investment in social capital,[26] is coherent with the ideology of motherhood as the unrestricted dedication to the well-being of those one serves (Schmalzbauer 2004). In my hypothesis, the fact that my findings indicate that this pattern of behaviour was most obvious among Dominican heads of household is related to the type of family interaction that prevails in these households and its importance in Dominican sociodemographic structure.

The child-raising period was over, meaning that the problems that arose referred more to concerns over their offspring's possible marital disagreements, success or failure at work, financial difficulties or the grandchildren's needs. The mother's active role had therefore been weakened in general terms but was still present. Even at this late stage, two of the Dominican women made the radical decision to bring their youngest children to Madrid as an extreme measure to try to change their behaviour after they had refused to go on studying. The mothers' aim was to 'put them out to work' to prevent them from 'going astray', in other words, getting into crime.

Collective care management practices, governed by cultural notions of reciprocity, now include looking after one's aged parents, who often suffer from chronic, degenerative diseases. Critical events, such as the severe illness or death of some of them, require a large collective effort in terms of both material resources and affective support and, if possible, physical presence despite the political borders. After being told of her mother's imminent death, Julieta, a forty-eight-year-old women who left the country to put an end to many years of domestic violence, did not think twice about returning to Mexico. Shortly afterwards, she undertook the dangerous journey across the desert for a second time. Among the Dominican women, collective care management not only included the circulation of resources between Madrid, New York and Santo Domingo but also a fourth country, Venezuela, where some of them had had previous migratory experience and where some had left some of their offspring.[27] In affective terms, grief over the separation caused by migration has led to a certain resignation, yet other forms of loss persist, such as the death of one of the parents in the absence of the migrants,[28] which tends to cast doubt on the entire migratory project. The impossibility of providing them with face-to-face care is a source of considerable suffering.

Migratory policies leave a distinctive mark on long-distance family interaction, not only by restricting people's mobility, since most of the immigrants in this stage are legal residents, but because of the effects of the duration of the family reunification process on affectivity (Cohen 2000), a process that takes much longer in the United States than in Spain, particularly if the applicants have had to overcome the status of illegal alien. A lengthy separation with little or no opportunity for face-to-face interaction may give rise to processes of defamiliarisation and strangeness among family members (Bonizzoni 2011). This scenario occurred for the family of Raquel, a Mexican immigrant who became a legal resident, who had been living in New York for thirteen years and had been separated from her husband for seventeen out of the thirty-four years they had been married due to migration. The husband left for a year when the first child was six months old, and twelve years went by before she was able to cross the border with all their children as irregular immigrants. Two years later, she returned to Mexico with her four children since they were unable to make ends meet in New York. When, due to the migratory reform of 1987 (Immigration Reforrmand Control Act), they regularised their migratory status, she and her children met up again with their husband/father in New York. Meanwhile, twenty-five years had elapsed, and thirteen had gone by since the father had last seen his youngest child.

Afterwards, three of her four children did not adapt to the U.S. way of life and soon returned to Mexico on their own. Raquel says that after so many years of separation, not only did she and her husband become strangers to each other, but also, despite the family achieving legal residence and managing to travel to be together, she feels there is a lack of 'that connection', the love that should exist between parents and children, and that a lot of resentment remains:

> They always respect him [referring to the father] but I feel that there is a barrier of love. . . . In other words, the family has been emotionally destroyed.
>
> In the long run, when your children grow up, instead of thanking you for the enormous effort you made, they feel resentful.

In the context of the families in the study, this case is undoubtedly extreme yet emblematic of the various aspects that may be assumed by the transnational family life of labour migrants on the lower rungs of the social structure, migrants who experience powerful restrictions on their movement and interaction. The pain and distancing caused by prolonged separation coexist with the pride and satisfaction of having escaped from poverty and provided children with a minimum opportunity for an education.

## Migratory Systems and Care Circulation

The data show that the possibilities of mobility and interaction through the transnational social space are relatively greater for the Dominican than the Mexican families belonging to low socioeconomic strata, even though they are geographically more distant. Similar results have been found in Ecuadoran migration to both countries (Spain and the United States) (Herrera 2008). Among Dominican families, there is greater face-to-face interaction through the circulation of persons, as well as possibilities for family reunification, partly because of the greater ease of becoming legal residents.[29] The fact that international Dominican migration is inserted in more than one migratory system[30] multiplies the points of contact between relatives in the transnational sphere and the possibility of taking advantage of the opportunities for insertion in the labour force provided by these markets.[31]

As expressions of Latin American international migration, the flows from the Dominican Republic to Spain and from Mexico to the United States are part of two different migratory systems: the one linking Latin

America and Spain as part of the European Union and the one linking the same region to the United States, where Mexican migration plays a particular role. In the context of the European Union, Latin American migration to Spain also has a special place. Spanish migratory policy displays an attitude of positive discrimination towards Latin American immigrants, borne out by the fact that: (1) bilateral agreements with various countries have been signed to channel flows[32]; and (2) Latin Americans are able to achieve naturalisation in a shorter time. By virtue of traditional colonial links, Latin Americans have the privilege of being able to obtain Spanish citizenship within two years, provided they are able to prove continuous legal residence in the country.

Conversely, the United States displays a radically different attitude towards Mexican immigration, which can be described as overt criminalisation. Since 1993, enhanced border enforcement has been a key element of U.S. migratory policy, which was reinforced after the events of 9/11 when the U.S. Mexico Border became a target in the U.S. war against terrorism (Cornelius 2001; Waslin 2009).[33] This strategy helped weaken the eminently temporary and rural pattern of migration that had hitherto characterised the flow of Mexican migration into the United States, according to which migrants annually returned to their places of origin. The consequences of this strategy include: (1) the steady rise of arrests and the deaths of migrants trying to cross the border; (2) rechanneling the flow towards the east; (3) the higher cost and physical risks associated with illegal entry; and (4) the higher rate of permanent settlement among undocumented migrants (Cornelius 2001, 664–676). Beyond the internal factors of domestic policy, these measures can be explained by the place Mexico occupies as a border country of the main pole of attraction in this migratory system and the double role of the Mexico–U.S. border: the pivot of the anti-terrorist strategy and a wall of contention keeping out transit immigrants from other countries.

The U.S. migratory policy is based on a settlement model with emphasis on family immigration: Direct blood links with the resident population are the main criteria for admission (Moulier and Papademetriou 1994; Calavita 1989).[34] Paradoxically, however, there are few (or infrequent) effective possibilities of legal entry into U.S. territory for the type of working-class immigrants I am analyzing. This is not only due to the high proportion of Mexicans with an irregular immigration status, but also because of the complicated admission system requiring blood links with legal residents and citizens, which follows a strict hierarchy, as well as the fact that the set number of annual visas per country for non-citizens may involve waiting times of ten years or more (Parreñas 2005a). The waiting period is much greater for immigrants from countries whose demand for reunification far exceeds the annual quota of approximately 20,000 visas per country, as happens with Mexico.[35] Conversely, Spanish migratory policy, promoted by the European Union, is based on labour migration (Moulier and Papademetriou 1994). Precisely because they were admitted as workers (or obtained legal status to enable them to work), within the short space of a year, immigrants can make use of the right to family reunification, provided they are legal residents.

It seems obvious that the most important effect of both migratory systems on family life lies in the different migratory status of the majority of (unskilled) labour immigrants encouraged by both countries and its impact on the possibility of family reunification: More than 70 percent of Dominicans are legal immigrants whereas between 60 and 70 percent of Mexicans are illegal. Forcing migrants into illegality, with few escape routes, undoubtedly reduces their chances of constructing a decent family life and envisaging a horizon of reunification in the nearby future.

In the context of the overlap between migratory policy and security policy and by virtue of the strongly asymmetrical nature of Mexico and the United States as border countries, geographic proximity somehow strengthens the obstacles to affective proximity in the construction of transnational family life. Thus, the acute asymmetry between the two countries translates into greater social and affective distance for those who interact through them. If we accept that in the global environment mobility is a factor of stratification (Bauman 1998), then this is relatively more unequal in the migratory system in which the Mexican immigrants in the study participate.

## CONCLUSIONS

The care circulation practices of transnational families from Mexico and the Dominican Republic have significant similarities that probably lie in the fact that they are labour immigrants with relative socioeconomic homogeneity. Sending remittances, frequent communication and the shared management of collective welfare are distinctive features of this interaction. The succession through the different stages of the family life cycle show the dynamic nature of care circulation: *Grossomodo,* the regular sending of remittances, increases in the early and consolidation stages and decreases in the advanced stage. Once they reach this phase, the mother assumes the role of grandmother, and the demands for support from the migrant's family generally decrease. The priority for care and attention is now given to elderly parents, although children never leave mothers' affective sphere. For transnational families living in Spain, the possibility of achieving family reunification increases over time.

Although remittances (both monetary and non-monetary) are sent less often or reduced, concern over relatives' well-being and the desire for connection remain. Telephone communication is the omnipresent means of interaction between migrants and their families, beyond the stage of the family cycle that they are in and the role they play (daughter, mother, grandmother). The dramatic drop in the cost of international calls—a by-product of globalisation—has turned them, in Vertovec's (2004) happy turn of phrase, into the 'social glue of migrant transnationalism'.[36]

The differences in family structure between Mexico and the Dominican Republic, in terms of the greater presence of women-headed households in the Caribbean country, not only create greater financial dependence in the households of origin on the migrants' precarious international work, but sometimes also on the intergenerational reproduction of this dependence. Even more important are the differences in policy between the migratory systems into which the two migratory flows are inserted. For specific reasons linked to geopolitics, the historical links between the nations of origin and destination, economic and specific political factors, currently place more restrictions on the mobility and exchange of Mexican transnational families from low socioeconomic strata.

Relying on a care circulation perspective undoubtedly enriches our perspective of family life in transnational social spaces since it sheds light on the endurance of social interactions based on relations of reciprocity. It also prevents us from looking just towards one end of the *continuum* of transnationality, either the host or sending country. However, it entails the risk of overemphasising harmony and continuity. Therefore, in applying the lens of circulation, we must be sensitive to the various axes of asymmetries that pervade transnational social spaces, stemming from either migratory policies or the realms of gender, generation and ethnicity.

## NOTES

1. These interviews form part of a broader research project, *Migration and Female Labor Markets in the Context of Globalization. A Comparative Perspective*, financed by the PAPIIT (IN303006) program of the National University of Mexico. The project seeks to compare the labour insertion into domestic service of Dominican women in Madrid versus Mexican women in New York.
2. The concept of transnational motherhood was put forward by Hondagneu-Sotelo (2001) and Hondagneu-Sotelo and Avila (1997) to refer to the situation in which immigrant domestic workers (nearly always Latin Americans) took care of the children of U.S. families while their children remained in their countries of origin. By global chains of affect or assistance, Hochschild (2000, 131) understands 'a series of personal links between people across the globe based on the paid or unpaid work of caring'. These chains are usually formed by women, although in unusual cases by men alone. They usually start in a poor country and end up in a rich one. For a critique, see Yeates (2005b) and Part A, this volume.
3. In the case of Iraq and Afghanistan, they are refugees.
4. These levels certainly do not reflect the variety of elements that intervene in the delimitation of transnational family space, but I believe that they summarise the most important variables present in this population.
5. Between 60and 80 percent of Mexican immigration to the United States is undocumented. By 2008, it was estimated that there were approximately 39.2 million immigrants, 30 percent of whom were undocumented and more

than half (i.e., 58.8 percent [7 million out of 11.9]) of whom are Mexican (Passel and Cohn 2008). In Spain, the percentage of illegal Dominicans was approximately 23.6 percent in 2001 (Domingo and Martínez 2006).

6. In New York, a limited number of interviews were conducted with women immigrants employed in the industrial sector (factories) as a means of controlling the inferences regarding the domestic service labour market.
7. On the basis of data from the 1991 Regularization Survey 1991, Oso (1998, 238) points out, the 'Dominican Republic has the highest proportion of workers with dependents (84%). It is a type of migration consisting primarily of female heads of household'.
8. In 2008, 58.6 percent of Mexicans who had lived in the United States for fewer than ten years were men (Caicedo 2010).
9. In addition to the United States and Spain as the first and second most important destinations, Dominicans workers immigrate to a number of countries, including Italy, Switzerland, Holland, Belgium and Germany. Conversely, aproximately 90 percent of Mexican international migration heads to the United States (INEGI 2009], ; Ariza and Portes 2007).
10. Maguid (2008) notes that the data should be viewed with caution due to the problems of estimating international emigration on the basis of national censuses.
11. For this purpose, I used a simplified version of the Economic Commission for Latin American and the Caribbean's (ECLAC) operating classification for the family life cycle. Thus, women in the early and expansion stage, which I will simply call the early cycle from now on, have children under age thirteen. Those women in the consolidation phase have children between the ages of thirteen and eighteen, while those at the advanced cycle have children over age nineteen. In fact, Eclac combines the mother's age with that of the youngest child, whereas I only use the last criterion.
12. More than one hundred interviews were conducted in the project: Fifty semi-structured interviews were carried out with immigrant workers in the two destination cities; another twenty-five interviews were conducted with key informants (NGO representatives, teachers, priests, mayors, lawyers, institutions for dealing with minors, members of civil society); twelve were carried out in the places of origin with the relatives of women who had previously been interviewed in Spain and the United States; and more than thirty informal interviews with non-relatives were carried out in the places of origin. A criterion of sociodemographic heterogeneity guided the selection of immigrants. An attempt was made to diversify them in terms of age, marital status, length of migration and condition of motherhood, among other aspects. All the interviews were carried out by the author.
13. Although many of the immigrants performed some form of paid care work, since they were virtually all domestic workers, in this chapter, I chose to restrict the focus of analysis of care relations to those that took place within the transnational families to which they belong to avoid making the analysis excessively complex. This aspect would have included other heterogeneous factors in the comparison.
14. By non-monetary remittances, I mean the sending of material goods (from food to gifts and clothes) as opposed to monetary cash. The sending of such remittances has always accompanied transnational family practices, although it has been somehow overlooked by the focus on monetary flows.
15. The mobility of practices and ideas throughout the transnational social space differs from Levitt's (2001) notion of social remittances since the exchange takes place in both directions on the continuum and not only from host-to-sending-country communities.

16. In the event of more than one migratory displacement, the most recent one was analyzed.
17. For both women, engaging in migration was a solution to what seemed to be a future without alternatives: failure to enter university and episodes of domestic violence in Gertrudis' account, and the narrowness of the marriage market and unemployment in the case of Marisol. For the sake of privacy, all names have been changed.
18. Within Dominican migratory culture, anyone who leaves the country is expected to support those left behind since it is assumed that the migrant's socioeconomic situation has improved. People who do not do so are morally sanctioned.
19. To assess families' degree of transnationality, I have used the criterion of whether one of the immediate relatives (siblings, parents, children) lived in another country and whether, at the time of the interview, they provided some form of support to the nucleus of the family in the place of origin or among themselves.
20. Anastasia, born in Mexico, had two younger children whom she had with her husband in the United States after a lengthy separation due to migration. The other two daughters stayed in Mexico with her mother-in-law.
21. In the case of the Dominican women, the children lived with their ex-husbands in the homes they used to share or, in the case of one child, alone but supervised by the migrant's son-in-law and a domestic worker. As for the Mexicans, they lived with the mother's parents-in-law or the migrant's maternal family.
22. These data emerge in the interviews with women and those with key informants at institutions responsible for looking after children in Mexico's main sending communities.
23. Jerónimo, a Mexican boy interviewed in the state of Puebla whose mother had emigrated alone many years earlier, reported that for a long time during his childhood, he was unaware that his mother had sent him money regularly. He and his siblings were never told, which led the mother to make the decision for the children to live by themselves.
24. This finding parallels the endless breadwinner responsibilities found byFresnoza-Flot (2009b) among Filipina domestic workers in Paris.
25. From the point of view of people close to Beatriz, her children had turned out 'ungrateful' since even after they had grown up, they continued to ask her for financial assistance, instead of helping her, even though she was no longer young and had worked for them her whole life.
26. I am in debt to María Eugenia D'Aubeterre for this observation.
27. Venezuela was an important destination of Dominican international migration during the years of its oil boom, particularly during the 1970s.
28. Four out of the eight migrants at this stage of the family cycle lost one of their parents when they were outside the country.
29. Spanish family reunification forms part of the norms established for the protection of families within the framework of the European Human Rights Agreement. Foreigners who are legal residents may request reunification with their spouse, children under age 18 (both biological and adoptive) and economically dependent family members of the previous generation, provided they have spent at least a year in Spain, are authorised to live there for at least another year and have the financial means to support them (Fernández 2002; "Legislación de Extranjeros" 2005; Díaz 2009).
30. A migratory system includes a particular combination of types of flows of population between countries of origin and receiving countries, the rules that govern these flows and the institutionalised reactions or counter-reactions

of the organisations that seek to maintain or eliminate them (Moulier and Papademetriou 1994).

31. The Dominican international migrants in the study participated in three migratory systems: from Latin America to Spain (European Union), from Latin America to the United States and within Latin America (flow between Dominican Republic and Venezuela).
32. Agreements have been signed with Ecuador, Colombia, Morocco, the Dominican Republic, Poland, Rumania and Bulgaria (San Martín, 2006).
33. Some of the technology that forms part of the 'concentrated border enforcement' strategy along the Mexico–U.S. border such as the infrared night scopes that detect migrants by their body heat dates from the Vietnam War (Cornelius 2001, 663). Measures with a negative effect on the U.S. Latino community after 9/11 include: (1) new changes of address requirements, (2) state and local police enforcement of federal immigration law, (3) restrictions on identification documents, and (4) worksite enforcement (Waslin 2009).
34. Of the 946,142 permanent residence visas granted in 2004, 65.6 percent involved family links. According to Wasem (2005), four main principles govern U.S. policy on permanent residence: (1) family reunification, (2) admission of immigrants with particular skills for which there is a demand, (3) protection of refugees, and (4) diversity of admissions requirements by country of origin.
35. Mexico is the country with by far the largest number of relatives on the waiting list: 1,381,896 in the 2010 tax year, followed by the Philippines with 535,750. For that year, the number of annual visas per country was 25,620 (http://travel.state.gov/pdf/waitinglListItem.pdf, last retrieved on 5 August 2011).
36. Vertovec (2004: 219–220) notes that , between 1995 and 2001, calls from Mexico to the United States grew by 107 percent, calls from the United States to Mexico grew by 171 percent and calls from United States to the Dominican Republic grew by 189 percent. The overall volume of international calls climbed from 12.7 billion in 1982 to 154 billion in 2001 (Vertovec 2004).

# 5 A Macro Perspective on Transnational Families and Care Circulation

## Situating Capacity, Obligation and Family Commitments

*Laura Merla*

Nacho migrated to Perth, Western Australia, in 1989 under a political refugee program together with his pregnant wife and three children aged seven, five and three. In El Salvador, Nacho had worked as an anaesthesiologist in a children's hospital, and his wife had managed a small coffee shop. The refugee program included financial and practical support from the Australian government, in the form of housing, unemployment benefits and English classes. Nacho was informed that he needed to go back to university and pass English tests as a prerequisite for the recognition of his qualifications. Because his English was too poor and he needed money, Nacho renounced his profession and took a low-paid cleaning job while his wife stayed at home to look after the children. Later she also took a low-paid, part-time cleaning job that allowed her to care for her children after school, and Nacho became the (unpaid) pastor of a Spanish-speaking Church while still working as a part-time cleaner. His mother still lives in El Salvador and only receives a small pension that does not cover her expenses, and he manages to send her monthly remittances despite limited financial resources. Nacho is one of the few Salvadorans that I interviewed who communicates with his mother on the Internet. He chats with her every single day, and he also calls her on the phone three times a week because he likes to hear her voice. Mother and son exchange advice and emotional support at a distance. Nacho has never been able to visit or invite his mother and his half-brother. The reasons for this include, among other things, prohibitive costs, visa issues, and an inability to access long paid leave.

In 1999, Natalia, a single mother who worked as a receptionist, accepted the invitation from her Belgium-based aunt to move to Belgium. She travelled alone, leaving her three children (ages ten, seven and five) in the care of her mother Josefina. She didn't require a visa to enter the Belgian territory, but after ninety days, she became an irregular migrant. She found an undeclared job as a domestic worker that allowed her to send weekly remittances back home. She remained involved in the emotional, practical and personal care of her children by calling her mother and children on the phone several times a week. Those discussions were also the occasion to exchange emotional support and practical advice with Josefina. In 2001, she repatriated to El Salvador because she couldn't stand living apart from her children, but she travelled back to Belgium two months later with the intention of saving enough money to bring them to Europe. Over the years, she has been able to bring her children to Belgium, as well as two of her brothers, who occasionally work in the building sector. Natalia continued to send regular remittances to her mother and call her every week. Because of their lack of employment, her brothers Marco and Arturo were unable to regularly send their mother money. Arturo called her several times a week, while Marco only called her once a month mainly because he felt guilty for not playing a substantial role in her financial well-being. In 2009, Gloria, Josefina's eldest daughter who lives in the United States, financed her mother's visit to Belgium. Josefina was meant to spend only a few months with her family, but she had been in Belgium for more than a year when I interviewed her. She was staying at Marco's apartment, providing and receiving personal, practical and emotional support to and from her children. Josefina wanted to move back home, but Natalia, who was granted a five-year visa in 2006 as a result of marrying a Belgian, was trying to get her a visa, which would also grant her access to social security and public health services in Belgium.

These case studies are drawn from comparative research on transnational care practices of Latin American migrants living in Australia and Europe.[1] The study focused on migrants who occupy a low qualified and/or low remunerated position in Australia and Europe despite coming from a mix of working-class and professional backgrounds in their homeland. Data collection in Australia and Belgium comprised forty-four life-history interviews in the participants' native language and participant observation with Salvadoran migrants living in Perth, Western Australia and Brussels, Belgium (nineteen men and twenty-five women). One of the main aims of this project was to analyse and compare the impact of the institutional context of two different receiving societies (Belgium and Australia) on migrants' capacity to care for ageing parents across borders.

In this chapter, I will discuss the usefulness of situating the care circulation framework (Part A, this volume) in a migratory context by discussing the interconnections between institutional contexts and capacity, obligation and negotiated commitments (Baldassar et al. 2007). I will show that care arrangements that result from a dialectical relationship between these three elements are influenced by migrants and their kin's respective positioning in the migration, welfare, gendered care and working-time regimes of their societies of origin and destination.

## UNDERSTANDING THE IMPACT OF INSTITUTIONAL CONTEXTS: A FRAMEWORK

The various contributions to this book highlight that the circulation of care within transnational family networks is a key element for the maintenance of 'familyhood' (Bryceson and Vuorela 2002a, 2002b) and cultural belonging. In the context of globalisation and increased geographical and virtual mobilities, combined with population ageing, transnational caregiving is becoming a common feature of a growing number of families. Once we recognise that transnational families represent a significant category in typologies of contemporary family forms, it becomes necessary to address the implications of mobilities and care circulation for social policy. The idea of a 'situated transnationalism' (Kilkey and Merla 2013) highlights that the specific contexts of both receiving and sending societies play a major role in shaping actual and potential care circulation.

Bonizzoni and Boccagni (Chapter 3, this volume) underline the importance of understanding the constraints and resources available to transnational family members, in both their home and host countries. According to the authors, these details help explain variations in the shape and outcomes of long-distance caregiving arrangements, as well as their evolution over time. Bonizzoni and Boccagni identify several factors of key importance, including infrastructures and technologies, immigration policies, migrants' integration in the labour market as well as cultural constructions based on age and gender, to name just a few.

Research has indeed shown that the institutional contexts of both the home and host societies play a key role in shaping the resources and constraints of transnational family caregiving (Al-Ali 2002; Baldassar 2008a; Baldassar, Baldock and Wilding 2007; Fresnozat-Flot 2009b; Zechner 2008). In collaboration with Loretta Baldassar, and in order to provide a framework for understanding the inequalities that arise from different institutional contexts and their influence on migrants' capability to care for their relatives, I have conceptualised care within transnational families as a capability that is affected by three sets of factors (Merla 2012a; Merla and Baldassar 2011). The first set includes mobility (being able to travel) and communication (being able to communicate and send items across borders), which are the major channels through which care circulates within transnational families. The third set comprises paid work, later renamed 'finances' (Kilkey and Merla 2013) (having access to sufficient financial resources), education and knowledge (for instance, having the opportunity to learn how to use ICT and having one's qualifications recognised in the host country) and time-allocation (being able to dedicate time to caregiving exchanges), which provide the necessary resources for mobility and communication.

Social networks (having access to social networks in the home and host societies) play a mediating role between the first and third sets of factors, as networks of friends, relatives, neighbours and so on can help migrants and their kin overcome difficulties related to limited access to resources for mobility and communication (Merla 2011). Access to and use of all these resources are strongly influenced by the host and home countries' formal and informal policies, such as visa regulations, leave policies and development of infrastructures.

In order to get a fuller picture of the policies involved and highlight the critical role of national contexts, Majella Kilkey and I (Kilkey and Merla 2013) have drawn on the various strands of 'regime' scholarship to specify the institutional contexts within which the resources necessary for caregiving exchanges within transnational families are in part constituted. We have identified four regimes as relevant. First, the migration regime, 'characterised by immigration policies—rules for entrance into a country (quotas and special arrangements), settlement and naturalisation rights, as well as employment, social, political and civil rights' (Williams 2010, 390) and which also includes migration cultures in home and host societies. Second, the welfare regime, which defines a system of welfare provision (Esping-Andersen 1990). Third, the gendered care regime, which aims at capturing who is responsible for care, the nature of state support for non-familial care, and provisions for care leave (Williams 2010) as well as dominant national and local discourses—'care cultures'—on what constitutes appropriate care (Kilkey and Merla 2013; Williams and Gavanas 2008) and gender equality expectations and outcomes associated with care arrangements (Pfau-Effinger 2000). Finally, the working-time regime defined to 'include the set of legal, voluntary and customary regulations which influence working-time practice' (Rubery, Smith and Fagan 1998, 72). Policies around the regulation of cross-border transport, including its availability and affordability and around the quality and accessibility of the communication infrastructure, are also important.

For each regime, we have identified relevant parameters for the circulation of care in transnational families. These are specified in Table 5.1.

These different regimes and policies, which have specific features in different home and host countries, interact to create particular contexts that facilitate or hinder the circulation of care within different types of transnational families. The level and form of involvement in caregiving—and receiving—of each member of a transnational family network, and the ease with which they are able to participate in these exchanges, are partly shaped by their position within the migration, welfare, gendered care and working-time regimes of their home and host societies, as well as their access to transport and communication technologies. Regimes influence people's migratory status, insertion in the labour market, social entitlements, access to education, rights to take time to care or be cared for as well as cultural

*Table 5.1* Care Circulation: Institutional Contexts*

| *Institutional Context* | *Relevant Parameters* |
|---|---|
| Migration regime | Exit/entry/residency rights for migrants and family members |
| | Policies governing migrants' and their family members' insertion in the labour market: conditions on labour market access, rules on recognition of 'foreign' qualifications, training and professional reorientation<br>Regulations governing migrants' and their family members' incorporation in the welfare regime: migrants' entitlements to social benefits and services |
| | Migration cultures: norms around appropriate (family) migration strategies in sending societies, the overarching approach to migrants in receiving societies |
| Welfare regime | Quality of social entitlements to benefits and services in areas related to: health, income, housing and education |
| | Rules on the portability of entitlements across national borders |
| Gendered care regime | Policies around the right to time to care: care leave, reorganisation of daily working schedules<br>Rules on the location of dependants recognized in the right to time to care |
| | Policies around the right to receive care: services and financial support for those with care needs |
| | Gendered care cultures: norms around appropriate gender division of labour and appropriate forms of care for dependants |
| Working-time regime | Policies around the regulation of working-time practice: regulation on maximum working hours and holiday entitlement and their coverage across all sectors of the labour market and all work contracts |

* This is a short version of the table that comes from Kilkey and Merla (2013).

and gendered norms regarding the definition of appropriate care and of who should perform this care. These impact on their freedom to circulate within transnational family networks for care purposes and to participate in caring from a distance. People's 'situations' within these regimes also vary according to key factors such as gender, class, ethnicity, age and position in the migration and family cycles (see Chapter 4, this volume).

Baldassar et al. (2007, 204) define transnational caregiving as 'a dialectic encompassing the capacity of individual members and their culturally informed sense of obligation to provide care, as well as the particularistic kin relationships and negotiated family commitments that people with specific family networks share'. This dialectic is equally pertinent to an analysis of care circulation. In this chapter, I will discuss the usefulness of the situated caregiving capabilities framework presented above for understanding the influence of institutional contexts on the three aspects of this dialectic, drawing on my own research and on the various contributions to this volume.

## INSTITUTIONAL CONTEXT AND CAPACITY

As I mentioned earlier, for members of transnational families, being able to be mobile and communicate with kin are the main conditions that allow participation in care circulation. The framework helps better understand the relative lack of physical mobility that is characteristic of Nacho, Natalia and their kin's caregiving exchanges. The impact of the migration regimes is clear. The mobility of Natalia's family arises from the absence of a visa requirement for El Salvador citizens who enter Belgium with the intention to stay a maximum of ninety days. Those who stay for longer periods of time and who can apply for family reunion because their relative holds a valid permit must prove that they are dependent on the person with whom they wish to reside. Since 2006 and 2007, they must also prove that their sponsors can accommodate them, have sufficient means of subsistence 'to ensure that they do not become dependent on the Belgian welfare system' (SPF Affaires étrangères 2011) and have obtained a health care insurance policy. If family reunification represents the main source of migration in Belgium, family members other than spouses and children only represent a minor proportion of beneficiaries (Lodewyckx, Timmermans and Wets 2011). In their study of a sample of 9,298 beneficiaries of family reunification in Belgium between 2000 and 2005, Lodewyckx et al. found that only 4 percent were older than age fifty-five, and fewer than 1 percent was reunited with a daughter or son (including in-laws) (Lodewyckx et al. 2011). Those who cannot apply for family reunification because their relative is an irregular migrant become irregular migrants themselves, which means that they will have no access to public health and social security in Belgium. Irregular migrants who wish to visit their families back home face the risk of not being able to return to Belgium.

In this context, migrant children tend to remain in Belgium and engage in long-distance caregiving, whereas ageing parents who can afford to travel with the support of their extended family networks regularly visit their children in order to give and receive care. This is very different from the Australian case, where the mobility of all the actors involved is extremely limited. The lack of mobility of Nacho's relatives is explained in large part by restrictive visa regulations. In the Australian migration regime, El Salvador citizens require costly visas and health insurance, both of which are more expensive for elderly people in particular (for more details, see Chapter 12, this volume).

Many contributions to this volume confirm the primary importance of migration regimes for the lives of transnational families in general and for the circulation of care in particular. The conditions under which kin circulate within family networks—and the possibility of such movements—are highly dependent on visa regulations and family reunion schemes. Needless to say, border crossing and settlement represent different experiences depending on whether one is an undocumented or a legal migrant. Ariza (Chapter 4, this volume) shows that undocumented Mexican migrants living in the United States face greater restrictions to mobility and family solidarity compared with Dominican legal migrants in Spain, a situation that she partly attributes to differences between the migratory systems of the two host countries. Spain's relatively friendly migration policies towards Latin American migrants, based on positive discrimination, involves easy access to citizenship, freedom to cross the Spanish border and easier access to family reunion schemes than the much more hostile attitudes predominant in the United States towards Mexican migrants, who often have no other choice than to cross the border illegally and have no access to family reunification.

There are also important differences between legal migrants. Each type of visa entails a particular series of rights and obligations that can facilitate or hinder the circulation of care and impact the type and direction of flows of support within transnational families. In the case of Indian students in Australia (Chapter 11, this volume), not having access to welfare benefits means that they must rely on their distant families for financial support. Not knowing whether they will get a job and be able to successfully apply for family reunion in Australia also makes it difficult for them to make future plans. The interrelation between migration and family is vividly illustrated by the case of a former student who has a permanent visa in Australia but who considers migrating to Canada where family reunion is easier. These examples contradict the assumption, commonly found in migration literature, that geographic mobility is predominantly triggered by 'rational economic', profit maximisation motives, by showing the existence of other motives such as the need to give or receive care—a point made by Baldassar, Baldock and Wilding (2007) and Ackers and Dwyer (2002, 152; see also Merla and Baldassar 2010b).

As a refugee, Nacho was immediately granted a permanent visa and faces no legal restrictions to borders crossing. What comes into play here is his positioning in the welfare/labour market nexus. In Australia, Nacho faced downward social mobility because of a lack of proficiency in English and of recognition of his qualifications. This resulted in being downgraded to low-qualified, low-paid jobs in the cleaning sector, and it also led Nacho's wife to postpone her return to the labour market to look after their young children. As irregular migrants, Natalia and her brothers had to accept low-paid and time-demanding jobs, and she struggled to improve her situation after gaining a temporary visa. Martens and Verhoeven (2006) point to the ethno-stratification of the Belgian labour market where foreign-born workers, and non-Europeans in particular, have lower opportunities for good employment conditions and access to certain types of professions and sectors, a stratification that can also be observed in the Australian labour market (Colic-Peisker and Tilbury 2006). Since the late 1990s, the demand for migrant workers in Belgium has increased in highly flexible, illegal and low-paid jobs in the construction industry, catering and domestic services (Bribosia and Rea 2002; Caestecker 2006).

Mobility is also restricted due to a difficulty to set aside time for travel, which is also related to a migrant's positioning within working-time and gendered care regimes. In both countries, irregular and short-term workers like Nacho, Natalia and her brothers are excluded from policies that regulate working hours and holiday entitlements. Their labour market positioning also excludes them from time to care provisions such as long-service leave (a three-month paid leave accessible to employees with ten years of continuous service) in Australia and time credit (a one-year paid leave accessible to employees after working at least twelve months for the same employer) in Belgium. In Australia, working migrants can accumulate their annual paid vacations and travel once they have saved enough time to make a long visit home, an option that is not available in Belgium. As Palmas and Ambrosini (2008) outline, it is particularly difficult for domestic workers who bring their children to Europe to balance their child-rearing and working obligations. These tensions also reduce the possibility for women like Natalia to make visits for eldercare purposes.

## INSTITUTIONAL CONTEXT AND OBLIGATION

Building on Blackman, Brodhurst and Convery's (2001) argument that welfare regimes predispose societies towards particular configurations of social care for eldery people, Baldassar (2008a, 271) states that cultural notions of obligation in transnational families 'are influenced by and in turn influence existing and historical patterns of social structures and service provision in the countries of relevance'.

This statement invites us to consider the interrelationships between culture, institutions and practices, which particularly come to the fore in the migratory context. Grillo's (2010) work on diversity regimes in multicultural societies, in particular his discussion of the interrelationships between moral orders and the politico-jural domain, is particularly helpful. He proposes to consider (diversity) regimes as politico-jural domains (or sets of formal and informal rules and regulations) informed by, backing up and (re)producing moral orders, defined as 'beliefs and values that provide guidelines (or imperatives) for right and proper conduct' (Grillo 2010, 26). Although this conceptualisation derives from a discussion of cultural diversity, I would argue that it can also be applied to other types of regimes. Indeed, the migration, welfare, gendered care and working-time regimes are all informed by, back up and (re)produce dominant (hegemonic) moral orders. Norms and values represent a central element of these regimes, together with policies and regulations. The four regimes that influence the circulation of care within transnational families are informed by particular notions of the family as a moral order that 'provides guidelines or rules for constituting relations between kinsfolk and affines, and between men and women (across gender and generation), and for identifying their transgression' (Grillo 2010, 27). Hegemonic—and patriarchal—normative conceptions of the family set guidelines for the gender division of paid and unpaid work and the form that this division takes. This normative vision is reflected in the various regimes—for instance, the working-time regime may include formal and informal regulations that encourage part-time work in highly feminised sectors/professions, thus reflecting and (re)producing what Lewis calls a 'male full-time earner–female part-time carer' model (Lewis 2001). The interrelations between moral orders in the family domain and institutionalised sets of regulations are captured by the notion of 'gendered care culture', which form an integral part of gendered care regimes, and by the notion of 'migration cultures' in migration regimes. The latter are informed by, and (re)produce, normative conceptions of the family that influence, between others, acceptable/desirable migration strategies in sending societies and construct acceptable/problematic migrants in receiving societies.

It is important to keep in mind that various moral orders coexist in a given society and vary across time and space (at the local, regional, national and international levels) as well as across social classes, ethnic groups and so on (Grillo 2010). The migratory experience exposes individuals and families to different and sometimes contradictory notions of obligation to care, which are informed, and sometimes constrained, by the welfare/gendered care regimes of both home and host countries.

The idea that children should support their parents financially, practically and emotionally is widespread among the Salvadoran population, all classes and genders included (Benavides et al. 2004). Sons and daughters have a strong sense of duty to care for their ageing parents, and this sense does not fade with distance (Merla 2010). This is related to the characteristics of El Salvador's informal-familialistic welfare regime, where the state is absent and extended families carry the full burden of care duties and play the role of production units and social protection networks (Martínez Franzoni 2008). Only 20 percent of the population has access to state-sponsored health care services (Martínez Franzoni 2008), and 50 percent of Salvadorans ages sixty and over entirely rely on family and community support (Guzmán 2002, 14). Institutional care in El Salvador is not available, nor is it considered a desirable option by Natalia and Nacho's mothers, in either their home or their children's host countries. Nacho's rapid acceptance of professional downgrading is also related to a reluctance to become dependent on social benefits (also noted by Santos 2006), which in turn is related to the low level of social protection offered by El Salvador's welfare regime.

El Salvador's care regime is highly gendered: Women assume the quasi-exclusive responsibility of unpaid work in general and care in particular (Martínez Franzoni 2005). This explains why Nacho's wife postponed her entry in the Australian labour market in order to care for her young children despite financial difficulties. It also explains why Natalia asked her mother, and not her children's father, to look after her children when she migrated to Belgium.

Gender differences are less obvious when we look at Salvadoran men's participation in long-distance elder care. My study of Salvadoran transnational families actually challenges the assumption that women are the main actors of caregiving exchanges in transnational families (Merla 2010). Here, gender does not entirely determine variations in the form and degree of Salvadoran men's involvement in care exchanges with ageing parents, except for hands-on care during visits, which is more common among women than men. In Australia, some men are the main coordinators of the support provided to their ageing parents. They are in constant communication with their distant kin and provide important levels of emotional support (Merla 2010). Other factors come into play, such as birth order (being the eldest) or family structure (not having any sisters). These factors have also been acknowledged in the literature on geographically proximate family networks (Attias-Donfut, Lapierre and Segalen 2002; see also Chapter 8, this volume). In addition, the Belgian case shows that sons' involvement in financial support can be compromised by an increased difficulty to find paid work in the host society. As Natalia's brothers note, it is more difficult for men to find an undeclared job in Belgium than it is for women because the demand for domestic workers is higher, and controls are less frequent than in the building sector, where they unsuccessfully tried to get a job.

Legal frameworks play a decisive role in the definition and recognition of family obligations (Attias-Donfut et al. 2002). Different gendered care–migration regimes nexuses produce different types of transnational families. This is partly based on the definition of family that underlies migration regimes—a definition that is in turn influenced by a prioritisation of parenting over elder care obligations. Transnational motherhood is more common in Belgium than Australia because the latter country is characterised by a gendered care–migration regimes nexus that makes the importation of foreign live-in nannies difficult, and the migration regime 'tends to produce families in which migrants live with their children but are separated from ageing parents' (Chapter 12, this volume). None of the Australian migrants who participated in the study that informs this chapter has experienced transnational motherhood or fatherhood, except for one case where a father migrated to Australia with his second wife and left his children behind, but these children were already living in the United States with their mother, who had sole custody. But Australia and Belgium's migration regimes are based on a similar assumption that elderly migrants represent a burden for social security and health systems and largely exclude them from family reunion schemes. These schemes are based on a construction of family as a nuclear household composed of adult parents and their dependent children. Notions of obligation and filial duty towards ageing parents are not recognised (see also Merla and Baldassar 2011).

Migrants' culturally informed notions of obligation and appropriate forms of care for dependants are also challenged by the welfare/gendered care regime of receiving societies and the moral orders that underpin them. As Grillo (2010, 27–28) notes, 'migration is an important catalyst for changing perceptions of self and other and forces (re)interpretation of beliefs and practices', which the author partly relates to the pressure that receiving societies and their institutions exert on migrant families. The clash can be quite important for migrants moving from societies characterised by familialist regimes to more 'individual-oriented' welfare systems in receiving societies (Blackman 2000, 181). In this context, migratory projects can go through a tension between real or desired increased autonomy and the reaffirmation of family obligations and duties. People migrate for a variety of reasons, including family care obligations and duties (Merla and Baldassar 2010b). But the confrontation with a receiving society, where autonomy and individualism challenge family duties, can lead migrants to reconsider their own investment in the circulation of care. Research on Italian transnational families has shown that this confrontation can create tensions between the expectations of left-behind kin and first- and second-generation migrants' vision of familial interdependencies and appropriate/desirable responses to care needs (Baldassar 2007a; Zontini 2010; see also Chapter 10, this volume). Intergenerational tensions may also appear in situations where ageing parents who reunite with their children in the host society come to realise that their offspring are unable to care for them in person because their children's perceptions of appropriate care have changed, because they do not wish to prioritise caring over paid labour or because they do not have sufficient access to work/family balance measures (Wilding & Baldassar 2009).

Within multicultural societies, the interarticulation between 'alternative (subordinate) familial regimes and moral orders associated with immigrants and minority ethnic populations of migrant origin' and dominant (hegemonic) moral orders is constantly negotiated (Grillo 2010, 31). This means that globalisation and migration can in turn challenge dominant models in receiving societies, as is exemplified by current debates on care options for ageing migrants in Europe. There is a growing concern that service provision in receiving societies will not meet the expectations and needs of migrants and their relatives. For instance, a Belgian study highlights Moroccan migrants' reluctance to use institutional care, as this is considered a form of abandonment and a source of shame within this community (Moulin et al. 2006). The Salvadorans whom I interviewed in Australia and

Belgium were critical of their host countries' aged care cultures and did not consider institutional care as an acceptable option (Merla 2011).

Migration, globalisation and transnationalism have led to significant social transformations in both receiving and sending societies (Vertovec 2009, 158), which affect moral orders and practices. The circulation of care within transnational families influences these changes. Ariza (Chapter 4, this volume) conceptualises the circulation of care in the transnational space as a two-way flow between home and host communities that involves, among other things, the mobility of ideas, images and practices (Chapter 4, this volume). Members of transnational families who are engaged in reciprocal care exchanges participate in the circulation of norms around appropriate care, filial duty and family solidarity at a global level. These transnational exchanges provide family members who have never migrated with a 'personal repertoire comprising varied values and potential action-sets drawn from diverse cultural configurations' (Vertovec 2009, 69). Research still needs to fully address the transformative potential of the transnational circulation of care within families, not only on host communities, but also on home communities, in terms of practices, moral orders and policymaking (also highlighted in Chapter 8, this volume).

## INSTITUTIONAL CONTEXT AND NEGOTIATED FAMILY COMMITMENTS

Negotiated family commitments form the third element of Baldassar, Baldock and Wilding's (2007) definition of transnational care. This notion was developed by Finch (1989a) and Finch and Mason (1993) in their study of geographically proximate families living in the UK. Negotiated family commitments are the result of the gradual emergence of an understanding of what certain people in the family would do for other kin members, so that when a need arises, it becomes obvious that a particular person will be the one to provide the necessary support. As Finch (1989, 201) puts it, 'every negotiation between members of the same family, about whether a particular kind of support is to be provided, draws upon a history of relationships and commitments in that particular family, and anticipates a future'. Elements such as the history of the relationship, personal reputations developed over time and accumulated commitments play a central role in these negotiations.

Family commitments are not fixed but subject to constant (re)negotiations. Expectations, investments and practices change over the family, individual life and migratory cycle (see Chapter 2, this volume). Migration significantly impacts, and potentially disrupts, individual biographies and family relationships and can lead to renegotiations of family commitments and care arrangements. For the Salvadoran migrants I interviewed in Belgium and Australia, participating in care exchanges at a distance was considered a way of continuing the role they had played before migrating. Nacho started contributing to the family budget when he was a teenager and continued to support his mother financially, but also practically and emotionally after he got married and left the house. The migration experience reinforced his sense of obligation to care for his distant mother, as he tried to compensate for his 'physical' absence by sending remittances and chatting with her every day. Several migrants said they would probably communicate less often with their ageing parents if they had not migrated. Geographical distance makes the need to keep family ties alive more pressing (Bryceson and Vuorela 2002), and exchanging care across boundaries is a key way of maintaining a sense of familyhood (Goulbourne et al. 2010; Baldassar 2008a).

Migration led to downward social mobility for the Salvadorans I met in Perth, and this impacted on their participation in the circulation of care, which led to renegotiations of family commitments. People who migrate are exposed to a new structure of opportunities and constraints that can modify their capacity to provide particular forms of care. Roberto, who had a comfortable situation in El Salvador where he worked as a manager, was the main provider of financial support to his mother, but he had to pass on this role to one of his brothers because his cleaning job in Perth did not provide him with sufficient funds to send regular remittances. Al-Ali (2002) notes in her study of Bosnian refugees living in the UK and the Netherlands that women (and, to a lesser extent, men) who struggle to find qualified jobs in their host country and/or to integrate new social networks tend to compensate a sense of isolation by strongly investing in maintaining a relationship with relatives and friends back home. The strong investment in the circulation of care of several Salvadoran migrants I interviewed can similarly be interpreted as a way of dealing with a feeling of isolation and loneliness, of compensating professional, material, social and/or personal problems (in both Australia and Belgium) and ultimately creating/maintaining a positive sense of self as a 'good' son or daughter who fulfils her or his filial duties (see Merla 2010).

Migration can also challenge the balance of power within (transnational) families. Power relations are central to negotiation processes, and these cannot be understood without reference to structural conditions and moral orders, which affect the bargaining power of family members involved in formal or informal negotiations of care duties. Patriarchal power increases men's capacity to impose certain tasks on women, such as domestic and caring tasks (Finch 1989a, 200). Within many societies, family relationships are governed by structural models of power relations that link authority with masculinity and are interconnected with the sexual division of labour (Connell 1987). As Pessar (2005, 7) notes, access to paid work and state services can help immigrant women gain more control over household decision-making and expenditures, whereas men 'commonly experience a decrease in relative authority and privilege within households, workplaces, and the wider community'. In my study, women's relatively easy insertion in the (informal) Belgian labour market as compared with men located them as key providers of financial support and gave them extra weight in care-related decisions, whereas men experienced their reduced capacity to send remittances as a source of shame that led in some cases, such as Marco's, to the adoption of a low profile in the family network.

Migrants also face new expectations that may not correspond to their real situation and place additional burden on their shoulders. Several male and female Salvadorans complained about left-behind family members who tended to overestimate their financial situation and place high expectations on them, which deprived them of the possibility of using financial problems as a 'legitimate excuse' (Finch 1989a, 210) for reducing or ceasing to send remittances (Merla 2010).

## CONCLUSION

As Baldassar (2008a, 270–271) notes, 'all migrants and their transnational family members are located in particular places at particular times and their caregiving practices are variously affected by this "territorialisation"'. In this chapter, I have tried to demonstrate the usefulness of 'situating' migrants and their kin's caregiving exchanges by discussing the interconnections between institutional contexts and capacity, obligation and negotiated commitments. I have shown that care arrangements are influenced by migrants and their relatives' respective positioning in the migration, welfare, gendered care and working-time regimes of their home and host societies.

The use of the term 'influenced' is by no means accidental. Institutional contexts can make it easier or harder for actors involved in transnational family networks to circulate particular types of support, but practices are not automatically determined by structures of opportunities and constraints. I would like to stress here the importance of combining an analysis of practices related to the circulation of care at the macro, meso and micro levels (also argued by Baldassar 2008a). I have shown elsewhere that social capital, in the form of social networks in both home and host societies, can help migrants and their kin overcome obstacles related to difficult access to caregiving related resources, such as finances, education or time (Merla 2011, 2012b). Natalia assisted several migrant families in Belgium, providing them initial accommodation and helping them find a job. Members of the network that she re-created in Belgium exchange useful tips on cheap communication, and those who travel back home regularly deliver gifts and remittances to their friends' relatives. Family networks also represent an important resource for migrants and ageing parents. Josefina could only be reunited with her children in Belgium thanks to her daughter Gloria, who financed her trip. Gloria had recently applied for a permanent visa in the

United States and thought it would be easier to visit her relatives in Belgium rather than trying to reunite the whole family in El Salvador or the United States. This example attests to the capacity of migrants to circumvent obstacles to family solidarity that are specific to a certain institutional context by mobilising family members located in a more favourable environment (see also Merla 2012b). I would argue that actors can work the system a great deal precisely because different forms of care circulate in multiple directions within transnational families and provide them with the necessary resources to participate in these reciprocal exchanges of solidarity.

The experience of circulating care in a transnational context reveals that constraints coexist with agency and fluidity. The migration experience in particular challenges expectations, meanings and practices in the realm of families, affecting individual actors, wider kin groups as well as communities of origin and destination. The transnational circulation of care, that is, multidirectional flows of emotional, personal, practical and financial support via the circulation of people, ideas and material objects, has consequences that go beyond individual households and wider family networks: They can potentially play an active role in the 'creation, re-creation and transformation of cultures' (Herrera Lima 2001, 91, cited in Vertovec 2009, 64) as well as sociopolitical institutions.

## ACKNOWLEDGMENTS

I am grateful to Ralph Grillo for his helpful comments.

## NOTES

1. This research was financed by the EC 6th Framework Programme–Marie Curie Outgoing International Fellowship (MOIF-CT-2006–039076 Transnational Care). This chapter reflects only the author's views. The European Community is not liable for any use that may be made of the information contained herein. This chapter is also informed by a research on 'Transnational Care-Giving in the Belgian Context: An Analysis of the Intra-familial Dynamics at Play in the Exchange of Care Between Adult Migrants and Their Parents' financed by the Belgian Federal Science Policy under the EC 7th Framework Programme (Return Mandate).

Part C

# Gendered Care Circuits

## Exploring Absence Beyond Mother–Child Dyads

# 6 Migration and Care

## Intimately Related Aspects of Caribbean Family and Kinship

*Karen Fog Olwig*

The 'global care chain', a term coined by the American sociologist Arlie Hochschild (2000), has been used to describe the asymmetrical chain of care exchange that emerges when Third World women migrate in order to care for children in the Western world, leaving their children behind to be reared by relatives, friends or neighbours. While there is no doubt that this 'chain' of relations reflects a world system of severe inequality, focusing only on this clearly negative aspect of care work migration nevertheless does little justice to the complex system of social relations and cultural values in which such care relations are embedded. It is thus problematic to analyze this chain in terms of fixed notions of proper family relations in which the biological mother cares for her biological children because these values can vary both within and between societies.

Drawing on ethnographic research among Caribbean people, I analyze how relations of care are practiced and given meaning within the context of migration. I argue that for Caribbean women, particularly in the lower classes, care work migration does not involve a unidirectional flow of care extending to privileged families in the West. Rather it is part of a circulation of care (Part A, this volume) that is integral to family and kinship in Caribbean societies. This circulation of care, furthermore, is often associated with considerable physical mobility through the life course, beginning with children moving to other homes, where they help with various chores in exchange for their upkeep, and continuing with young women's migrating to obtain the material basis of the care of children and elderly relatives who are left behind. Finally, there is a return migration to the family home to look after care-dependent relatives or migration to various destinations to provide care to close relatives and/or to receive care. From a Caribbean perspective, migration and care are therefore intimately linked and should be interpreted as a way of doing family relations in a mobile world of unequal social and economic opportunities.

## INTRODUCTION

In the literature on female migration, there has been a strong focus on women in the economically undeveloped south who leave their own children behind in the care of others in order to care for other people's children in private homes in the economically privileged north, thus freeing the privileged parents of these children to pursue their own careers. This form of migration has been regarded as being highly problematic for the caregivers. As the term 'global care chain' suggests, the displacement of caregiving challenges the prevalent 'ideal of biological mothers raising their own children' because it makes it difficult for migrant women, who have left their biological children in the care of others, to maintain their position as mothers in the families left behind (Hondagneu-Sotelo and Avila 1997, 548). The mothers are thereby forced to struggle to retain their social identity as proper, caring mothers through remittances, presents and phone calls as well as sustained efforts to visit whenever possible (Hondagneu-Sotelo and Avila 1997; Constable 1999; Parreñas 2001b; Dreby 2008).

Although migration researchers generally agree that migrant care workers often endure long working hours for poor wages, some have questioned the preoccupation with the special plight of migrant mothers, as reflected in the notion of the care chain. Cati Coe (2008) has thus argued that much of the research on female migration has been influenced by the sociocultural context within which it has been carried out, which is primarily migration from the Philippines or Central America to Western destinations. These areas maintain a strong ideology of the nuclear family, a residential unit of husband, wife and their joint children, where the wife's primary role is caring for the children and the home. Other parts of the world, such as West Africa and the Caribbean, she states, do not share this ideology but are known for their 'flexible family arrangements that may or may not have developed in relationship to patterns of travel or migration' extending back in history (Coe 2008, 226). In Ghana, where Coe has carried out research, such arrangements include extensive practices of child fosterage among relatives or with better-off non-kin (Coe 2008). She found that, only recently, as a result of Pentecostal missionary activity, has the notion of the nuclear family become an ideal in Ghana, primarily among young people. This, in turn, seems to have led to more critical views of long-distance parenting amongst children left behind.

In the Caribbean, a dual family system that is similar to that in Ghana, which involves wide-ranging, fairly open kin relations as well as the more exclusive nuclear family, can be found. Here the ideal of the nuclear family is more deeply entrenched due to this area's long history of colonisation and Christian missionising, which has resulted in this family form becoming a societal ideal associated with upper or middle-class status in Caribbean societies (Wilson 1973; Smith 1996). In the lower classes, however, extensive networks of kin relations, tied to flexible gender roles and strong traditions of physical mobility, prevail (see e.g., Olwig 1985, 1993, 2007). Studies from Ghana as well as the Caribbean thus show that, while the 'ideal of biological mothers raising their own children is widely held' (Hondagneu-Sotelo and Avila 1997, 548), it is by no means universal. It is therefore important to be attuned to different ways of constructing family and kinship historically, socially and culturally and how this may be linked to notions of care and migration.

This chapter analyses how relations of care are practiced and given meaning within the context of Caribbean migration and how these relations are shaped by, and shape, notions of family, kinship and motherhood. The framework of circulation of care (Part A, this volume) offers a productive way to examine how these relationships evolve through time as various parties interact via the exchange of care. While most of the literature on care migration has examined how care workers experience leaving their families in order to work abroad, here I will explore the relationship between migration, care and kinship from the perspective of the Caribbean sending societies rather than that of Caribbean migrants abroad. I will focus on the former British West Indian island of Nevis, with particular emphasis on the 1980s. This was a time when Nevis—like most British Caribbean societies—had experienced, since the 1950s, massive outmigration involving women as well as men.

## CARE—NOTIONS AND PRACTICES OF FAMILY RELATIONS

In the Caribbean lower classes, those forms of relatedness that we may term the family are defined by what Hymie Rubenstein (1987, 233) refers to as a 'folk model' that 'merely states that *family ought to live loving* and that this should be expressed by help in time of need: the lending of money when a person is *broken*; the giving of food when a person is hungry; and moral or emotional support in crisis situations'. This rather loosely defined notion of the family, Rubenstein (1987, 233–234) adds, results in 'an elastic, open-ended kindred system permitting adjustment to changing circumstances' and characterised by 'replaceability, personalism, and permissiveness in affiliation' (see also Bauer and Thompson 2006, 14; Barrow 2010). Within anthropology, there has been increasing interest in the ways in which notions of relatedness are established through 'statements and practices' revolving around, for example, 'feeding, living together, procreation, emotion—elements which are themselves not necessarily bounded entities but may overflow or contain parts of each other or take new forms' (Carsten 2000, 3, 34). This means that being a mother, for example, may take varying forms depending on the situation of particular individuals, just as the position of 'mother' may be assumed by varying persons depending on who undertakes the associated responsibilities. In this construction of family and kinship, I suggest, the circulation of care between individuals plays a key role.

In her book *Globalizing Care Economies and Migrant Workers*, Nicola Yeates (2009, 5) suggests that the notion of care should be broadly defined so that it 'covers a range of activities to promote and maintain the personal health and welfare of people,' including 'cooking, cleaning, shopping and general maintenance work' as well as 'income-generating activities necessary for provisioning'. Among Caribbean people, I will show, family relations are closely associated with the giving and receiving of care but not in the sense that a particular genealogical position in a family determines what kind of care is owed to, or expected by, specific relatives. Rather, the nature of family relationships emerges through the exchange of care. Furthermore, I will argue that in the Caribbean lower class, where the material basis of life is limited, this circulation of care is often associated with considerable physical mobility through the life course. It begins with children moving to other homes where they help with various chores in exchange for their upkeep and continues with young women migrating to provide the material basis for the care of children and the elderly in the family home left behind, and family reunification of dependent relatives in the migration destination of resourceful close relatives or return migration to care for elderly or ill relatives. From the perspective of people from the lower strata of Caribbean society, migration and care are therefore intimately linked and should be interpreted as a way of doing family relations in a mobile world of unequal social and economic opportunities.

## CHILDHOOD

The notion of care is strongly associated with the responsibility to help children who are not able to manage on their own and are therefore dependent on others. Children need to be *raised* from their position of dependency to one of self-sufficient adulthood, and this entails a long process of care. Such care has been seen as fundamental to the exchange relations that are foundational to human society. Thus, Marshall Sahlins (1972) has proposed that the mother's unconditional care for her infant is the archetypical image of 'generalised exchange', the giving of something with no expectations of any returns—at least not in the immediate future (see also Part A, this volume). According to Shellee Colen (1989a, 84), for Caribbean women, 'regardless of class, childbearing and child rearing are major sources of respect—a crucial component of West Indian social relations'. If child care is given with no consideration of immediate financial reward, it is thus expected to confer a reputation for being a good mother. Indeed, a precondition for being respected as a mother is caring properly for the child.

Many children, however, are not reared primarily by their biological mother. Children born to single mothers usually live in the maternal grandmother's household. This grandmother, or another female relative in the home, often assumes primary responsibility for looking after the child, while the biological mother works to support the child, especially if little support is forthcoming from the biological father of the child, as is often the case. As a result of this arrangement, the child may come to regard the grandmother as the 'mother'. Such a mother–child-like relationship between an everyday caregiver and a child may also develop when the biological mother has migrated for employment and another person is providing the daily care for the child.

Mother–child relations are not just shaped by the physical presence or absence of the biological mother in the natal home. It is common throughout the Caribbean, as in Ghana, for children to live for periods of time in another home.[1] Such temporary or long-term fostering of children takes place for a complexity of reasons. Frequently mentioned reasons are the biological mother's difficulty providing for the child, especially if she has many children and receives little support from the father(s) of the children, and the desire to offer a child the social and economic opportunities to be had in a more well-to-do home or an urban area with better educational facilities. Children, however, are not only viewed as a drain on a home's resources; they are also regarded as an important source of help (see e.g., Rubenstein 1987, 246–247; Olwig 2012a). From a young age, girls are usually required to help with cleaning, cooking, washing and child minding in the home, whereas boys are expected to clean the yard, look after animals and fetch water. Furthermore, both boys and girls are supposed to run errands, such as buying something at a nearby shop or bringing a meal or provisions from the kitchen garden to family or friends in the community. Children therefore contribute extensively to the broad range of care activities taking place within the home and exchanged between different homes. For this reason, it has also been common for children to grow up in the home of childless relatives or friends as well as the elderly who might be in special need of help.

When a child is placed in another person's custody/care, this person assumes the rights and obligations inhering in the parent–child relationship, as long as the child stays with the foster parent. If foster parents rear children for an extended period of time and treat these children in a parent-like manner, a kin-like tie will often develop, and the foster child may become regarded as a child of the foster parent. Child fostering may not entail a formal agreement between two homes, however, but rather be the outcome of various informal practical solutions to everyday challenges. This is especially the case when it takes place between homes already linked by close kinship. An example from my ethnographic research on the Leeward Island of Nevis illustrates this. It concerns the childcare relations between Mama Smith,[2] as she was fondly called by the villagers, and her daughter Mary, who together had raised eight children and one grandchild. Mary, who lost her husband when the children were still young, was living down the road from Mama Smith, but as Mama Smith explained, the children grew up between the two houses because 'the grandmother helps the daughter rear them when they get along well':

> I looked after all of them, because when Mary was going anywhere, she left them with me. Otherwise, Glenda and Sam [two of the grandchildren] lived here with me.

[How did that come about?]

Well, you see, only me myself was living here, so they stayed with me, to keep me company.

[You also said something about rearing Susie [a great granddaughter left behind at one year of age when the mother joined her husband in England]]

Well, her mother did not leave her with me; she left her with the grandmother [Mary]. But Mary and Esther and Tania [two of Mary's daughters] got sick at the same time, so Mary sent to call me because the same Susie, she was small. And when I went, they all had the measles. So I brought Susie up here that she shouldn't get the measles from them. And then she stayed here with me from then, she didn't come back. Mary never came for her to say send her back. So she was here, until old; went to school and everything.[3]

When Susie's mother attempted to send for Susie, after she was settled in England, Susie refused to go, saying that she preferred to stay with her grandmother on Nevis.

Whereas local informal child fostering arrangements among relatives and friends would not be perceived as migration, fostering outside the local community clearly can be conceptualised as care-related migration—care in the double sense that the children are expected to be looked after, provided with the material means of existence and given the opportunity to go to school in exchange for providing the domestic services (cleaning, minding of small children and running of errands) customarily performed by children for adults. In some cases, however, children will be regarded, and treated, by the receiving family as a servant rather than a child. Such asymmetrical relations seem to develop most often if the receiving family has experienced some social and economic mobility and therefore is eager to demarcate its superior social status. Thus, a discrepancy can exist between the sending and the receiving families' views of the agreement. The sending family may be under the impression that the child will merely help in the home, as all children are expected to do, and continue to attend school, whereas the receiving family may regard the child as a source of domestic labour, leaving little or no time for school. Esther, born on Nevis but partly reared by distant relatives on the neighbouring island of St. Kitts, spoke with great bitterness about this experience:

I was 14 when . . . my mom sent me to a family. . . . The agreement was that I was to go to school, but I didn't. . . . She was the middle class, high colour, more up. She could mix with bigger folks, the white people, the doctors and those kinds of people. . . . I just did as I was

> told, I washed the clothing, cooked the food, looked after their needs, and that was all. I was not allowed to play with the child [in the family], because it could not play with the servant. My parents were not there to see me treated in that way. I had a really lonely life when I was a kid. That is why I am so shy now.

Child fostering in the home community can also lead to unhappy experiences, but here it is easier for children to return home or receive some protection from relatives nearby if they are treated badly. This is illustrated by Sharon, who grew up with her grandparents. She related that her grandmother was temperamental and beat her frequently. Nobody wanted to interfere, however, because the grandmother fed and clothed her properly and sent her to school and church on a regular basis. Besides, some disciplining (i.e., beating) of children was regarded as necessary, although the grandmother's treatment of the child was viewed as rather excessive. Most felt, however, that Sharon's situation was acceptable, especially in light of the limited support she received from her biological parents, who had migrated to England and the Virgin Islands, respectively. Sharon therefore was stuck in the home. She dealt with her difficult situation by spending as much time as possible in the nearby home of her maternal grandparents, where she enjoyed the company of a large, friendly extended family that included aunts and cousins as well as her maternal grandparents.

While both Sharon and Esther disliked their living arrangement intensely, Sharon learned to live with it by developing close relations with her maternal relatives, whereas Esther, who was away from her family on Nevis, described her life on St. Kitts as 'really lonely' and the cause of her later difficulty engaging in social relations with other people. These examples point to the importance of having a network of relatives and friends who care for one's well-being. Such networks are not just important to foster children but are a vital resource for all children. Thus, children will often seek to establish strong ties to resourceful homes where they can receive the care they may be missing in the home where they are living—whether better and more plentiful food, personal attention, the company of other children or the opportunity to go to school. Interestingly, they often initiate such external relationships by offering to help with cleaning, cooking or looking after animals, the sort of 'care' in the broad sense of the word that makes children a valuable resource in homes.

The exchange of children between homes has been characterised as a key element of Caribbean family and kinship. Colen (1989a, 85) thus describes fostering as 'an extension of the activities, relationships, and values associated with motherhood in West Indian culture. It carries rich meanings and creates webs of interdependent ties in which social and economic resources are shared across time and space through the temporary transferral of parental rights in children'. At a quick glance, this quote may give the impression that child fostering involves a community of loving, sharing and caring among relatives and friends, with the able freely and happily assisting the less able. As I have shown, however, children are not only viewed as dependants who need to be nurtured through the sharing of social and economic resources. They are also regarded as a social and economic resource that can be shared. This attitude exposes children to possible exploitation, but it also enables them to develop their own networks of social relations. Children therefore should not be viewed as merely passive objects of adult engineered exchange between households. Indeed, a vital aspect of growing up in Caribbean society is the development of a network of one's own that can both mitigate the worst effects of poor treatment in the home and offer possible paths towards social and economic opportunities as young people move towards adulthood.

## ADULTHOOD

While the Caribbean has an established tradition of people leaving for areas of greater social and economic opportunity, which dates back to the abolishment of slavery in the mid-1800s, it experienced unprecedented migration to Europe, North America and Caribbean areas of economic development after the Second World War. Nevis is no exception to this. When I began to do research on Caribbean migration in the late 1970s, the state of St. Kitts-Nevis was experiencing some of the heaviest outmigration in the Caribbean (Mills 1985, 1–2). Most of these migrants were young people; indeed, migration and the coming of age had come to be seen as closely linked. As a young Nevisian woman explained, 'When you grow up on Nevis, you wait for your turn to leave the island. It is usually the oldest one who leaves first, and then the next ones according to age'.

Studies have noted that the Caribbean migration tradition is sustained by a prevalent narrative of the successful return—the migrant who does so well abroad that it is possible to return with sufficient economic means to build a large house and live a life in comfort in the community of origin (Byron 2005, 215–216; see also Philpott 1968; Bauer and Thompson 2006). My research suggests that this is a gendered narrative, related mainly by men who aspire to social and economic mobility through employment abroad. A female migrant rather emphasises the importance of being a good daughter, sister, aunt or mother who migrates for employment that will enable her to improve the condition of life of the family left behind (Olwig 2005, 2012b; see also Colen 1989b, 172; 1989a, 84). This urge to help the family is further fuelled by the female migrant's awareness that the family helped her migrate. Venetta, who left Nevis for England during the 1950s, explained:

> I came to England because my parents suggested it. I had no work, and my parents said that they didn't want their children to work as "hard in the blazing sun" as they had done. . . . I was the first one to leave in

> the family, and my family got the £65 together for my passage. They sold some sheep, borrowed from an uncle, and friends and family gave a little. My auntie in America sent me clothes. I didn't have a clue what to expect in England, I only hoped to get work to help my parents. All I could think about was to help my parents who worked so 'hard in the blazing sun'.

Thus, she migrated as the caring daughter (cf. Yeates 2009, 5), endeavouring to earn an income that would generate the funds necessary to improve the welfare of the family left behind.

Women who leave children with family or friends when they migrate feel an even stronger obligation to help the family. In fact, when a family helps a young mother to migrate, by both giving passage money and providing care for children left behind, it does so with the clear understanding that she will send support to the family. Such migration is not viewed as a failure of the mother to care for the child. As Colen (1989a, 85) notes in her study of Caribbean domestic workers in New York, 'West Indian women migrate to New York to provide for their families as a normative aspect of motherhood' (see also Philpott 1973, 120).[4] A conscientious mother does not stay behind with her children struggling to obtain the most basic means of life. She migrates in order to ensure and improve the material and social welfare of the children as well as the relatives who are providing the everyday physical care for them. The migration of mothers therefore usually leads to the development of what Basch et al. (1994, 83–84) have termed 'transnational networks' of family relations extending between the place of origin and migration destinations with children as the basic 'building block'. These networks involve 'gifts of money and goods, the minding of migrants' children and the care of their property' as 'the symbolic and material enactments of transnational family relationships'.

It was quite apparent from fieldwork conducted on Nevis during the 1980s that local family life was deeply embedded in wide-ranging networks of relations extending to Britain, North America and various Caribbean destinations. Most young adults were working abroad, and many of the local households consisted of elderly grandparent(s) and young grandchildren, often with one person from the adult generation present to help run the home, usually a younger daughter. Arlene's home can illustrate how this arrangement may develop through time.

The home consisted of Arlene, her mother, three of Arlene's children and two children of Arlene's sister, who was working in Puerto Rico. Another sister was living on St. Thomas with her husband and children. Arlene had also lived on St. Thomas but decided to move back to Nevis, where she had three children with a man who was living close by in the village. She opted to stay in her mother's home, however, to avoid having 'too many children', as she explained. When she returned to Nevis, she left a young son, born on St. Thomas, with his father because he was capable of supporting him, whereas she would have experienced difficulty rearing her son without the father's support, which would be uncertain given the distance. She explained that she felt sure her son was treated well because her sister on St. Thomas was keeping an eye on him.

Arlene's sister on St. Thomas left her two children with her mother, when she first migrated, but she sent for them as soon as she had established a new home abroad with her husband. She sent two boxes—one with food and one with clothing—to her mother's home on Nevis whenever a boat was going from St. Thomas to Nevis. 'She is really sending to her mother', Arlene explained, 'because she took care of her children when my sister was on St. Thomas without them, and now she is showing her gratitude to her mother by sending things to her, thanking her'. The sister in Puerto Rico had not managed to send for the two children she left behind because she was an undocumented immigrant. This also meant that she had not been able to visit her family on Nevis, including her children ages sixteen and nineteen, for the ten years she had been away because she would not be able to return if she left Puerto Rico. She sent generous support, however, in the form of regular remittances and three to four boxes every year. Arlene proudly added that when her sisters first began to send these boxes, people were asking whether they were going to open a shop because they received so much.

As Arlene's account demonstrates, family relations are characterised by pragmatic considerations concerning how to ensure the support of dependants, such as Arlene's son, who grew up with his father on St. Thomas, and the children of the absent sisters, who were left with the grandmother so that the sisters could seek work abroad. Arlene's return to her mother's house can also be seen as a practical arrangement because it meant she could help her mother care for the grandchildren left behind. At the same time, Arlene and her children were assured a good material standard of living because the absent sisters would be supporting the mother's home. Indeed, the presence of the migrant sisters' children in the mother's home was not regarded as a burden but as insurance of receiving regular remittances and material goods. As Arlene said of her sister in Puerto Rico, she 'is so good at sending because she has the two boys with her mother that she supports'. Caregivers on Nevis were quite aware that the children played a key role in this system of support, and it was therefore common to send a photograph of the children to parents abroad at every birthday and to make sure the children wrote thank you notes when they had received gifts from them.

The exchange relations between family members were not only of material importance, they also had moral significance because they were evidence of a strong and well-functioning family. Thus, while Arlene was pleased that the home received enough supplies from abroad to ensure the material welfare of the family, she also noted with great pride that the neighbours had remarked on her sisters' generosity. Most families who received abundant remittances from abroad made improvements on the house—building an addition to accommodate the many children, constructing an indoor bathroom, purchasing modern appliances like a refrigerator, stove and washing machine and acquiring a television. Such a well-maintained, modern house was clear testimony to caring and loyal relatives abroad. The strength of dispersed family ties was also displayed when the schools began after the summer break and the children were able to show up in new uniforms, well equipped with all the necessary school supplies. It was also demonstrated on Sundays, when migrant children and other relatives living in the home attended church and Sunday school wearing the latest fashions from abroad (see Olwig 1993).

Although it is apparent that family networks extending to far-away migration destinations had become an integral part of life on Nevis, the official institutions on the island, such as the schools, the churches and the welfare office, were rather critical of the effects of migration on the local society. When I interviewed teachers and welfare officials, they complained that some absent mothers had rather flimsy childcare arrangements, which meant that the children were basically left to fend for themselves. Also, some parents sent little or no support to the family caring for their children. If no local solution could be found to the problem, the welfare office contacted the immigration authorities in the country of the mother's migration destination. In this way, it succeeded in having several mothers deported from the nearby Dutch island of St. Martin, but it had less success in the U.S. Virgin Islands because many of the negligent migrants were undocumented and therefore beyond the reach of local authorities. Both teachers and welfare officers acknowledged, however, that migration provided the only way out for many Nevisians. As the head of the welfare office explained:

> When children are of age, they must leave the house. They cannot just stick around. If they are not qualified for civil service or teaching, migration is the only way to get a good steady job. The parents don't want them around either, because this is expensive . . . [and] the children themselves also feel that they must earn, they can't depend on their parents.

They therefore were not against migration, as such, but rather irresponsible migrants (primarily mothers) who did not make adequate care arrangements for their children and who failed to send support to family left behind.

It was a different matter with the churches, especially those of a fundamentalist Christian persuasion. For them, a proper childhood belonged within the nuclear family, where the mother shows her love for her children by personally caring for them. The 'danger' of leaving children behind was vividly illustrated by the preacher in the local village church I attended during fieldwork. Thus, in her sermon, she elucidated the notion of an 'outcast', used in a Biblical parable to characterise a harlot, by relating a story about a local girl who was left by her migrant mother in the care of her grandparents. The grandparents were so poor, the preacher explained, that the girl had to steal in order to get something to eat. She therefore became an 'outcast' and, like the harlot, ended up being accused of things she had not done. If the church condemned irresponsible mothers who left their children in the care of others, it celebrated the mothers who stayed on the island tending their own children. This was particularly apparent at a special service held on Mother's Day, when mothers were invited to sit in the front of the church, and gifts were given to the oldest and the youngest mother, to the mother with the most children attending church and to the largest extended family in attendance that included husband, wife and children. Also, children whose mother was present were asked to give her a kiss.

This service, however, generated a heated discussion among the villagers. One woman, who had no children of her own but had cared for the children of her emigrant siblings, said that she always wanted to get up when mothers were acknowledged because she had raised so many children. Another woman, a single mother who lived with her children in a large extended family, noted dryly when the largest extended family in church (that included a husband) received its reward, 'It is too bad my husband doesn't happen to be present'. Several also said that they felt sorry for the children of migrant mothers who were reminded of their mother's absence when they had nobody to kiss in the church. These women were faithful members of the church and subscribed in principle to the ideal of the nuclear family of father, mother and children living in their own home. Yet for them, and for most of the women in the congregation, this ideal was rather abstract and had little to do with the far-ranging and flexible networks of relations that sustained them and were central to their life on the island.

## OLD AGE

In their study of Jamaican migration, Bauer and Thompson state (2006, 205), 'What help was given to the old depended—as with Jamaican kin relations more generally—very much on whether any feeling of reciprocal obligation had developed'. The exchange of care through time, I suggest, plays a central role in the development of a sense of responsibility towards the elderly. As noted, grandmothers are generally mentioned as the most common care providers for migrants' children, a role that is often a continuation, and further elaboration, of the key part they play in the raising of the children of daughters before the daughters migrate. Caribbean grandmothers, however, also care for grandchildren who are born abroad but sent back to be reared in the migrant parents' society of origin. This 'return' migration takes place to a great extent, as Philpott states (1973,

138), because children are a liability abroad where they make it difficult for mothers to engage in wage employment, whereas they can be viewed as an asset in the place of origin where they provide company for the elderly and help with domestic work. When a daughter stays behind to help manage the home and care for the migrants' children, her contribution to the home should ideally be acknowledged by the migrant siblings, for example, by letting her 'inherit a choicer or larger piece of land and/or, possibly more important, the house' (Philpott 1973, 127). Care for the elderly, therefore, leads to a certain continuity in the home base in the community of origin, at least as long as the elderly stay behind. This continuity is essentially grounded in the intergenerational circulation of caregiving over time that shapes patterns of mobility and immobility. Mama Smith's life trajectory illustrates this.

Mama Smith, who was in her 80s when I interviewed her in 1981, related that she was only two years old when her mother died and that she therefore grew up in her grandparents' home. Her grandmother died when she was fifteen, her grandfather died two years later, and she then contemplated emigrating:

> I was to go to Cuba, but my aunt told me that I must not go. And it was good I didn't go, because after her husband died, I had her and the [aunt's] children to look after. . . . If I went along she would have had nobody to look for her, you see? When she took sick I carried her to the hospital. . . . She died there and I buried her.

I later asked Mama Smith whether she really was glad that she didn't go anywhere, when everybody else was leaving the island. It seemed to me that one of the aunt's eight children could have cared for the aunt, but Mama Smith explained:

> I am glad, because after my mother died, she helped my grandparents rear me because I was young [when I lost my mother], so then I could look after her.

Mama Smith thus felt that she had just as strong an obligation to help her aunt as had the aunt's children because the aunt had helped care for her as a child. Besides, she added, the aunt's children who had migrated to St. Kitts did their share of helping:

> They did help their mother. But I am telling you that they went to St. Kitts to work, and I being up here. . . . They helped because they sent money to the mother. I, being here, looked after her.

Mama Smith later cared not only for her own two children, she also, as noted, helped rear her eight grandchildren and a great grandchild. When the grandchildren began to work abroad, they reciprocated by sending regular remittances and boxes of food and clothing to their grandmother. The two grandchildren, who had lived with Mama Smith for several years, also sent money to build an addition to her small house. As the grandchildren established their own families in the U.S. Virgin Islands, Mama Smith's daughter began to spend much of her time in the Virgin Islands in order to help with child minding. When Susie, the great granddaughter who had been living in Mama Smith's house, left the home to marry a Nevisian in the U.S. Virgin Islands, the family pleaded with Mama Smith to join them there, but she refused, saying that she wanted to live and die on Nevis. The family then arranged for a woman in the village to help her on a regular basis. Mama Smith emphasised that she was not hired to work for her: 'Whatever little I have got I give her. So she does not ask for this price or that. Whatever I give her, she takes'. This was, she explained, because the helper and Mama Smith were 'family', the helper's grandfather and Mama Smith's grandmother being 'two sisters' children'. The implication was that because of this family tie, the helper was not motivated by a desire to make money but by the wish to help care for an elderly relative (cf. Leinaweaver 2008, 90–97). Although the family basically had left Mama Smith all alone on Nevis, it had managed to create a network of supportive family relations so that she was happy about her situation:

> Look, I reared them, and now they keep me up, because they send me food, they send me clothes, they send me money. I reaped my reward, you understand? You sow good seed, you reap good fruit.

Not all the elderly left behind on Nevis benefited from such responsible care arrangements. In the village where I conducted fieldwork, I encountered elderly individuals who were more or less left to fend for themselves and had to manage with the few dollars they received from the welfare office and the limited help they received from neighbours. Such neglect of parents was generally condemned, and if it became known among fellow Nevisians in the migration destination that a particular person was ignoring a parent, especially a mother, strong pressure was put on this person to make amends. Philpott (1973) gives an example of such pressure in his study of Caribbean migrants in London. It concerns a man who failed to send remittances to his mother because he was making payments on a van. When a fellow islander heard about this, he said, 'Man, you na pass through you van. You pass through your mother' (Philpott 1973, 178).[5] Because of the flexible family relations, however, there might at times be disagreement with regard to who were owed remittances from migrants. The welfare officer, for example, recalled a case where they had written to the migrant son of a destitute elderly woman on Nevis, asking him to send economic aid to his mother. He replied that he had supported his mother, but that she had died several years back—apparently referring to the woman who had reared him rather than his biological mother, who had been too poor to do so.

## CARE WORK MIGRATION VIEWED THROUGH A CARIBBEAN INTERPRETIVE FRAMEWORK

I have shown in this discussion how care relations have constituted a central nerve in Caribbean family relations, presenting individuals with obligations as well as expectations concerning the giving and receiving of social and economic support. Such intergenerational circuits of care have been extended in space as various opportunities have been explored in new places, resulting in dispersed networks of interpersonal ties. When viewed from the perspective of such family networks and through the framework of care circulation, the migration of single mothers for care work abroad is not viewed as an aberration or a challenge to the family, as long as they arrange adequate everyday care for their children and other dependants left behind, send generous support and remain in regular contact through letters, phone calls and/or visits (cf. Barrow 2010). Indeed, migration and being a responsible family member are regarded as closely linked because it is often through migration that individuals are able to fulfil the obligations that they have towards the network of people they identify as their family. This is clearly brought out in the narrative of the good relative who leaves to help the family that is, as I have argued elsewhere, dominant amongst Caribbean migrant women (Olwig 2012b; see also Constable 1999). If Caribbean women are willing to participate as migrants in a global care chain of unequal social and economic relations, this is, to a great extent, because this chain of relations is integrally linked to an intergenerational Caribbean network of care that gives meaning and purpose to such engagement.

The social significance of women's migration as a means to help the family left behind does not mean that such migration is without problems. At an emotional level, according to Bauer and Thompson (2006, 91), 'for migrants of all ages, the realignment of close family relationships, both partings and reunions, continues to be a primary pain—on both sides'. They add, however, that the 'strongest feelings of loss and loneliness' were remembered by those who joined their parents abroad as teenagers, while 'childhood experiences of complex large households . . . were strikingly positive' (Bauer and Thompson 2006, 91, 192). My research generally corroborates their findings. While children had varying experiences being left with grandparents and joining parents, most had positive recollections of living in large extended families. Indeed, one person even claimed that it made no difference to him whether his biological mother or another adult reared him. This is a reminder not to project emotions associated with the Western nuclear family on migrants and relatives left behind, who may subscribe to different notions of the family (cf. Coe 2008; see also Chapter 7, this volume). The difficulties associated with care-related migration have thus not so much revolved around the breakup of the mother–child tie but rather concerned malfunctioning family relations grounded in divergences between local expectations and global realisations of family obligations. Such problems may be particularly apparent during periods of massive out-migration, such as Nevis experienced from the 1950s to the 1980s. This analysis, therefore, points to the need to develop a broader approach to familyhood, care and migration that does not just focus on the moralistic predicament of biological mothers who leave their own children to care for the children of strangers. Rather, it is necessary to explore the complex interrelationship between the exchange and circulation of care and the development of notions of relatedness and the ways in which this interrelationship is played out and attributed with meaning in societies where mobile livelihoods have become an important way of life.

## NOTES

1. For a more in-depth discussion of child fostering and its relation to migration, see Olwig 2012a.
2. All the names are pseudonyms.
3. I have modified Mama Smith's Nevisian dialect to conform generally to standard written English.
4. Apparently the U.S. immigration authorities did not realise this. A young woman on Nevis thus told me that her application for a U.S. tourist visa had been rejected because she did not own land or have any children on Nevis. The American authorities, therefore, did not think that she had sufficiently strong ties to Nevis to guarantee that she would return to the island. But as the Nevisian woman explained, women with children would be the most likely to overstay their tourist visa to find wage employment in the United States.
5. In standard English, 'Man, you weren't born by a van. You were born by your mother'.

# 7 Ghanaian Children in Transnational Families

## Understanding the Experiences of Left-Behind Children through Local Parenting Norms

*Miranda Poeze and Valentina Mazzucato*

The migration of parents to more-developed countries is often motivated by the prospect of securing a better future for their children at home. However, the physical distance between a parent and child necessitates a reordering of care arrangements and raises questions concerning the emotional impact of parental migration for left-behind children (D'Emilio et al. 2007; Mazzucato and Schans 2011; Whitehead and Hashim 2005). In particular, in Western societies, it is believed that intimacy between parents and their children can only be created through physical proximity and that physical separation interrupts healthy childhood development. However, in many societies, caregiving and parenting norms allow for a more flexible and inclusive notion of parenthood, with caring for a child being not only the responsibility of the biological parents but also that of the extended family network (see also Chapter 6, this volume). In such societies, physical separation between a parent and child is socially accepted and, at times, even favoured. We argue that the presence of such normative principles of parenting results from the circulation of care (Part A, this volume) for children amongst a wider network of actors than only the biological parents and that such principles, together with how care is enacted, will impact the way children perceive their transnational care arrangements.

Few studies have examined the impact of the cultural contextualisation of parenting on left-behind children's perceptions of living in transnational families (Mazzucato 2013). Furthermore, the African continent has remained underexplored in the vast literature on transnational families (Grillo and Mazzucato 2008; but see Åkesson et al. 2012; Bledsoe and Sow 2008; Kastner 2010) and rarely is the focus on the perspectives of children (Coe 2008). We seek to address these gaps through a study of fifty-four Ghanaian children's oral accounts of their experiences in a transnational child-raising arrangement. As we analyse these accounts, we interpret the experiences of left-behind children in relation to local parenting norms.

## NUCLEAR FAMILY IDEAL AND PHYSICAL SEPARATION

Previous qualitative studies amongst transnational families from Southeast Asian and Latin American sending contexts have emphasised that left-behind children suffer emotionally when they are separated from their parents (see Dreby 2007; Parreñas 2005a). Parreñas (2005a, 120) argues that children left in the home country by their migrant parents express 'a lack of intimacy, feelings of abandonment, and a commodification of mother-child bonds'. Although these negative feelings were alleviated by the support of family members and children taking into account that the parents' absence was for the welfare of the family, the emotional suffering was considered to be profound.

Negative outcomes on left-behind children have mainly been explained by gender role expectations that are particular to family norms that hold the nuclear family and 'intensive mothering' as prerequisites for a stable childhood development (Bernardes 1999; Erel 2002). The biological parent is expected to perform all caregiving tasks, necessitating geographical proximity between the parent and child (Bowie 2004). When a parent moves abroad, the child is negatively affected because his or her situation departs from the proximity prescribed by the nuclear family ideal. In particular, when a mother moves abroad, children suffer from the physical separation. Regular phone calls and the sending of remittances cannot fill the geographical gap and the distance poses challenges for the mother to fulfil her role as the primary caregiver (Hondagneu-Sotelo and Avila 1997; Parreñas 2005a). Although it is acknowledged that feelings of loss can be alleviated when other female members of the family serve as the main caregiver (Åkesson et al. 2012; Parreñas 2005a; Smith et al. 2004; Suárez-Orozco et al. 2002), the caregiver's role is seen as limited given that nurturing tasks are exclusively reserved for the biological mother. Thus, the suffering of children in transnational families in which the mother has migrated abroad is explained by the principles of the nuclear family ideal (i.e., love and care necessitate proximity with the child) that cannot be fulfilled in transnational family structures.

Although studies focusing on the effects of father migration on children are scarce (but see Chapter 9, this volume), the few such studies reveal elevated cases of teen pregnancies, alcohol and drug abuse, robbery and emotional distress as a result of communication problems and a lack of emotional intimacy between the children and their fathers (D'Aubeterre 2000; Parreñas 2008). Here, it is also argued that non-proximate forms of care (e.g., remittances, phone calls and return visits) cannot foster the development of an intimate relationship between a father and child, ultimately resulting in a lack of care provision for the child. One study found less negative effects of parental migration on children living in Mexico, but this was compared with families in which the father was away due to divorce (Nobles 2011).

## SOCIAL ACCEPTANCE OF PARENT–CHILD SEPARATIONS

The importance of parental physical proximity in the upbringing of a child, also called biocentrism, has been a dominant concept in the discourse on kinship and parenting in Euro-American societies and has influenced researchers' approaches when dealing with these issues. The idea that all children need face-to-face contact with their biological parents for intergenerational intimacy to emerge and that nurturing tasks can only be successfully carried out by biological parents undermines the fact that familial relationships and related emotions are cultural constructions and thus does not do justice to the culture-specific aspects of caregiving and parenting (Bowie 2004; Schneider 1984). Nonetheless, such a static and exclusive definition of parenting has dominated many studies on transnational families and the impact of parental migration on left-behind children.

Parental ideologies and definitions depend on the local context (Cole and Cole 2001) and influence the way that children feel about their caregivers and the care that they receive. In contrast to Euro-American societies, observations made in the Caribbean, Latin America and West Africa show that it is socially accepted for families to separate and for children to circulate between family and non-family members (Goody 1982; Isiugo-Abanihe 1985; Leinaweaver 2007; Pilon 2003). In these countries, child fostering is a common practice, with children transferred between their natal homes and the households of others for at least part of their childhood and for a variety of reasons. Here, childcare is not centred on the core household but is considered a collective endeavour in which other kin and non-kin actively participate (Alber 2003; Goody 1982).

Ghana is one of the countries in which social parenthood and child fostering are important childcare practices (Goody 1982; Hashim 2005). Although modern-day realities have led to changes in the Ghanaian family structure with a decline in kin support in child raising, particularly in urban regions (Oppong 2006), according to the 2008 Ghana Demographic and Health Survey, still 18.6 percent of all children under the age of eighteen are fostered (Ghana Statistical Service 2008).

The norm of social parenthood and the practice of child fostering bring into question the ideal that all parenting tasks are the sole responsibility of the biological parent and the assumption that the child and parent always need to be in close proximity of each other. However, this is not to say that parent–child separations are always unproblematic. The first studies conducted on child fostering in West Africa in the 1970s and 1980s focused on the importance of child fostering in terms of its social and economic functions (Goody 1982) but not in terms of its impact on children. In a more recent study based in East Cameroon, Notermans (2008) observed that foster children were more critical about child fostering than their parents, most notably as a result of tensions arising in the everyday lives of the children.

While child fostering creates a context of 'normality' with regard to being raised by a non-biological parent and living geographically separated from the birth parent, the transnational context presents different conditions under which parent–child relationships develop at a distance. International migration creates differential access to material and financial resources, it brings with it different expectations of the roles of parents and caregivers on the upbringing of the child (Mazzucato 2011) and modern communication technology renders possible parental involvement in upbringing from afar (Madianou and Miller 2011), all of which combine to impact children's experiences. Conditions abroad as well as pre-migration, such as the ability of the parent abroad to send remittances, the quality of the relationship between the migrant parent and the child's caregiver, the quality of the relationship between the parent and child before the departure of the migrant and the socioeconomic positions of the migrant and the caregiver also affect children's experiences of parental migration. Figure 7.1 depicts the way in which pre-migration and situational factors related to the conditions of migration interact with cultural parenting norms to influence children's emotional experiences. In this chapter, we focus on the frequently neglected aspect of parenting norms in affecting the emotional experiences of left-behind children.

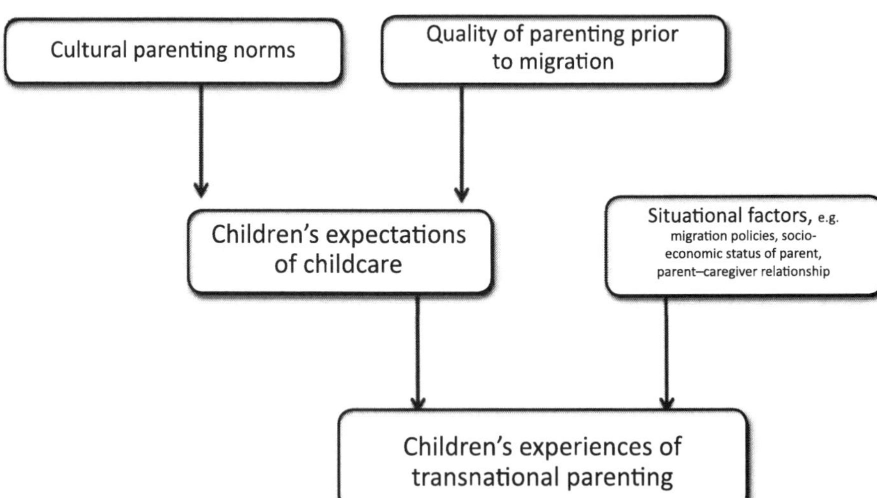


*Figure 7.1* Influential factors on children's experiences of transnational parenting.

## RESEARCH METHODS

In-depth interviews were conducted over a three-month period in 2010 with fifty-four Ghanaian children and adolescents aged twelve to twenty-two, who had either one or both parents living in a Western country at the time of the interview. The children were selected from a larger survey of Ghanaian school children (N = 2,670) carried out in four different localities in mid-2010 as part of the 'Transnational Child Raising Arrangements between Ghana and the Netherlands' (TCRA) research project.[1] Children were selected for in-depth interviews from Accra (n = 25) and Kumasi (n = 29), both of which are urban regions known for their high ratio of migration to the West, as indicated by remittances received from abroad (Mazzucato et al. 2005). The main criteria for selecting the children were based on TCRA type, that is, having a mother abroad (n = 17), a father abroad (n = 25) or both parents abroad (n = 12). By studying these three family configurations, we took the diversity in the structure of transnational families into account. We selected both boys (n = 21) and girls (n = 33) who attended either junior high schools (JHS) (n = 24) or secondary high schools (SHS) (n = 32). We strove to incorporate diversity in the number of caregiver changes experienced by the children and the children's emotional well-being as measured by the Strength and Difficulties Questionnaire (Goodman et al. 1998).

A majority of parents of the selected children were residing in the United States and the United Kingdom. Other parents resided in Germany, the Netherlands and Italy. Table 7.1 shows that for the majority of cases, parental migration took place when the child was between the ages of six and thirteen. Fathers were more likely than mothers to leave the children before the age of six. Children who had at least a father abroad were younger and separated from their parent for a longer period of time compared with children who had at least a mother abroad. In our sample, the majority of caregivers were female and kin (see Table 7.2).

The interviews were conducted at schools during breaks or after school hours. We sought permission from the schools to interview the children. The school setting was perceived as a place where children would feel safe and free to voice their opinions without the influence of caregivers or other adults. Each interview lasted between forty-five minutes to one and a half hours and was recorded with the child's permission. The interviews were subsequently transcribed and analysed with the aid of the qualitative data software Atlas.ti.

Although some child-centred studies call for 'child-friendly methods', such as drawing, we found, in line with Notermans (2008), that in-depth interviews in a formal interview setting were most effective in terms of allowing children to express themselves. In contexts such as Ghana, where it is common for children and adults to occupy different spheres in their daily lives, the formal interview setting aligned most closely with children's ideas

*Table 7.1* Number of Children by TCRA Type, Age at Separation and Length of Separation

| *TCRA Type* | *Children's Age at Separation* | *Years of Separation* 0–5 | 6–10 | >10 | *Total* |
|---|---|---|---|---|---|
| Father abroad | 0–5 | 0 | 1 | 7 | *8* |
| | 6–13 | 3 | 12 | 1 | *16* |
| | >13 | 1 | 0 | 0 | *1* |
| Mother abroad | 0–5 | 0 | 0 | 3 | *3* |
| | 6–13 | 7 | 4 | 0 | *11* |
| | >13 | 3 | 0 | 0 | *3* |
| Mother and father abroad | 0–5 | 0 | 1 | 8 | *9* |
| | 6–13 | 1 | 1 | 0 | *2* |
| | >13 | 1 | 0 | 0 | *1* |
| Total | | 16 | 19 | 19 | *54* |

*Note*. The length of separation and age at separation reflect the departure of the first parent who migrated.

*Table 7.2* Caregivers by TCRA Type and Sex

| | *Caregiver* | | | | | |
|---|---|---|---|---|---|---|
| | *Left-Behind Parent* | | *Family Member* | | *Non-Family* | |
| *TCRA Type* | *Mother* | *Father* | *Female* | *Male* | *Female* | *Male* |
| Father abroad | 21 | 0 | 4 | 0 | 0 | 0 |
| Mother abroad | 0 | 6 | 10 | 0 | 1 | 0 |
| Mother and father abroad | 0 | 0 | 9 | 2 | 1 | 0 |
| Total | 21 | 6 | 23 | 2 | 2 | 0 |

about ways to express themselves to adults. Younger children attending JHS showed occasional difficulties in describing and explaining their emotions. When this occurred, we probed further, asked for examples and gave children ample time to think about their answers.

Issues addressed during the interviews related to the quality of their care relationships with the parent(s), caregiver and people in the wider care network before and after the migration of the parent. Questions were asked about the departure of the parent, the arrangements made for care, the type of care received before and after departure, positive and negative experiences in the care relationships and changes and continuities in the children's relationships with their overseas parents and within their care arrangements.

Given the exploratory nature of the study, we interviewed many children from diverse situations to gain a wide array of children's experiences in transnational families. Future work would benefit from more in-depth methods and interviews with children's parents and caregivers to enable a greater understanding of the material conditions of the child's living arrangements and thus deeper insight into situational factors on children's emotional experiences (Figure 7.1). In this study, we do not address situational factors; instead, we focus on the gamut of children's experiences and seek to understand these experiences through the lens of cultural parenting ideologies and the framework of care circulation.

## CHILDREN'S EXPERIENCES OF LIVING IN TRANSNATIONAL FAMILIES

### Feeling Cared About

The gender role expectations that children have for parents who move abroad typically reflect cultural parenting ideologies. These expectations inform the way in which children interpret the behaviour of their migrant parents. Children expect their migrant parents to maintain an active role in their upbringing, but the care that a migrant father and mother provides does not necessarily need to be geographically proximal. Below, we recount how children expressed feeling cared about by their migrant parent and pay particular attention to the differences between the children of migrant mothers versus fathers.

When describing their feelings about a father's departure and their feelings of closeness with him, children first referred to the way in which their father was or was not providing for their material needs. Children felt positively about their father's decision to move abroad especially when they expected an improvement in their material conditions, which could manifest in the form of luxurious gifts, such as laptops and cell phones, but also in the form of money for school fees and the prospect of a family house. In addition, being able to ask for and be given anything the child desired was considered an important advantage of having a father abroad:

*Emmanuel:* When he was here, he wouldn't buy these things but would have said that it is waste. But when he went there [abroad], and when I told him, 'dad, I want this', then he would send it.
*Interviewer:* So everything you ask for, he sends?
*Emmanuel:* Yes, and that makes me happy.

*(Emmanuel, seventeen years old)*

In some cases, a father's increased ability to provide material care was described as an improvement in the relationship:

*Interviewer:* Has the relationship with your father changed in any way since he left?

*Seth:* It is the same . . . and even better.

*Interviewer:* How?

*Seth:* The money he has given me, he has increased it, and the things he has been buying for me here, when they went there [abroad], they have increased these things too.

*(Seth, twenty-two years old)*

Children can feel loved and cared for by the father despite the geographical distance, and migration with the prospect of remittances can even increase these feelings of being loved. However, the association of fatherly love and care to finances also means that feelings of neglect and disappointment may arise when the father does not provide materially for the child or does not do so to the extent that the child expects. Meredith (thirteen years old) complained that the material care from her father living in the United Kingdom was limited to her school fees and believed that he was providing more for her half-siblings, who were living with him. This thought compelled her to ask her father on the phone whether he loved her half-siblings more than her. Francisca saw her relationship with her father as not good in terms of the lack of regular remittances:

*Interviewer:* So now the relationship with your father, since he is gone for eight years, how do you see this relationship?

*Francisca:* It is not good.

*Interviewer:* Why is that?

*Francisca:* Sometimes he has not been sending us money for two or three months.

*(Francisca, fourteen years old)*

A father's absence in a child's life in the form of absent material care was even met with anger, as in the case of Poomah, especially when the relationship with the father had been weak before departure:

> I think one day I was in school when he called me and I asked, 'who is this?', and he told me, 'it's your dad'. Then I asked him, 'what do you want from me'? He was annoyed that I asked him what he wanted from me, and I said, 'yes, you have not been catering for me since I was born from JHS to now SHS, so what do you want from me that you are calling me'? So I just cut the line. *(Poomah, eighteen years old)*

In cases where the migrant father played an active part in the child's life before departure, it was easier for a child to understand his father's lack of material provision. For these children, a lack of material care was unlikely to motivate a severance of the relationship with their father. However, they did mention disappointment and a lack of fatherly love and care.

For Francisca, her father's lack of material provision made her feel reluctant to take care of her father in the future, indicating the reciprocal nature of the parent–child relationship:

> He doesn't take care of us. At first I said that I would not take care of him when I grow up, but my mother said that is not good, I should take care of him. *(Francisca, fourteen years old)*

Children described the quality of care received from their migrant mothers in different terms. Migrant mothers are expected to provide emotional care. From the interviews, it became clear that the physical absence of the mother was not necessarily problematic in terms of providing emotional care and for children to feel loved and cared about. Mothers were able to maintain their emotional caring role from a distance through regular communication:

> I'll say that she was always with me, even though she was not here . . . because she called me frequently. . . . I like her so much because like, if I need anything I tell her, if something is bothering me, I tell her. Because she has been there for me all the time, that's why. *(Kwabena, eighteen years old)*

Consequently, feelings of neglect and abandonment can result when mothers do not provide the emotional care expected by their children during phone calls. For example, Barbara's mother sent remittances on a regular basis through Barbara's aunt and caregiver. However, her mother had not contacted Barbara since she left for Austria five years ago. This situation became a source of complaint for Barbara:

*Barbara:* Sometimes I just forget about her, that I have a mother. The woman I am staying with [mother's sister], she treats me better. She cares about me. So sometimes I easily forget about my mum.
*Interviewer:* So you feel like she doesn't care about you?
*Barbara:* To me no. Mmmmm . . . somehow.
*Interviewer:* Why is that?
*Barbara:* Because since she travelled, she has not called me. She doesn't call me at all, unless I have to call her. She will never call me.

*(Barbara, seventeen years old)*

In addition to providing emotional care, mothers also need to take care of the material conditions of the family, especially when the father is absent due to death or divorce, which is a common situation in Ghana. According to the Ghana Statistical Service (2008), 7 percent of women are divorced or separated and 2.1 percent are widowed. From the interviews, we can see that many fathers do not play an active role in financially providing after divorce. Children perceive the need for single mothers to take on this extra parenting task and consider migration as a way to help them accomplish this. Jackeline, whose parents were divorced and whose father did not contribute financially to the family, provided the following explanation for the migration of her mother:

> She said she was going to work so that she can take care of us, that's why she had to leave and I said, 'ok, if she is going to work she can go' because when she was in Ghana, she had nothing to do, she was just sewing some people's clothes and they paid little for that. That's why she was going, to take care of us. *(Jackeline, twelve years old)*

As a result of such household dynamics, financial care was considered an important component of the children's evaluation of their relationship with their migrant mothers. Nonetheless, the inability of the mother to respond to financial needs of the family did not tend to produce feelings of neglect or abandonment because children typically expect this role to be fulfilled by the father and consider financial care to be a burden on the mother, given the perceived difficulty for women to secure an income.

Although migrant fathers are mainly expected to focus on material care, and migrant mothers are expected to focus more on emotional care, children do value the social and emotional care that they receive from migrant fathers. For example, Sara explained she felt that her father was caring for her when he asked about her school performance:

> I think it is a good thing [that he asks about her educational performance]. Even at a time when he was not talking about it, I started to feel, 'why is my daddy no more thinking about me'? So when he asked me of my studies again, I became very happy, and it makes me feel cared for and loved. *(Sara, seventeen years old)*

Phone calls are important ways to provide social and emotional care across geographical distance (see also Baldassar 2008b; Merla 2010). Children value the opportunity to express their feelings, talk about personal issues, receive advice and be asked about their school performance and the care they receive from the caregiver. When care is not provided during phone conversations, as in the case of Ivana, negative feelings can arise:

> [The conversations are] always about money, money, money . . . I've written to him [father] before . . . and I really, really poured my heart out. But when he called, I don't know whether he didn't want to talk about it because he only asked me about school, academics and stuff. That was all. *(Ivana, eighteen years old)*

In addition to frequent phone calls and remittances, return visits from both the mother and father add to feelings of being cared about. Return visits provide children with an opportunity to spend time with their parents in person and share experiences that cannot be realised over the phone. Such visits were even more important if the child had no visual memory of the parent, as was often the case for children whose migrant fathers had left when the children were very young. For example, Vanessa met her father for the first time when she was thirteen years old on his first return visit. Although Vanessa was only able to spend one week with her father, she described this period to be one of the happiest times in her life and felt closer to him after meeting him physically:

*Interviewer:* How would you describe the closeness? Because in one week, how close can you be?

*Vanessa:* Whenever he went out I went with him. We were always together. We look alike, I am the photocopy of my father. We walk the same, everything. Even when he came, he didn't trust anyone, but he could even leave his own purse with me and go out. I did everything for him when he was here for that one week.

*(Vanessa, sixteen years old)*

Children can also feel disappointed in their parents when they fail to make return visits, as shown by the case of Benjamin:

*Benjamin:* Last time he called me I was angry.

*Interviewer:* Why?

*Benjamin:* Because I feel bad for not seeing my father for about twenty years now, so I don't feel happy, and I tell him every time he calls, and he says he will be coming. The main motive that I was angry was that he lied to me that he will be coming [to Ghana] in December last year and he didn't, so I never return his calls, I haven't called him again.

*(Benjamin, sixteen years old)*

Thus, while children may hold different expectations for migrant mothers and fathers, both parents are expected to maintain an active role in the upbringing of their child. However, the care provided by the migrant father and mother does not necessarily need to be provided in geographical proximity. Through the sending of remittances, regular phone calls and return visits, children can feel that their migrant parents are caring for and about them. The acceptable nature of non-proximate care is grounded in parenting ideologies that allow parenting tasks to be transferred to caregivers other than the biological parents.

## The Transfer of 'Motherly' and 'Fatherly' Tasks

When children talked about their relationship with the caregivers, in cases where this was not the left-behind mother or father, they often described the caregiver as treating them like his or her own children. Comments such as 'she is like a mother to me' and 'she treats me like I'm her own child' were heard regularly during the interviews. In their explanations, children referred to the care that a biological mother would give her child, as shown in Sylvester's descriptions of his stepmother, who took care of him while his father was abroad:

> She was trying to be like our mother, so anything we ask of her, she does, and she does anything for us. The things we need, she normally talks to our father and tells him the things we need so that our father will provide it for us. *(Sylvester, seventeen years old)*

When a caregiver provides motherly care in the absence of the biological mother, children no longer need to experience a lack of parental care as a result of migration and the physical distance between the parent and child. Gottlieb, feeling sad about the departure of his mother five years ago, explained:

> The stepmother I am living with, she treats me like a real son, so now I live very comfortably. I take her as my own mother, so I don't feel like if this guy is having his or her mother around, I don't miss her [biological mother], I know I have a mother who loves me. *(Gottlieb, thirteen years old)*

In these cases, when the child felt that the caregiver was fulfilling the role of a mother, children often referred to the caregiver as 'mother'. Nonetheless, the biological mother has not been replaced by the caregiver; rather, the definition of mothering has been broadened to incorporate other people. This was further illustrated by Gottlieb when he described his relationships with his biological mother and his stepmother:

> I am more close to my mum [in the UK] because she is my mother, but my stepmother, she is . . . she is now my mother. She has taken like the position of my mother in my heart now, but still my mum is the one I really love, really!

Kwabena's comments also show how a caregiver can take over some of the biological mother's caring tasks to help alleviate the effects of her absence:

> When I was with my aunty, she made me feel . . . she was not treating me bad, so that I'll miss her [mother]. She was treating me good, so like, I see everything as normal because most of the time, my aunty was there for me. *(Kwabena, eighteen years old)*

Thus, although the relationship with the biological mother is still perceived as unique, caregiving is not exclusively reserved for the biological mother. Nonetheless, because the caregiver is considered to be just helping out in the structure of the transnational family, children do not regard all of the care tasks to be transferrable to the caregiver. Most importantly, the caregiver is not expected to provide financially for the child, which is considered the responsibility of the biological parents.

In the Ghanaian context, it is not only the primary caregiver who plays an important role in the provision of care. Other persons in the care network can also perform motherly and fatherly tasks and be considered additional parents. In this way, care can be seen to circulate through extensive networks of kin and friends. In the following excerpt, Henrietta describes the role of her father's brother in her upbringing:

*Henrietta:* I've taken him to be a father.
*Interviewer:* Why is that? What kind of things does he do for you?
*Henrietta:* He encourages me and he calls to check on me when I'm in school, he behaves like a father to me, and he treats me like his own children.

*(Henrietta, seventeen years old)*

In particular, male figures in the wider care network are involved in the disciplining and physical punishment of left-behind children. Obeying and showing respect for adults in society are important duties of Ghanaian children, and those who disobey or disrespect any adult can be physically punished (Twum-Danso 2009). Also children themselves see advice and physical punishment as necessary ingredients on the journey to adulthood. In fact, children feel cared for by the adults who perform these tasks and would not consider it problematic if care tasks of this nature are delivered by a person other than their biological parent or caregiver. Emmanuel, whose father was abroad and lived with his mother, provided the following explanation:

*Emmanuel:* Both of them [father and mother], anyone can call him [father's friend].
*Interviewer:* And then he would come to the house?
*Emmanuel:* Yes, to talk with us.
*Interviewer:* To talk?
*Emmanuel:* Ok, we are grown now so he doesn't discipline [physically beat] us anymore.
*Interviewer:* And before?
*Emmanuel:* He used to cane us.
*Interviewer:* Can you give an example of some of the things that he would come for, like some of the trouble you would make?
*Emmanuel:* When they sent me [to buy something] and I didn't go. Then he would come, they would talk to him about me, and then he would cane me.

. . .

*Interviewer:* How did you feel that this man was disciplining you?
*Emmanuel:* I knew him, so I took it. I knew him closely, so I took it like that. We call him our father. We've taken him as our father, so I wasn't having any problems with that.

*(Emmanuel, seventeen years old)*

When accepting discipline from people other than their biological parents, children compared the amount and means of disciplining to the way in which their biological parents used to discipline them. The care provided by their biological parents was their frame of reference. A deviation from this could be perceived as problematic by the children:

*Interviewer:* What are bad things about having your mother abroad?
*Ralph:* She has a brother. I don't like him. He beats too much. He likes beating.
*Interviewer:* Why does he do that?
*Ralph:* I don't know.
*Interviewer:* He comes to your house sometimes and beats you?
*Ralph:* Yes, he beats us.
*Interviewer:* Is it your mother who tells him to go to the house or he just comes?
*Ralph:* He just comes to the house. But now he stopped.
*Interviewer:* Why?
*Ralph:* Once, me and my brother ran away from the house and my mother spoke to him and told him to stop and then he stopped. . . . Once, after classes, I came home late, and then my phone, the battery was low, so I couldn't call. I came, and he called and told me that he would come and lash me. I phoned my mother and told her that he is coming to lash me. She phoned him and told him not to lash me. And then he came! He came to lash me! He is the oldest, so when my mother told him not to come, he told her she should go away, she should not disturb him. He would come to lash us.
*Interviewer:* And your father didn't do that before?
*Ralph:* No.
*Interviewer:* But isn't it normal for parents to discipline their children?
*Ralph:* It is normal for parents to lash their children. But it was too much, he was overdoing it.
*Interviewer:* And when your mother was here he didn't come to beat you?
*Ralph:* No.

*(Ralph, fourteen years old)*

Whether a care task is considered a 'fatherly' or 'motherly' care task depends on the activities the person is performing instead of the sex of the person.

Kwame's (age sixteen) father used to take care of his son's material needs while his mother was abroad. After his father's death, his father's sister in the United Kingdom took over these financial tasks:

*Kwame:* I feel like she is my father now because she provides the school fees for me.
*Interviewer:* So why would you not say that she is like a mother to you?
*Kwame:* I'm not saying that she is like a mother to me because I feel like my mother is alive, my mother is performing all the duties as a mother, and she is the one performing other duties as my father, so I consider her as my father.

*(Kwame, sixteen years old)*

Due to a combination of care provided by different persons in the child's care network and the acceptance that not all parenting roles have to be fulfilled by the biological parents, children come to accept their transnational caregiving situation as normal. Due to the availability of multiple mothers and fathers, parental migration does not necessarily lead to a perceived lack of parental care. It is even impossible to distinguish between the experiences of children with one parent abroad and those with both parents abroad because in all of these cases it is the combination of care provided by the migrant parents, caregiver and wider care network that determines a child's experiences.

Although life in a transnational family is supported by cultural norms of parenting, it can also cause children to feel pressured to hide the fact that they miss their migrant parent for fear that these feelings might be seen as a critique of the care that is received from their caregiver, as Sheila described:

> My aunty, I didn't want her to see it. Maybe sometimes, when I'm feeling sad, I'll go and sit at a place where no one will see me, and then when I finish crying, I come back because I don't want her to think that maybe, maybe because my mum has left, maybe she's not taking care of me . . . so I am doing it in private.*(Sheila, twenty years old)*

Physical separation due to parental migration does not necessarily lead to negative experiences for the child when tasks are performed well by all of the parties involved. However, the care provided by caregivers and persons in the wider care network is not always sufficient. The presence of the caregiver's own children was often cited as a source of negative experiences. Children complained that most of the money sent by their parents ended up being spent on the care of the caregiver's own family. As a result, there was not enough money for school fees and supplies. In several cases, children even had to miss school for extended periods of time. As children are often unaware of the exact amount of money that their parents are sending and the agreements that their parent and caregiver made concerning remittance distribution, caution must be exercised when drawing conclusions based on children's accounts alone. Nonetheless, our interviews revealed that left-behind children felt neglected as a result of unequal financial care provision for the children of the caregiver and themselves. Caregivers were also reported to make significant demands on left-behind children, especially the girls, in terms of taking up household chores and babysitting the caregiver's own children. These demands shifted the focus away from education and resulted in lower school performance. Children also felt neglected when they were beaten excessively and blamed for everything, as Abigail experienced in the house of her aunt:

> Anytime we the children we do something [wrong], even though they [the children of her aunt] will be at fault, she will blame me for it and insult me, she never liked me. *(Abigail, sixteen years old)*

Conflict between the parent and caregiver is another cause of insufficient care from the caregiver. When the conflict is not resolved and the parents have no means to relocate the children, it can have a negative impact on the quality of care provided to the child. Josephine explained that the situation changed for the worse when her aunts, who were taking care of her, got into a conflict with her migrant parents. Although she did not know the source of the conflict, she experienced the impact it had on the care she received:

*Josephine:* Something came between my parents and my aunties.
*Interviewer:* What came between them?
*Josephine:* I didn't really get it. . . . I was in school, so I didn't really get the story. When I went home, my daddy was complaining about my aunties, but I didn't get the story well. So now, our aunties are not on free terms with us, like at first.
*Interviewer:* How are they relating with you?
*Josephine:* Now everything is changed. First, when we needed something . . . they gave it to us. But right now, if we need something, they want us to tell our daddy to bring it; if not, then they are not going to give the thing to us. . . . They get angry at any time, and sometimes, if there's no food in the house, no one wants to cook the food for us to eat. They are doing things on their own.

*(Josephine, sixteen years old)*

Not only do children expect their migrant parents to maintain an active role in their upbringing, they also expect their parents to ensure a good quality of care. When children suffered from poor experiences with the caregiver, they complained about it to their migrant parents over the phone, expecting their parents to improve the situation. Expectations of mothers and fathers did not differ in this regard. When left-behind mothers took care of the children, children complained to the migrant father when they perceived the care provided by their mother as inadequate and expected their fathers to improve the quality of care. When migrant parents did not respond to such complaints, children often found themselves in prolonged periods of inadequate care and emotional distress. Some children even threatened their overseas parent by claiming that they would run away from home if the situation did not improve.

## Children's Ideals of the Nuclear Family

We have argued that the norm of social parenting in Ghana can help children perceive their life in a transnational family through a positive lens. This is especially true when good care is provided by all of the involved caregivers, including the migrant parent. However, children also expressed a longing for the nuclear family ideal, particularly in situations of inadequate care. The wish to live with both parents was based on the assumption that living with biological parents would automatically improve their care arrangements. Another manifestation of children's desire for a nuclear family was observed in the children of divorced parents. For these children, a return to a nuclear family represented their longing for their biological parents to be on good terms with each other and, in turn, for there to be fewer financial problems and better communication with the migrant parent. However, it may not be necessary for all persons to live in the same household. With one parent abroad and one parent in the household with the children, a nuclear family situation could still be accomplished if everyone is willing to talk to each other on good terms during regular phone conversations.

Moreover, children expressed a desire for physical proximity with their migrant parent. The main motivation for this desire was children's expectation that their relationship with their parents would become closer if they could live together:

*Interviewer:* So do you think that if your father had been in Ghana for all those years, if he hadn't gone abroad, do you think your relationship with him would have been different?
*Emmanuel:* Yeah, I think so.
*Interviewer:* In what way?
*Emmanuel:* That we would have gotten a lot closer.
*Interviewer:* In what way, because you say that you are still close to him?
*Emmanuel:* Like feel him. Now I can't feel him. Sometimes I think about talking to him face-to-face, but I can't talk to him face-to-face. I have missed him.

*(Emmanuel, sixteen years old)*

This 'feeling' of the parent's presence could not be developed through short return visits, remittances and phone calls:

*Frank:* I miss him a lot; I have never been able to stay with him for even 2 months.

*Interviewer:* So what do you miss if you haven't seen him for more than 2 months in a row?

*Frank:* Father caring, I want to feel father caring.

*Interviewer:* What is that, 'father caring'?

*Frank:* Like you will be at home, and during weekends, your father will be taking you out and advising you and telling you some old folk tales and so many things but I don't feel it now.

*(Frank, sixteen years old)*

The ideals of a nuclear family that underlie these feelings and experiences can be attributed to similar ideals propagated by the Pentecostal church, which has been influential on children in urban Ghana (Coe 2008; Chapter 6, this volume). We found that schools were often the place where children missed the physical presence of a parent the most. In particular, visiting days at boarding school and parent-teacher meetings were cited by children as moments when they would see parents come to visit and take care of their schoolmates. This sense of longing for the physical presence of the parent was observed more frequently in Accra, where children typically live in small households, than in Kumasi, where children typically live in larger households and are surrounded by larger care networks. Relative to the Accra children, the Kumasi children were also visited more often by people other than their biological parents.

## DISCUSSION AND CONCLUSION

In this study, we interviewed Ghanaian left-behind children living in transnational families in which one or both of the parents migrated to 'the West', analysed their experiences and explored the best ways to explain this phenomenon. We proposed a model that interprets the experiences of left-behind children through the lens of societal norms on parenting. Our data showed that the experiences of left-behind children are influenced by their expectations about parenting, which derive from the social norms of parenting, the way care is circulated and enacted and their experiences with their parents prior to migration. In Ghana we did not see that children experience transnational family life as their parents' failure to fulfil a social ideal, as reported elsewhere in the world (Bernhard et al. 2009; Parreñas 2005a). Instead, the norm of social parenthood resulted in a general acceptance among left-behind children that care can be provided by a non-biological parent caregiver and wider care network, evident in the 'circulation of care' (Part A, this volume), even in the absence of parents due to migration. The flexible and inclusive childcare and family norms in Ghana help children to cope with and even value their lives in a transnational family context.

Different expectations exist with regard to fathers versus mothers. Fathers are overwhelmingly expected to provide financial care, with children perceiving financial provisions as the mode of care associated with their fathers. However, children also value acts that show emotional and social care from their fathers. In contrast, mothers are mainly expected to provide emotional care. Given that many children belong to households headed by a single female in which the mother has the responsibility of being the financial provider, children come to perceive the mother's migration as necessary for financial reasons and appreciate her financial provisions. Parents can provide emotional care from abroad through regular phone calls and return visits, as left-behind children do not see the absence of physical proximity in the provision of emotional care as necessarily problematic. The reason relates to the Ghanaian context in which social parenthood constitutes an important mode of caregiving. In this context, the biological parent is not expected to be solely responsible for all parenting tasks, and children see it as acceptable for the caregiver and others to perform certain parental tasks that the biological parent is unable to perform as a result of physical separation. Whereas biological parents are expected to maintain their parental roles from abroad through securing good care arrangements for the child and showing care through remittances, phone calls and return visits, children tend to accept it when certain 'motherly' and 'fatherly' tasks are taken over by other people. Having multiple mothers and fathers helps parental care to circulate—despite the physical absence of the biological parents.

While care circulation allows children to accept and value aspects of their transnational living arrangements, the quality of care is also important in determining how a child will perceive such arrangements. Not all care arrangements function well, and not all children feel as though they are receiving adequate care. In the case of transnational fathers, the most important factor concerns the lack of material care, although a lack of emotional care can also induce feelings of parental neglect. Mothers who do not provide emotional care create sadness in their children. In addition, left-behind children who feel maltreated, exploited or neglected by their caregivers in Ghana tend to suffer emotionally, socially and educationally.

Technologies enhance the circulation of care (see also Chapter 5, this volume). Despite the distance, parents were still able to provide care and guard their role as primary authority figures through regular phone calls, return visits and remittances. Likewise, children felt most cared about by migrant parents who sent regular remittances and made frequent phone calls in which they were asked about personal issues and given advice. In contrast, a lack of return visits, remittances or phone calls could keep a child in a state of longing for his or her migrant parent.

It is interesting to compare child fostering, a longstanding form of care circulation that is a common practice in Ghana, with the transnational child-raising arrangements described in this chapter. Child fostering practices, such as social parenthood norms, create a context in which it is socially acceptable to be raised by people other than biological parents. This situation differs from some other contexts and parts of the world that have been described in the transnational family literature (Bernhard et al. 2009; Parreñas 2005a). However, we also note important differences between local child fostering and transnational child-raising arrangements (Øien 2006). Bledsoe (1990) noted that biological parents were not expected to intervene after foster parents started to care for their children. This was because a good upbringing entailed some hardship ('no success without struggle'). For this reason, parents were unlikely to intervene even in negative child fostering situations. Whereas proper disciplining is also part of what children in the context of transnational child raising perceive as good childcare, parents are expected to, and do, intervene in the case of poor child-raising arrangements due to the unique reasons for fostering in this context and the expectations regarding a biological parent's role in caring from afar. Local child fostering is often a situation in which a parent who is less well off entrusts the care of his or her child to a foster parent who is better off (Verhoef, 2005). In contrast, in a transnational child-raising context, the migrant parent is seen as 'better off' than the local caregiver, thereby creating the expectation (on the part of the child and local caregiver) that the parent will be involved in the upbringing, at least in the form of material support. Furthermore, cheaper flights and modern communication technology, such as cellular phones and the Internet, make it possible for migrant parents to give advice to and be involved in the emotional care of their children (see also Baldassar 2008b). At the same time, geographical distance makes it more difficult for migrant parents to check on their children's situation through regular visits. This all results in different forms of care circulation than in local child fostering arrangements, where care in transnational arrangements is expected to circulate both transnationally and locally. This creates an interplay of expectations that are based on social parenthood norms in which a local network of people provide the day-to-day material and emotional care for children and in which the nuclear family and biological parents, specifically, have old as well as new expectations on them resulting from their migratory project. More research in this area is necessary to help us better understand how local child fostering norms can facilitate transnational child-raising arrangements and how child fostering differs from transnational child-raising arrangements in terms of expectations, rights and responsibilities of the various actors in the care arrangement.

Furthermore, we have seen in this chapter that local norms of parenting are neither static nor comprehensive. As argued by other scholars, nuclear family ideals are also present in Ghanaian society through processes of urbanisation (Oppong 2006) and modern religions (van Dijk 2002). We noted that when children experienced a lack of quality care in Ghana or divorce, they could begin to consider the nuclear family as an ideal. The coexistence of both the societal norm of social parenthood and the ideal of a nuclear family help us understand why children's experiences of living in a transnational family tend to be so complex and at times ambivalent.

Nonetheless, it is clear that the norms of social parenthood help Ghanaian children in their transnational family life and that migration does not necessarily imply a deterioration of the level of care provided for the left-behind children remaining in the home country. This study showed that the manner in which children experienced the separation from their biological parent tended to be mediated by their expectations with regard to their migrant parents, their caregiver and others in the care network. These expectations were guided by social parenthood norms and shaped within a context in which child fostering is common.

## NOTES

1. www.tcra.nl

# 8 Men's Caregiving Practices in Filipino Transnational Families

## A Case Study of Left-Behind Fathers and Sons

*Asuncion Fresnoza-Flot*

## INTRODUCTION

The aggregate demand in the service sectors in developed economies results in the dynamic migration of Third World women. This phenomenon implies a 'care drain', as these women are the ones 'who normally care for the young, the old, and the sick in their own poor countries' (Hochschild 2003, 17). Many of them are mothers who leave their families in their country of origin, and their migration has been the object of scientific inquiries in recent years, including investigation of the care arrangements they make in their own country (Hondagneu-Sotelo and Avila 1997; Raijman et al. 2003; Moran-Taylor 2008). Women kin members and eldest daughters are often cited as caregivers to migrant mothers' households, which represents one part of the 'global care chains' connecting migrants and non-migrants through paid or unpaid care work (Hochschild 2000). As suggested by recent studies, fathers in some migrant families also accomplish housework and childcare as do women family members (Pingol 2001; Shinozaki 2012; Sørensen 2004a), but the caregiving practices of fathers and sons in chains of care remain largely unexplored.

Using the analytical lens of care circulation (as proposed by Baldassar and Merla, Part A, this volume), this chapter elucidates the caregiving practices of male members in the households of migrant mothers through a case study of Filipino fathers and sons left behind: What forms of care do these men provide to other family members? What factors influence their level of involvement in caring? In what ways do their caregiving practices affect their individual lives and those of other family members? Addressing these questions is expected to shed light on the gendered dynamics of migrant mothers' transnational families and also on the process of their social reproduction. Fisher (1994, 677) points out the importance of such a study in order 'to develop a new appreciation of the caring capacities of men', as 'there are circumstances where men accept the obligation to care, undertake intimate personal care, and derive identity and reward from their caring work'.

Focusing on one of the unexamined aspects of the 'transnational domestic sphere' (Gardner and Grillo 2002), this study lies at the intersections of migration, family and men's studies. Here, caregiving in the family setting refers to the unpaid activities provided by and directed towards one or more family members 'encompassing both instrumental tasks and affective relations' (Abel and Nelson 1990, 4). It results in an interdependent relationship, which may be symmetrical or asymmetrical, between the caregiver and the care receiver (Waerness 1984). Feminist scholars consider caregiving as part of 'reproductive labour', that is, activities necessary for the daily maintenance and (re)production of people: for example, 'purchasing household goods, preparing and serving food, laundering and repairing clothing, maintaining furnishings and appliances, socialising children, providing care and emotional support for adults, and maintaining kin and community ties' (Glenn 1992, 1). Such 'care work' is mostly associated with women and implies physical, mental, emotional and even symbolic labour (Abbott and Wallace 2000; Anderson 2000). This chapter takes into account these dimensions of reproductive labour to examine the caregiving practices of left-behind Filipino fathers and sons.

There are no official statistics available regarding the number of husbands or children of Filipino migrant women left behind in the Philippines. Data gathered by non-governmental organisations (NGOs) and advocacy groups suggest that there are about nine million left-behind children in the country, a number equivalent to 27 percent of the total Filipino youth (Reyes 2008). Public concerns about their well-being arose in the 1990s when Filipino overseas migration became increasingly feminised. In Filipino families, reproductive work (including caregiving) is traditionally performed by women and productive labour by men. Because of this gendered division of labour, most migrant women rely on their daughters or other women among their kin to perform care work in their households. However, Filipino men, specifically the husbands and sons of migrant mothers, also provide varying degrees of care to their families, and their caregiving practices have been overlooked in most previous studies.

Here I start by revisiting the literature on migrant parents' transnational families to understand the nature and character of care work in these social units. This is followed by a short presentation of my data-gathering methods and of some sociodemographic characteristics of the persons interviewed. The next sections are devoted to the exploration of the case of fathers and sons left behind. The chapter concludes with some future research tracks related to caregiving in migrants' households.

## CAREGIVING IN TRANSNATIONAL FAMILIES WITH MIGRANT PARENTS

Family and kin caring, either long distance or proximate, is a strong component of transnational family dynamics, which reflects the 'feeling of collective welfare and unity' (Bryceson and Vuorela 2002b, 3) that dispersed family members maintain towards each other. In such care obligations and practices, male and female family members contribute differently to family functioning, mostly following the gendered norms in their household.

The 'transnational motherhood' (Hondagneu-Sotelo and Avila 1997) of migrant mothers has been well documented. Prominent care strategies include regular communications with their children, remittances and gifts, family visits and care arrangements with other women in their home country (Parreñas 2001b; Raijman et al. 2003; Schmalzbauer 2004; Madianou and Miller 2011). The migration status (regular or irregular) of migrant mothers plays an important role in determining the relative intensities of these practices: Because they cannot visit their families, undocumented mothers communicate and send gifts more frequently than documented ones (Fresnoza-Flot 2009b). Migrant women also maintain kinship ties through phone calls, remittances, home visits, family gatherings and financial assistance during difficult moments (Alicea 1997; Zontini 2004a). As daughters, these women provide care to their elderly parents, moving them to their immigration country or simply by mobilising their kin networks at home to ensure the well-being of their parents (Baldassar 2008a; Merla 2011). All these care practices underline the overlapping family obligations of migrant women and their continuous subordination in the family.

Unlike migrant mothers, migrant fathers' transnational family caring has rarely been examined. The relatively scarce data available show that these men involve themselves in childrearing via financial support, visits, gifts and phone calls (Dreby 2010; Nobles 2011; Parreñas 2008; Pribilsky 2004). Compared with migrant mothers, migrant fathers tend to focus more on providing financially for the needs of their family and less on communicating with their children (Parreñas 2008). They also perform kin work, but mainly in the form of financial support, thereby affirming their breadwinning role in the family. Hence, the ways in which migrant mothers and fathers express their care towards their families reflect their gendered perception of family obligations and highlight the forms of care that dispersed family members provide to one another: financial assistance and moral, emotional and practical support (Baldassar et al. 2007).

Caregiving arrangements in the households of migrants differ depending on who migrates. When the father goes abroad, the mother assumes the bulk of domestic responsibilities, acting as both a mother and a father to the children (Parreñas 2005a). On the contrary, when the mother or both parents migrate, children are generally put under the care of a member from the immediate or extended family (Chamberlain 1998; Save the Children 2006). In some cases, non-relatives are asked to look after the children. Some children take care of themselves as they are left on their own (Lahaie et al. 2009). A few studies, particularly in the Philippines, have shown that fathers sometimes provide full-time care for their children (Asis et al. 2004; Pingol 2001). Other fathers participate less in reproductive labour and are generally assisted by female family members (ECMI-CBCP/AOS-Manila et al. 2004).

Acknowledging the caregiving skills of these women, the migrants sometimes request their assistance and make them migrate too, as seen in the case of 'transnational grannies' (Plaza 2000) and 'flying grandmothers' (see Chapter 12, this volume).

Recent studies have shown the impact of transnational caregiving on the lives of migrant parents. For instance, migrant mothers experience distress and ambivalence and feel pressured to work hard to sustain the needs of their children (Fresnoza-Flot 2009b; Raijman et al. 2003). However, their transnational mothering strategies also reinforce their motherhood and make them 'good mothers' (Avila 2008). Similarly, despite the stress brought about by their productive activities, migrant fathers become good family providers and caregivers for their children notably upon home visits (McKay 2010).

To sum up, the transnational family arrangements discussed above are gendered and dominated by women, reflecting the 'inequalities in transnational families' (Dreby and Adkins 2010). What remains to be explored in transnational caregiving is its reciprocal character that some studies have only recently started to examine (e.g., Baldassar 2007a, 2007c; Merla 2011; Zontini and Reynolds 2007). In the case of migrant mothers who fulfil intensive long-distance caregiving, little information exists on how their family members at home care for them in return and how these members' caregiving practices affect their lives and those of other family members. In addition, many studies on migration tend to focus on the productive and reproductive work of migrant women and on the situation of their children left behind. As a result, the role of men who are left behind and their perspective on transnational family caring have long been overlooked. For instance, the lesser involvement of fathers in reproductive work has mostly been approached from other family members' points of view. As Mazzucato and Schans (2011, 707) argue, 'To get a complete picture of transnational family life, it is important to add fathers to the picture, not just on the sideline but as main actors'. This is also the case of left-behind sons, whose caregiving practices remain unclear. The viewpoints of all family members are crucial to understanding the social reproduction of transnational families.

## METHODOLOGY

The data presented in this chapter originate from a larger study of the transnational family dynamics of Filipino migrant mothers in France (Fresnoza-Flot 2009a). Adopting 'multi-sited ethnography' as an approach (Marcus 1995), I carried out fieldwork in France and the Philippines between March 2006 and January 2007. In France, I conducted observations, documentary research and semi-structured interviews with fifty Filipino migrants among whom thirty-five were mothers separated from their families. With the permission of these migrant women, I visited their families in the Philippines during my fieldwork in Metropolitan Manila and in the Tagalog-speaking region of the country. I carried out semi-structured interviews with forty family members.

The persons interviewed in the Philippines included six fathers, thirteen sons, fourteen daughters and seven kin members. The bigger number of women respondents in this sample suggests their engagement in the care arrangements in migrant Filipinas' households. Hence, in this chapter, I examine the perspectives of fathers and sons while taking into account the role of women family members. Concerning the group of fathers interviewed, most of them finished tertiary education and were in their forties at the time I met them. Except for one, who had retired due to health problems, all these men were professionally active. Five respondents confided that their wives decided first to work abroad and that they were only consulted afterwards. Only one had encouraged his wife to emigrate as a solution to their financial problems (caused partly by his wife's family always asking them for money). Other fathers disagreed at the beginning with their wife's decision to migrate but later on decided to let them go, thinking about the future of their children. However, these men explained that if they had found an opportunity, they would have preferred to be the ones going abroad. Among the six fathers interviewed, four were entrusted by their wives with the responsibility of taking care of their children and their house whereas the other two were left with caregiver(s) from their extended family.

Most of the thirteen sons interviewed were young adults, single and unemployed (i.e., financially dependent on their parents). Even some respondents who had already graduated from college still depended on their parents' financial assistance (including one who was already married). When their mothers emigrated, nine sons were less than ten years old, and the other four were between the ages of eleven and nineteen; eight of the sons interviewed were aware that their mother would be working abroad whereas the five others only understood it afterwards when told by their father or a close relative. All the respondents, except in one case, were left under the care of a family member (either their father or someone from the extended family), at least initially.

## THE IMPROVED CARE CONTRIBUTIONS OF MIGRANT FILIPINAS' HUSBANDS

The migration of the mother modifies the rhythm and functioning of the family (Asis and Baggio 2003; Hondagneu-Sotelo and Avila 1997). In the case of the Filipino fathers interviewed, their wives' migration prompted them to improve their care contributions in the family as a coping strategy in their new situation characterised by conjugal separation.

Before their wives emigrated, the fathers interviewed only focused on productive work and performed few household tasks, mostly do-it-yourself activities (such as changing electric bulbs and repairing furniture). They explained that they participated 'a lot' in domestic chores just after their wife delivered a baby or when their children were small. After the departure of their wives, most of these men started to accomplish more reproductive work, including childrearing for two of them. The household chores they performed included dishwashing, shopping, housekeeping and cooking. What they considered a 'new task' was their remittance and family budget management, which contrasts with the situation of other left-behind Filipino fathers (Shinozaki 2012). For two fathers, disciplining and morally guiding their children represented another new role. All the fathers generally kept their wives informed via telephone conversations about family matters like their children's school performance. Nonetheless, they were the ones who directly dealt with the daily challenges of doing reproductive work. Juanito, a father of four and an upholsterer, described his caregiving experience after his wife migrated to France:

> When I wake up in the morning, I cook breakfast. After that, I prepare the table and wake up the kids. While they are eating, I boil water for their bath and prepare the food that my two daughters will bring to school for their lunch. After eating, they take a bath and prepare for school. As soon as they leave, I do shopping and cook immediately because I have two children who will come back home for lunch. I cannot go out to work until I am done with my household chores.

Aside from this, Juanito provided hands-on care for his youngest daughter in the early days of his wife's migration. He remembers changing her diaper, feeding and bathing her as well as putting her to bed while singing nursery songs. Juanito's care work can be attributed to the young age of his children: His eldest child was nine and his youngest was only a few months old when his wife left for France.

Another factor that prompts fathers to become involved in taking care of the children and the house is the absence of an available relative to fulfil this role. Renan (unemployed father of four) shared his experience when his wife migrated to Qatar and then to France: 'I washed our clothes and cooked for my kids. I didn't feel ashamed of that, because there was really nobody to wash clothes, I had no choice'. Renan's case is exceptional as other fathers interviewed emphasised the paramount role of some women in their family and friendship networks in accomplishing household chores and in looking after the well-being of their children. These fathers devoted less time to reproductive work in comparison with those who found themselves alone in fulfilling them partly because they tried to avoid conflict with kin caregivers to whom their migrant wives had entrusted the nurturing role in the family. Nevertheless, having a caregiver in the family did not always impede the father's participation in care work, which demonstrates his individual agency. Among the fathers whose households were cared for by other kin members, Juanito was the only one who ended up accomplishing the bulk of the reproductive work (including childrearing) after he grew dissatisfied with the caregiving practices of seven different persons from his extended family.

Taking care of the children requires physical work as well as emotional labour. In addition to their sadness due to conjugal separation, the fathers interviewed found themselves confronted by the physical and physiological changes their children undergo as they grow up. Those with daughters entering adolescence relied on the help of some women they knew, particularly regarding sexuality and other physical issues.

Like migrant fathers who express their affection towards their family through successful breadwinning (McKay 2010; Chapter 9, this volume), left-behind fathers also care for their children by fulfilling a productive role. All of the fathers interviewed, except Renan, who suffered the effects of a stroke, continue to financially support their families by being professionally active despite their wife's larger financial contribution to the family revenue. This allowed them to respond to immediate household needs and to avoid relying on their wife's remittance, which they considered to be their 'wives' money' (Fresnoza-Flot 2011). They allocated such 'money' to their children's education, the maintenance of their house and the family's larger projects, including possessing socially valued objects (land, cars and house). This suggests that their wives fulfil their care role in the family despite their absence, reinforcing the fact that they are good mothers. Such 'social meaning' of money (Zelizer 1989; Chapter 11, this volume) earned through maternal migration compels the left-behind husband to maintain his productive role. These husbands also make sure that their children have enough pocket money to meet their needs at school, a role normally accomplished by their wives. Moreover, some husbands invest part of their wife's remittance in real estate to offer a comfortable home for their wife when she returns for good and to prepare for the couple's old age.

Meanwhile, all the fathers interviewed tried to spend more time with their children by watching movies together, eating in restaurants, playing basketball with their sons or simply accomplishing household chores together. This confirms other studies showing the fathers' inclination to carry out physical activities with their children (Doucet and Merla 2007; Lamb 2000). Some of the fathers interviewed also tried to become more communicative with their children, which often surprised the latter. These changes in the attitude of the men after their wives migrated suggest that left-behind Filipino fathers are also capable (like their wives) of providing affective, material and symbolic care at home (Asis et al. 2004; Pingol 2001).

Furthermore, the fathers who were interviewed carry out transnational caring towards their migrant wives, especially during important family events such as their wedding anniversary, Christmas and New Year. Since international telephone calls are expensive in the Philippines, some fathers sent SMS messages or simply rang their wives' phones as a signal to call them. During telephone conversations, these men never forget to give advice to their wives, telling them to eat well, take care of their well-being and avoid working too much. Their emotional support to their partner can also be observed in some of the things they send to them. When cellular phone communication was not yet widely available in the Philippines, some fathers sent voice tapes to their wives to keep them updated about important events, notably concerning their children. At the time of the interviews, all the respondents explained their reliance on phone communication and their continuous sending of family photos to their migrant spouses. When they knew someone who was going to Paris, they would ask him or her to take some items for their wives such as letters, vitamins and medicines. Baldassar (2008b) describes these as ways of creating and maintaining 'co-presence' in transnational family relationships that reinforce feelings of emotional closeness and 'being there' for each other.

These transnational gestures of caring reinforce intimacy in spousal relationships. In fact, the state of such relationships often influences the care arrangements in migrant Filipinas' households, notably the wives' choice of caregiver and their husbands' participation in reproductive work. Among the six fathers interviewed, two had problematic relationships with their wives, who entrusted their children to the care of female kin members before their departure. Close intimate spousal relationships make it easier for some husbands to accomplish some care obligations, like Renan and Juanito. On the contrary, Lito (father of two and a carpenter), who had a disconnected-aloof relationship with his wife due to his suspicion of the latter's infidelity, performed few household chores and let his wife's kin take care of their house and children. The fact that his wife's kin as caregivers were defending her against his allegations also shaped his attitude towards reproductive work. However, regardless of the degree of participation in reproductive work of the husbands interviewed, it was obvious that their wives' migration had changed the way in which they accomplished their father and husband roles in the family.

## THE "UNSEEN" CARE PRACTICES OF LEFT-BEHIND SONS

Like some fathers who assume a caregiving role in Filipino transnational families, the left-behind sons of Filipino migrant mothers find their own way to contribute to the functioning of their households. Their greater involvement in emotional caring rather than in reproductive work shows the other face of the life of children left behind, that is, the reinforcement of intimacy in family relations, particularly in the mother–child dyad (Fresnoza-Flot 2009b).

Although most of the sons interviewed did not participate much in reproductive work, they performed emotional work towards their siblings:

giving advice, helping with school assignments or teaching moral values to younger siblings. Moreover, they emotionally supported their migrant mothers through various gestures. First, they sent their mothers greeting cards, photos, letters (albeit rarely) and things their mothers requested from them: medicine, Filipino films and foods (canned goods, instant noodles, pastries). Second, they expressed their gratitude towards their mother by studying hard, participating in household work or spending their monthly allowance in a reasonable way. Dino, age thirty-two, a medicine graduate and the eldest child in his family, saved part of his mother's remittances to buy a big house as a gift for his mother when she returned home. In fact, Dino had not seen his mother for eighteen years due to her irregular migration status in France. Third, and perhaps the most commonly expressed caring gesture of sons left behind, was their maintenance of regular communication with their mothers by phone and through the Internet. They generally called their mothers to inform them about family events, personal successes to celebrate or, in case of emergencies, when they required financial assistance. Like their fathers, the sons who were interviewed mostly sent SMS messages or rang their mothers' phones instead of calling them from the Philippines. The emotional caregiving of these sons exhibits their agency. This supports other studies which have also demonstrated that children can be caregivers as well as care receivers. For example, older children in immigrant households in the United States perform sibling caregiving aligned with the 'culturally informed family roles, responsibilities, and obligations' (Hafford 2010, 294).

Concerning reproductive work, certain factors influence the attitude of the sons interviewed. Birth order played an important role: Eldest sons usually performed more household tasks than younger ones. Other studies have shown that daughters, particularly the eldest ones, usually fulfil most of the reproductive work in migrants' households (Alicea 1997; Parreñas 2010; Toro-Morn 1995). Indeed, among the sons interviewed here, those who had no sisters or only young ones participated more in the reproductive work than the four who had elder sister(s). Joel, twenty-one years old and a college student, shared his experience with his three elder sisters:

> My sisters were the ones working in the house, while me, still small at that time, was only studying and playing most of the time. Sometimes, I helped my sisters cleaning the house and washing dishes. [. . .] I started to cook for our family only recently. Before, when I was in high school, I didn't cook at all, because my sisters had no trust in my cooking abilities.

Joel's case partly sheds light on the reasons behind the lesser involvement of sons in the accomplishment of reproductive work: The approval or disapproval of women members of the family regarding a son's fulfilment of certain household chores is certainly an influential factor. The tendency of migrant mothers to rely on their daughters, notably the eldest ones, to carry out care work vis-à-vis their siblings also plays a key role. Eldest daughters who were interviewed explained that their mother always reminded them to look after their siblings, which was often understood as saving them from the pressure of doing housework. Likewise, the presence or absence of available kin members to provide care for the household of a migrant mother represented another determining factor. Among the respondents, only two sons had no available kin members helping them at home: Joel and his sisters who lived in their house with nobody around after his mother left, and Eddie (thirty-three years old, married and unemployed) who became the caregiver to his father after his mother and siblings went to work abroad.

The age at the time of a mother's migration also determines her son's fulfilment of domestic chores and of care obligations towards other siblings. The four sons who were older than eleven when their mother emigrated took care of their siblings and participated in housework, whereas the other nine sons were only involved in a few household chores, such as sweeping the floor and setting the table. Those who had elder sisters remarked that the latter were the ones cooking, washing the dishes and ironing clothes—all 'instrumental chores' (Battaglini et al. 2002) that are considered in the Philippines as the realm of women. Kin caregivers looking after the well-being of the respondents contributed to such a gendered division of labour by deciding which domestic tasks should be performed by which children. Sons were most often not expected to work at home but rather to study hard. Caregivers often mediated migrant mother–child relationships by communicating regularly with the mother about her child's academic performance, health condition and behaviour. When problems arose, the migrant mother talked by phone to the child concerned and disciplined him or her verbally if necessary.

In addition, the absence of a father can motivate sons to involve themselves in care work: Five among the respondents talked about such experiences. Dino explained that he became the 'right hand' of his father, who was absorbed by farm work following his mother's emigration. Carrying out household chores posed no difficulty for him because his mother had trained him since he was in elementary school. When he, his three brothers and his younger sister went to Manila to study, he became the head of his siblings there. Aside from budgeting their mother's remittance, he took charge of dividing household chores, guiding his siblings in their studies and making important family decisions. His experience of sibling caregiving reflects the usual practice in the Philippines where parents normally delegate such responsibility to elder children in the family (Peterson 1990). Another case is that of Ramon, age forty-six, the middle child and a policeman, who, together with his two brothers, ended up taking care of themselves due to his father's extramarital affairs. Despite their mother's regular remittance, Ramon and his brothers did not hire any domestic help and instead accomplished the household chores by themselves. This attests to the agency of sons who are left behind and underlines how disconnected-aloof parental relationships affect the care arrangements in migrant families.

Aside from productive labour and extramarital affairs, illness and disability can also lessen a father's participation in care work, eventually pushing some sons to become caregivers. A migrant mother can also influence her son's decision to become a caregiver. For example, Eddie gave up searching for a job and started taking care of his father who suffered from a stroke. His migrant mother encouraged him to do so, reasoning that he was the only one among his siblings who was left in the country: His eldest brother and youngest sister were working in Saudi Arabia. Eddie and his family decided to live under the same roof as his father while his migrant mother and siblings regularly sent financial support to them. When remittances arrived late, Eddie borrowed money from his aunt who was living in a nearby city. When the money arrived, he paid his aunt back and sometimes took his father to visit other relatives. Such situations illustrate how care circulates between members of Filipino transnational families, involving various family members at different times and in different ways.

In addition to remittance and family budget management, most of the time Eddie ended up doing most of the care work alone as his wife maintained her own professional activity. On top of this, he was also looking after his baby daughter. Eddie described his role as being 'like housekeeper, housewife or househusband'. This situation was new to him because at the beginning of his mother's migration, his father was in charge of the house and performed most of the household chores. Eddie's case shows how care arrangements in a transnational family change over time and how care obligation moves from one person to another. In other words, over the course of their lives, individuals start as care receivers, then become caregivers and then again become care receivers from a certain age (Escriva 2005). Such circulation of care obligation can affect the lives of family members such as fathers and sons.

## THE IMPACT OF FATHER'S AND SON'S CAREGIVING

The caregiving role of men in the family context has been shown to be a stressful and challenging experience affecting their physical and psychological well-being (Doucet and Merla 2007; Kramer and Thompson 2002). In the context of the migration of Filipino mothers, the variable level of involvement of fathers and sons in family caregiving entails certain disadvantages and benefits.

For the fathers who were interviewed and became the major caregivers in the family, their new role triggered a radical change in their daily life rhythm, and consequently they experienced a 'time bind' (Hochschild 1997). For instance, Juanito, who maintained his professional activities, found his time divided between productive and reproductive work, resulting in stress and worries. Those fathers who received kin's support in doing care work also felt the sudden change in their lives. For example, even though his mother was helping him to take care of his children, Pedro remarked:

> In the past, every time I would go somewhere, as long as there were things to cook at home it wasn't a problem. It didn't matter when I would come back. It didn't matter if I wanted to go away for a month, as long as my children had something to eat. Now, I must go home every hour to look after them: 'are they fine?'

The fathers sometimes undertook paid employment to contribute to the family budget. On the one hand, this can be interpreted as a strategy to counter the feeling of sadness due to conjugal separation. On the other hand, a focus on productive labour by the fathers could also represent a way to confront the gender role reconfiguration in the family and their masculine identity crisis caused by their wife's breadwinning role acquired through migration (Fresnoza-Flot 2011).

Moreover, the accumulation of economic activities and the stress accompanying reproductive labour affected the well-being of the fathers, who most often neglected their health. Pedro remarked that since his wife migrated, he had not bought any new clothes for himself, while Rodolfo confided about his regular alcohol drinking sessions with his male friends.

Among the sons who were interviewed, most of those who received assistance from their extended family felt 'obliged' by their caregiver to participate in reproductive work, which according to the respondents eventually made them 'independent' and 'responsible'. Sons who provided care for their households felt their familial responsibilities increased, a situation that affected their professional lives. For instance, Eddie put aside his biology degree and postponed his plan to work abroad to become a full-time caregiver for his father and daughter. The feeling of being left alone to accomplish domestic chores and care obligations towards other siblings can also trigger 'deviant' attitudes. This is how Ramon explained his loss of interest in his studies, his escapades with his friends (drinking alcohol, smoking, partying) and his careless spending in the absence of his parents. Consequently, he was not able to finish his studies and only decided to go back to school after he started his own family. As Lahaie et al. (2009, 308) found, in their study of left-behind children in Mexico, 'children taking care of themselves (self-care) are three times as likely to experience behavioural and academic problems as children in other care arrangements'.

Coping with the 'undesirable' impact of the mother's absence on the children was emotionally difficult for all the fathers interviewed. They usually kept all family problems that they considered heavy and serious (such as children getting sick and being hospitalised) to themselves because they did not want their migrant wives to worry. They only talked with their wives about issues that required their wife's immediate attention, such as the teenage pregnancy of a daughter or a son's loss of interest in his studies. Similarly, all the sons interviewed concealed most of their problems from their parents, notably from their migrant mothers with the aim of preventing them from worrying. As a result, fathers and sons who were fulfilling a caregiving role were carrying all the emotional burden at home by themselves. This situation highlights the communication gap among members of transnational families: Migrants do not tell to their family everything that is happening to them in their receiving country (Bryceson and Vuorela 2002b; Fresnoza-Flot 2010; Schmalzbauer 2008; Baldassar 2007b), and their family members living in their country of origin do the same to them.

A positive impact of caregiving is that all the respondents earned respect and appreciation from their immediate family members. Migrant wives in separate interviews mentioned how their husbands' caring words alleviated their sentimental difficulties due to family separation. Among the spouses of the six fathers interviewed, three confided that their husbands became 'sweeter' and 'more thoughtful', saying more 'I love you' words than when they were together. The father's increased involvement in care work also caught the attention of their children who intended to take care of them in return. For example, Juanito's children were planning to work abroad when they grow up in order to support their father and mother in their old age. Caregiving sons also received recognition, particularly from their migrant mothers who during interviews in France were proud to show some of the things their sons sent to them: photos, greeting cards, letters and videos of family events. These things, which Baldassar (2008b) defines as creating a form of co-presence by proxy, appeared to be crucial for their emotional well-being, as they evoked a strong feeling of connection with their children. Moreover, a few respondents who became major caregivers for their families explained that their voice gained more weight in the family decision-making process. However, given that the migrant mother is often the principal or only breadwinner of the family, the final voice in familial decisions most often remains hers, especially when the decision to be made involves money. This empowerment of the mothers in their own households is made possible by the financial autonomy they acquire through migration (Mozère 2005).

The respondents, however, felt that their contribution (even small) in the fulfilment of domestic chores was not always recognised by their extended family. For example, Lito explained that his wife's kin criticised him as being 'fed by his wife' because he did not participate much in household tasks (even though he was working as a carpenter). Fathers who were largely involved in housework while working outside the home usually received no criticism from their kin. The sons who were interviewed who did not participate much in housework and sibling caregiving pointed out that the main concerns of their extended family were their school performance and their manners whereas those who contributed to reproductive work explained that their extended family recognised their efforts and showered them with words of admiration. For instance, Dino described how his extended kin looked up to him as a 'model' for his younger relatives, given his care role in his family and his postgraduate degree in medicine. This shows that the Filipino family can also be 'open' to changes in the gender order.

## CONCLUSION

Through the care circulation lens, this chapter brings to light the reciprocal care exchanges within Filipino transnational families with the case of left-behind fathers and sons as a reference point. This approach incites reflexivity with regard to the primary object of analysis and its connections with others. Unlike the global care chain framework that focuses on women's caregiving practices, the care circulation perspective framework (Part A, this volume) puts both men and women in the forefront of care-arrangement analysis. In this chapter, it sheds light on the variable participation in reproductive labour of male family members.

Left-behind Filipino fathers and sons experience care work in a more or less similar fashion. This care work has physical, mental, symbolic and emotional dimensions: using their body to perform household chores, using their mind to organise and plan their work schedule taking into account their other activities (studies, work outside of the family), considering care work as a way to fulfil family expectations and nurturing the psychological well-being of their family members. This is particularly obvious when it comes to the transnational emotional caring fathers and sons perform towards their migrant wife or mother. This demonstrates that caregiving is not unidirectional in Filipino transnational families: Each family member is linked to one another through material, emotional and symbolic gestures of caring; care receivers are also caregivers or can become caregivers later in time. Moreover, caregiving in the Philippine migration context is not exclusively 'women's work': Fathers and sons can also carry out caregiving tasks if it is necessary for the social reproduction of the family and for the well-being of its members.

Several factors explain the varying level of involvement in care work of left-behind fathers and sons. Caregiving appears most heavy during the initial stage of their wife's or mother's migration when children are young and dependent on adult care. Older children tend to carry out more reproductive work than younger ones, but this also depends on the availability of women's care in the household (kin member, daughter or sister): The absence of women entails a greater participation of fathers and sons in housework and childcare. The perspective of women family members regarding men's caregiving at home affect the latter's behaviour vis-à-vis care work: Favourable opinions stimulate participation. This confirms the observation of Gerstel and Gallagher (2001, 213) concerning men's kin caring, saying that caregiving is 'women's work because men's caregiving is contingent on the women in their lives. It is contingent on their wives, sisters, and daughters'. Nevertheless, in the case of the sons left behind, caregiving appears to also be contingent on their father: The absence of the father makes sons more involved in reproductive work.

As for migrant mothers, left-behind fathers and sons encounter constraints and obtain rewards while caregiving. The reorganisation of their individual lives is often accompanied by emotional difficulties such as loneliness. A few of them had to become full-time caregivers, which hindered their professional activities. Some fathers found themselves negotiating their new situation by accentuating their breadwinning role and engaging in several economic activities at the same time. However, most of the fathers and sons who were interviewed gained more voice in decision making as well as respect and recognition from their family and kin. Such effects raise new questions concerning the broader impact of the care practices of transnational families on their society of origin: Do they influence policymaking and public opinions concerning migration and the family? How do non-migrant families perceive and react to the caregiving practices in migrants' households? These represent some of the issues that will need to be addressed in future studies of caregiving in transnational families.

# 9 Polish Male Migrants in London
## The Circulation of Fatherly Care

*Majella Kilkey*

## INTRODUCTION

This chapter examines the experiences of migrant men through a fathering lens.[1] Utilising the framework of circulation as articulated by Baldassar and Merla (Part A, this volume), and in particular the ability of that concept to capture multiple care relationships, it offers a corrective to the tendency within research exploring the nexus between migration and caregiving within families—principally, global care chain research and research on transnational families—to do so predominantly through the experiences of women, and especially mothers. By focusing on the practices, meanings and projects of fathering in the context of men's migration, this chapter aims to examine whether and how fathering is reconfigured through migration. More specifically, it is concerned with establishing how fathering norms around breadwinning and active/involved fathering are reworked in the context of father migration and transnational fathering. Informing the discussion is an empirical study, which included semi-structured interviews with migrant men who worked for pay in private households in and around London, undertaking a range of male domestic chores—termed in the wider study 'handyman services'.[2] Data were gathered on a range of topics including those relating to the migrants' migration paths and ties with their homeland, their family biographies, their experiences of being a migrant in terms of work and family life and their understandings, projects and practices of fathering. The study centred on migrants from the Central and Eastern European countries that had joined the European Union (EU) in 2004 and predominantly on migrants from Poland.

The East-West intra-European migration flows that have developed in the context of EU enlargement have been conceived as being characterised by 'temporary circular and transnational mobility', and they are contrasted with the long-term linear migration and settlement that is considered typical of previous waves of inter-European (and possibly some intra-European) movement (Favell 2008, 703; see also Morokvasic 2004). In this respect, then, these migration flows are interesting ones to view through the lens of circulation. This is particularly the case in relation to the United Kingdom, which, as discussed further below, not only opened its borders to the citizens of the new Central and Eastern European EU Member States on 1 May 2004, but also its labour markets and, comparatively quickly, elements of its welfare system too. The chapter also explores, therefore, the implications for the practices and meanings of fathering, of movement, which is characterised by the potential for mobility and circulation. In doing so, 'the dynamics of the dialectical relationship between structure and action' (Introduction, this volume, 17) in configuring migrant men's father–care relationships, and particularly as these play out across the life course, become apparent. The lens of circulation, by focusing attention on what helps and hinders the flow of fatherly care in Polish migrant men's families, illuminates the importance of structures beyond the legal frameworks governing migrants' (and their families) entry and residency rights and also highlights the importance of situating understandings of transnational caregiving arrangements at the intersection of a complex set of institutional arrangements comprising migration, welfare, care and working-time regimes (Baldassar 2008a; Kilkey and Merla 2013; Chapter 5, this volume).

The chapter is organised into a further three sections. The first examines the positioning of migrant men within research around migration and caregiving within families. The second provides further detail on the migration case study that forms the focus of the chapter. The third presents findings from the empirical study, locating the participants' migration paths and their migration/family arrangements within the broader pattern of post-2004 Polish-UK migration before focusing on the men's migration experiences through the lens of fathering and circulation.

## MIGRATION AND CAREGIVING WITHIN FAMILIES: THE POSITIONING OF MIGRANT MEN IN RESEARCH

Early migration research was dominated by economic perspectives, which tended to construct migrants as non-relational and disembodied rational economic actors, who were implicitly, if not explicitly, also male (Hibbins and Pease 2009). Such a construction was both informed by and in turn influenced public policy, such that in migrant-receiving states migrants were predominantly conceived as individual units of labour, and their family needs were accorded little recognition.[3] Although it is debatable how much has changed with respect to policy, the same cannot be said of migration research, the gendering of which has contributed, among other things, to an acknowledgement of the social reproductive aspects of migrants' lives (Baldassar and Gabaccia 2011; Lutz 2010). Two bodies of research have been especially important in this respect: global care chain research and research on transnational families.

The concept of global care chains was developed to capture the new patterns of social relations accompanying the development of a global market for paid domestic and care labour (Hochschild 2000). The concept has served to illuminate the care deficits experienced by families and communities in 'peripheral' countries of the global economy when mothers migrate to work as domestics and carers in households of richer countries. It has also emphasised, however, the agency of migrant mothers who reconfigure traditional understandings of motherhood to incorporate their new roles and practices as breadwinners and to continue from a distance the emotional labours of mothering (see Hondagneu-Sotelo and Avila 1997; Huang et al. 2012a; Parreñas 2001b). The agency of migrants and their kin in reshaping care relations when the distance imposed by migration limits opportunities for proximate care is also a major theme of transnational families research. Much of its early work focused on how migrants provide care for elder kin members remaining in the 'home country' (see Baldassar et al. 2007; Baldock 2000; Bryceson and Vuorela 2002b; Gardner and Grillo 2002), although more recent research includes a wider range of multidirectional and intergenerational care relationships (see Kilkey and Merla 2013; Merla 2012a). The transnational families research has contributed in a range of ways to challenging economic paradigms of migration: For example, in highlighting that migration can be motivated by care responsibilities, it questions the construction of migrants as rational economic actors (cf. Baldassar 2007a; Merla and Baldassar 2010a). Recent research (Kilkey and Merla 2013; Merla 2012a) has further contributed to acknowledging migrants as relational and embodied by exploring how migrants' capacity to engage in transnational caregiving is related to whether and how national migration, welfare, care and working-time regimes recognise their care responsibilities (Chapter 5, this volume).

Commenting on the gendering of migration research in general, Hibbins and Pease (2009) observe that *female* migrants have constituted the main focus of study. Albeit to different degrees, this is also the case for global care chains and transnational families research. Discussing Rhacel Parreñas's (2001b) pioneering study of Filipina domestic workers in Rome and Los Angeles, Manalansan (2006, 241), for example, has argued that the global care chains literature tends to subscribe to 'normative universalising notions of gender scripts and domesticity', in which married mothers are assumed to be the only possible and logical links in the care chain. As Manalansan (2006, 240) also suggests, to the extent that global care chains research engages with the issue of men, it is solely as 'left behind fathers' who are invariably portrayed as 'pathologically prevented by cultural "tradition" from participating in domestic affairs'. This construction prevails despite evidence from other studies of Filipina labour migration that men's responses are more contextual, flexible and fluid (see e.g., Chapter 8, this volume; Asis et al. 2004; Pe-Pau 2003; Pingol 2001). Admittedly, there has been less of an exclusive focus on female migrants within the transnational families research. Thus, for example, in their seminal study of transnational elder care, Baldassar and colleagues (2007) include both female and male migrants in their sample. Moreover, they offer some reflections on the ways in which transnational care practices are gendered, with, for example, women and men found to conform to a traditional gender division of domestic labour when they provide assistance to elderly parents on visits to the 'home country'. That said, however, overall there is little explicit differentiation between women and men within the study. This is in part because, as the authors acknowledge, their specific focus was on relationships between parents and their adult migrant children (Baldassar et al. 2007, 224). It may also be because among their research sample, female migrants outnumber male migrants by a factor of between two and five depending on the national group; the remaining impression, therefore, is that it is women's experiences that are represented predominantly in the findings (but see Wilding and Baldassar 2009) .

One outcome of the tendency to focus mainly on female migrants is that the challenge to economic paradigms of migration research has not been extended to men to any great extent, and male migrants continue to be researched largely in relation to the workplace. As Kilkey, Plomien and Perrons (2013b) suggest, this has exclusionary potential because migrant men continue to be treated as economic units of labour at precisely the time when in many advanced industrialised societies there is a growing normative expectation, reflected in political and policy commentary (OECD 2007) and in stated male preferences (Hobson and Fahlén 2009), for men to be conceived as *embodied* workers, with family/care commitments alongside those of paid work.

## MIGRANT MEN BEYOND THE WORKPLACE: RECENT RESEARCH ON TRANSNATIONAL FATHERING

Such a shift is acknowledged in a growing body of empirical research that focuses to varying degrees of explicitness on transnational fathering.[4] Much of that research views transnational fathering from a breadwinning perspective, centring principally on how men 'make sense' of their migration experiences through the opportunities migration affords to provide economically for their families.[5] Thus, for example, Datta et al. (2009) and Pribilsky (2004), in their respective studies on male migrants in London and male Ecuadorian migrants in New York, find that to provide for the family was a key motive for the men's migrancy. Moreover, McKay (2007), in a study of Filipino seafarers, finds that the men emphasise their successful breadwinning, to both their families and wider communities, for strategic ends, seeking to counter the marginalisation and subordination they experience on the job as 'global south' migrant male workers. Such studies serve an important role in extending the challenge to the economic paradigm of migration research to men. They focus, however, exclusively on breadwinning and conceive breadwinning in unidimensional and instrumental terms. In doing so, they adhere to a rather economistic construction of fathering. Other work has taken steps to widen the lens through which transnational fathering is analysed. In a follow-up to her research on transnational mothers (2001b, 2005b), Parreñas (2005a, 2008) has undertaken a study of how children 'left behind' in the Philippines experience transnational parenting. Through interviews with young adults who had spent some of their adolescence in a transnational-family scenario, Parreñas finds that while transnational fathers perform the breadwinning and authoritarian roles prescribed by traditional gendered norms in the Philippines, in contrast to transnational mothers, they are less adept at providing emotional care and nurturance from a distance. When considering fathering beyond its traditional boundaries of breadwinner and disciplinarian, however, Parreñas seems to be analysing what the men do and do not do through a mothering lens. This is potentially problematic because, as the broader literature on fathering demonstrates, even primary caregiving fathers 'do not identify themselves as mothers or refer to the work they do as mothering' (Doucet 2006, 217); rather, there are 'distinctly felt qualities of mothering and fathering' (Doucet 2006, 217). One reason that Parreñas's (2008, 1060) study risks obscuring fathering practices of Filipino migrants, which stretch beyond the normatively prescribed, is that she does not speak to the fathers themselves, and as she herself acknowledges, it is possible that children's accounts may 'overlook certain caring labours that their migrant parents deem to be important indicators of intimacy, affection and dependency'.

This methodological limitation[6] is addressed in a further paper by McKay (2010) on Filipino seamen, in which he draws on the firsthand accounts of the men in order to explore more fully than previously the meanings they attach to the economic support they provide to their families. His findings confirm Parreñas's observations that Filipino transnational fathers emphasise above all else their commitment to being good providers. However, with parallels to Zelizer's (1989, 17) argument for a recognition of the 'extra-economic, social base' of money, McKay also argues that remittances and economic investments can have multiple meanings and can range 'along a continuum between simple economic provision and building more emotional connections' (see Chapter 11, this volume). Thus, for example, remittances might be seen as offering opportunities for families to buy physical reminders of the absent father, and financial investments in small businesses might enable men to spend longer periods at home with their children. Moreover, on visits home, McKay finds that some fathers provide active hands-on and nurturing care to their children as a deliberate strategy to strengthen emotional bonds. In such ways, McKay (2010, 16) argues that some migrant men are able to 'expand their actions beyond an exclusively provider role'.

The remainder of this chapter seeks to contribute to the literature outlined above on transnational fathering. In part, it does so by providing a new empirical case study. To date, the transnational fathering research has focused on a small number of national groups, especially on Filipinos. Gender norms and practices, including those relating to fathering, however, are not uniform across cultures (or, for that matter, across social classes and ethnic groups). Patterns of migration are also variable, differing, for example, in terms of distance, duration and legal status of the migrant. Such variations may also have a bearing on transnational fathering practices. It is, therefore, important to query the extent to which findings from a few case studies can be generalised to other contexts. In the following section, I introduce more fully the migration case study, which forms the focus of the remainder of this chapter—recent migrants to the United Kingdom from Poland.

## POLISH MIGRATION TO THE UNITED KINGDOM

Since Poland's accession to the EU, the United Kingdom has become the main destination country within Europe for Polish migrants (Fihel and Kaczmarczyk 2009). Between 2003 and 2010, the Polish-born population of the United Kingdom increased more than sevenfold, from 75,000 to 532,000 (ONS 2011). Labour migration has constituted the bulk of this migration, and by mid-2011, almost 450,000 Polish-born people ages sixteen and over were working in the United Kingdom (ONS 2011).[7] There has been intense political and academic commentary around current and future trends in Polish–UK migration. It seems that while numbers peaked in 2006 and 2007, they then fell off in the context of the 'global' economic recession and its differential impact on European economies (Perrons, Plomien and Kilkey 2010). There is also evidence of return migration to Poland (Finch et al. 2009), although its scale is contested (White 2011). Moreover, migration from Poland to the United Kingdom continues, with the number of Polish-born people working in the United Kingdom increasing by around 60,000 in the first half of 2011 (ONS 2011).

A number of factors account for the volume and speed of Polish migration to the United Kingdom post-2004. These factors include the high level of economic and social inequality between the two countries (Drinkwater, Eade and Garapich 2009), especially at the subnational level (Perrons, Plomien and Kilkey 2010). Also relevant is the presence in the United Kingdom of an existing Polish population, constituted originally by refugee settlement and governmental labour-market schemes in the aftermath of World War II, and subsequently by labour migration, largely irregular, following the liberalisation of Poland's border controls as a result of political changes from 1989 onwards (Kicinger 2009). While not a cohesive Polish 'community' (Garapich 2008), the existing population nonetheless provided a social network that could facilitate new migratory movement (Elrick and Brinkmeier 2009). A further factor is that the United Kingdom, along with

Ireland and Sweden, in contrast to the rest of the EU countries, adopted an open-door approach to EU8[8] labour migration following Accession. The United Kingdom immediately opened its labour market to EU8 workers, imposing registration with the Worker Registration Scheme (WRS) as the only condition. On entry to the WRS, workers were eligible immediately for a restricted range of social benefits, and following twelve months of continuous employment as a registered worker, they were entitled to European Economic Area (EEA) residency status, which extended eligibility to the full range of social benefits, including child-related benefits. EEA residency status also conferred a right of residence in the United Kingdom on the worker's family members, including ascendant and descendant dependent relatives regardless of their nationality. Since 1 May 2011, under EU law, any conditions attached to EU8 migrants in the United Kingdom have been lifted.

Debate also surrounds the character of Polish-UK migration, and specifically whether the pre-Accession pattern of predominantly youthful, individual and male migration (Morawska 2001) has persisted. Official data point to continuity in terms of age and gender, with those registering with the WRS being predominantly young (around 80 per cent ages eighteen to thirty-four) and male (56 per cent) (UK Border Agency 2009, 10). But WRS data only capture those registering to work; those arriving as 'dependants' and not seeking paid work are not counted (Ryan 2011). This also makes it difficult to measure the distribution between family and individual migration, a challenge exacerbated by the dynamic nature of families' migration strategies (Kilkey, Plomien and Perrons 2013b; Ryan et al. 2009), which as highlighted below is a characteristic of the respondents in this study. However, the available evidence suggests that while prior to 2004, the prevailing family migration strategy in Poland was one of male-breadwinner migration, whole-family migration, albeit staged, from Poland to the United Kingdom has become more common (for a review, see Kilkey, Plomien and Perrons 2013b). The tendency is partly accounted for by the distinctive features of the post-2004 migration regime for Polish (and other EU8) nationals: principally, the residency, labour market and welfare rights it accords them (Kilkey, Plomien and Perrons 2013b; Kilkey and Merla 2013). White (2011) also points to a growing preference in Polish society for whole-family migration based on shifting norms around partner relationships and fathering.

## THE CIRCULATION OF FATHERLY CARE WITHIN THE FAMILIES OF RECENT POLISH MALE MIGRANTS IN LONDON

The remainder of this chapter draws on data derived from twenty-two in-depth interviews conducted with recent Polish migrants in and around London in 2008–2009. Twenty of the interviews were with Polish men, and the remaining two were conducted with Polish women, both recent migrants to the United Kingdom; one was the wife and co-worker of one of the male participants, the other a co-worker. The majority (fourteen of twenty) of the men had arrived in the United Kingdom (although not necessarily for the first time) post-Accession. Of those, ten had had prior labour-migration experiences across 'Western' Europe. In this respect, there are resonances with the Central and Eastern European female migrants studied by Morokvasic (2004) who became 'settled in mobility' in order to secure family well-being. At the time of interview, six of the men's current stay in the United Kingdom pre-dated 2004. The majority of those had come in the years leading up to Accession, either on a tourist visa, but with the intention of staying longer than six months and finding work, or on a so-called 'self-employed' visa—a legal migration route to the United Kingdom for Accession-State nationals throughout the decade prior to EU enlargement, which Drinkwater, Eade and Garapich (2009) suggest had been especially popular with Polish citizens. For those with a pre-2004 experience of migration, irregularity was a common condition. At the time of interview, however, under the post-2004 migration regime in the United Kingdom for EU8 nationals, all were fully regular. The majority of men were uncertain about how long they would remain in the United Kingdom. This arose in part from the precarious economic conditions prevailing at the time of the interviews as a result of the economic recession that was taking hold in the United Kingdom. It also seemed to reflect the new potential for mobility offered by EU membership. As one father said:

> Who knows what will happen in a month, two or three? We are in the global village. The European Union gave us the possibilities to be everywhere at home. [Migrant Interviewee 09_father]

This father's sense of freedom in his mobility may be related to his stage in his family life cycle: He had three grown-up children, the eldest of whom were living in Poland and Ireland, and the youngest, a stepchild living with him in London, was seventeen years old. Other fathers, despite their desires, acknowledged constraints on their mobility, and these related predominantly to children's life stage and school career in particular.

As noted earlier, all of the Polish men interviewed were working in 'handyman services', and most defined themselves as self-employed.[9] Some of the migrants, enabled by English-language skills and a longer duration in the United Kingdom, had become owners of small handyman businesses, and reported earnings in the top 10 per cent of UK male earnings. Most of those interviewed, however, had earnings closer to the male median, and these were often achieved through multiple jobs demanding long hours. The men were mostly between ages twenty-five and forty-five years. They were equally divided between those who were fathers and those who were non-/not-yet-fathers. Although the following discussion draws predominantly on the interviews with fathers, the latter are included because not only did they offer valuable commentary on how their peers experienced migrant fatherhood, but their own migration stories were often bound up with future plans around family life and fatherhood.

## Migration/Family Arrangements

In their typology of caregiving arrangements within transnational families, Kilkey and Merla (2013) identify the potential for greater diversity in the spatial and temporal dimensions of the arrangements made by transnational families for their family life than tends to be captured in the global care chains and transnational families literatures. Their observation arises from recognition that both caregivers and care receivers can be migrants, that transnational families engage in both proximate and transnational caregiving, that care flows are multidirectional, that care relations are multigenerational and that caregiving roles and arrangements are dynamic across the life, family and migration cycles. Likewise, the migration/family arrangements of the Polish men interviewed evince considerable variability and dynamism and span almost the full set of arrangements identified in Kilkey and Merla's typology. At the time of interview, the fathers were distributed across three fathering situations—transnational fathers, migrant fathers with children present in the United Kingdom and migrant fathers with children both in the United Kingdom and 'back home'—although most had experience of more than one of those situations, highlighting the relevance of the concept of circularity to their caregiving arrangements. So, of the ten fathers interviewed, only one had arrived in the United Kingdom with any family members—his wife and child. Nine of the fathers had migrated alone, but reflecting the growing tendency for whole-family migration, five of those subsequently brought family members to the United Kingdom. This was usually staged—wife coming first, followed by children. During the period that both parents were in the United Kingdom, children were left in the care of grandmothers, usually maternal, who then went on to accompany children to the United Kingdom and/or visit for extended periods in order to provide care. For four of the fathers, there was no post-migration family reunification; all of those were already divorced before leaving for the United Kingdom, and their children tended to be older and were either independent of their parents and in the case of some had also migrated or were in the care of mothers. Of those four, however, three went on to build new families while living in the United Kingdom. Indeed, as is discussed below, post-migration family building was a common experience across all the fathers.

## Migration, Fathering and Breadwinning

In line with findings from survey data (Hobson and Fahlén 2009), the Polish men interviewed subscribed to an active hands-on fathering ideal and expressed a desire to be more involved and nurturing with their own children than their fathers had been with them. Thus, a father of four [Migrant Interviewee 19_father] commented, '[I]t's different, you know. I spend more time with the children. I give them more love. Definitely more love. I show more love to them because that's what I was missing'. His wife added immediately, '[Y]ou play with them'. That said, however, breadwinning was central to the Polish men's views of 'good fathering':

> A good dad is a person who above all puts the good of his family first and tries to guarantee them some kind of an existence, some kind of a good life, on a level, so that they never lack anything. (Migrant Interviewee 02_father)

As found in the study as a whole, the economic responsibilities of fathering were emphasised more by the Polish men than by the middle-class fathers whose households they worked in (Kilkey et al. 2013a; Perrons, Plomien and Kilkey 2010). That finding is not surprising given the poor economic circumstances that the former had experienced in Poland as a result of a combination of unemployment, low pay, job insecurity and an inadequate social safety net. Under such conditions, opportunities to be successful breadwinners were constrained:

> I was a mechanic and there wasn't much money for it. I was earning 200 zloty per week. Especially when the child was born, pampers, nappies were expensive because it cost sixty zloty for the nappies. Buying the nappies and some milk and my money was gone, you don't have enough. (Migrant Interviewee 10_father)

In this context, migration tended to be motivated by a desire to provide better for their families. For some of the fathers, the immediate challenge of 'making ends meet' dominated, whereas for others longer term goals, such as securing a *better education* or a *better future* for their children were emphasised; the latter was revealed by the one wife interviewed when she commented on the difficulties in Poland to be together with the children:

*Q:* Did you consider [father] going back to Poland instead of you coming over here.

*R:* No, we didn't even think about it because we couldn't afford it to be together. I mean, we could be together but to bring up children and secure their future, good education, school. (Wife of Migrant Interviewee 19)

The notion of migration as a 'sacrifice for the family' was present in accounts of a number of the men. Asked how he felt about his situation, one father, with children in Poland and the United Kingdom, commented:

'I don't really like England. In England I like the pound' (Migrant Interviewee 17_father). Those the men worked with spoke of the tendency of Polish migrants in London to compromise their own living standards in order to maximise remittances.

The successful breadwinning potentially secured through migration, however, could hold a meaning that went beyond the meeting of short- and long-term instrumental goals. Thus, for some of the men interviewed, it was intimately linked to the project of family building: 'We wanted to have another child and in Poland we couldn't afford it' (Migrant Interviewee 22_father). Interestingly, a number of non-/not-yet-fathers' plans for return to Poland were also bound up with the desire to start a family, but this could only be realised in the context of money saved during migration: 'I'm preparing a nest in Poland and I would like to go back. . . . I would like to go back in two years. In a few months I'm getting married. Then, we are going to think about children' (Migrant Interviewee 14_ non-/not-yet-father). Such plans highlight the importance of the life-course perspective bound up in the concept of circulation for understanding the care-migration relationship. Likewise, for those men whose children had remained in Poland temporarily, economic success in the United Kingdom was a precondition for family reunification, which among the study's respondents universally involved children and wives moving to London. Even for those whose position as transnational fathers seemed to be more permanent, material gain in the United Kingdom was seen as critical in facilitating contact with children: It allowed for the renting of more spacious accommodation, for example, so that children visiting from Poland could be hosted comfortably, and it enabled the fathers to make visits to Poland.

## Transnational Fathering Practices Beyond Breadwinning

Most of the fathers were or had spent a period or periods of time as transnational fathers, during which they undertook the various aspects of 'kin work'—'the work of keeping family links alive and creating a sense of family "togetherness" despite geographical separation' (Zontini 2004a, 1129)—that Zontini finds are utilised by transnational mothers, including remitting, sending gifts, transnational communications and reciprocal visits. As Baldassar (2008b) has argued, such actions help manage the emotions of missing and longing, which are common in transnational relationships by creating a sense of co-presence, which can be virtual (e.g., phone and email communications), proxy (e.g., gifts) or physical (e.g., visits).

And so it was, albeit to varying degrees, with the fathers in this study, even those whose children were grown up and those who had been living apart from their children prior to migration as a result of divorce. Thus, among the fathers, it was clear, for example, that the purpose of remitting could extend beyond economic support; it was also a means by which fathers could involve themselves in the everyday lives of their children and arguably fulfil other normatively prescribed fathering responsibilities, such as disciplinarian or role model of responsible breadwinner. Thus, in the month that he was interviewed, one father (Migrant Interviewee 09_father) had withheld his regular remittance to his seventeen-year-old son in Poland until his son opened a bank account. The father felt that putting the money in the bank would stop it 'burning a hole' in his son's pocket and help the son spend responsibly. The father expected the son to do this because this is how he manages his money. This and other such advice was communicated virtually via daily mobile phone conversations, or at least attempted ones, because the father reported that his son did not always answer. As other research documents (Portes, 2001; Wilding 2006), virtual communications have become easier and cheaper with the spread of ICTs, a development acknowledged by one father with prior migratory experiences: '[T]here was a time when from London to [name of town in eastern Poland] you had to call for four hours just to get through' (Migrant Interviewee 21_father). While a 'digital divide' exists between the United Kingdom and Poland (Eurostat 2010), this is not as great as in some other contexts (see Merla 2012a; Merla and Baldassar 2011), and fathers were adept at finding 'communication packages' that could accommodate disparities as is demonstrated by this father's arrangements:

> TalkTalk is a land line service you pay £21 a month and you get broadband [said in English and then in Polish] and phone. Up to 70 minutes is for free within the Union, the USA and Canada. I have a sister in Canada so I can call her and others, whoever I want to call. Not everyone has broadband but people in Poland have land lines. (Migrant Interviewee 09_father)

Poland and the United Kingdom are also comparatively close in terms of physical distance, and the more traditional sea/land option has been supplemented in the years following Accession by a rapid expansion in relatively cheap air travel between the two countries (Stenning and Dawley 2009), which facilitated reciprocal visits between fathers and children. So too has the post-2004 migration regime for Polish nationals in the United Kingdom: Fathers who had worked irregularly in the United Kingdom (and/or elsewhere) prior to 2004 spoke of how the risks associated with cross-border travel had disappeared, rendering them free to exchange visits with their children. Due to the children's ages, there was no need for physical hands-on care during visits; rather, fathers provided in person the advice and guidance that they undertook virtually outside of visits. Trips by teenagers to London also gave fathers the opportunity to contribute to widening their children's life experiences and could be conceived as part of a nurturing fathering role. The frequency and duration of visits varied considerably, however. Although the source of some of this appeared to lie in differences in the state of relations between fathers and children, or more commonly fathers and former partners, other factors were involved. In particular, a lack of money and/or time worked to constrain visits. Both problems were a product of the men's positioning in the UK labour market as predominantly self-employed service workers and had been exacerbated in the context of the economic downturn being experienced at the time of interviews.

While transnational fathers reported adopting a range of strategies to maintain ties with their children, fathers were not always satisfied with the quality of the relationships that ensued. For those (the majority) who had formed second families in the United Kingdom, there was a tendency to draw unfavourable comparisons with the quality of their relationships with children in Poland. Given the complexity of the family biographies, however, it is impossible to establish what independent role, if any, geographical distance plays in such perceived outcomes. Thus, divorce may have already loosened ties; the children in Poland were older than children in the United Kingdom, and men may approach second families with the benefit of experience and age, a situation found to contribute to different approaches to fathering (Kilkey and Clarke 2010). As Baldassar (2010b) has argued, emotions are also social phenomena, and those associated with migration must be understood within the 'culture of migration'. The public discourse in Poland around post-2004 migration has been largely negative, with contemporary labour migrants contrasted unfavourably with the political migrants of the post-World War II era (Garapich 2008). Migrating parents in particular have been subjected to criticism, with the term 'euro orphan' capturing the perceived social and moral costs of parental migration (Lutz 2010). Such public discourse did not escape the notice of the fathers in our study—'[A]t that time [2004] when parents left the country they were rubbish because they left the child' (Migrant Interviewee 19_father)—and may have contributed to framing their emotions around the effects on children left behind and their relationships with them (see Chapter 3, this volume). Those discourses and the emotions they engendered may have also contributed to the tendency observed in this study towards family reunification.

## CONCLUSION

Drawing on the framework of circulation as articulated by Baldassar and Merla (Part A, this volume), this chapter has sought to illuminate fatherly care in transnational families by examining the experiences of migrant men through a fathering lens. Parreñas (2008) has explained the paucity of research on transnational fathering in terms of the assumed normativity of father absence for breadwinning purposes. Yet the findings of the study reported in this chapter suggest that her explanation hinges on a rather unidimensional construction of fathering as synonymous only with breadwinning. Moreover, the findings add weight to McKay's (2010) argument that Parreñas's explanation also rests on a simplistic understanding of the breadwinning role, particularly in the context of migration and transnational family relations. Thus, the Polish men in this study, in line with a growing normative expectation and as reported by survey data on Polish fathers' preferences (Hobson and Fahlén 2009), expressed a commitment to a model of fathering that combined breadwinning with being involved with their children, both practically and emotionally. While their weak economic circumstances led them to place an emphasis on breadwinning, the meanings the fathers attached to breadwinning were reconfigured through migration and transnational family relations. Thus, successful breadwinning not only secured immediate and more long-term goals around financial security and children's well-being, it also facilitated more emotionally driven fathering projects, such as having more children and being able to be with children, by allowing for family reunification or reciprocal visits in the context of transnational fathering. Remitting, a key medium of caring and support in transnational relationships (see Chapter 11, this volume), provided a means of 'fashioning and refashioning meaningful social relations' (Zelizer 2005a, 223) between fathers and children separated by physical distance. In this way, the successful breadwinning facilitated by migration acted as a resource through which other fathering ideals could be *potentially* realised (cf. McKay 2010). While fathers were not always satisfied with the transnational relationships they had achieved with their children, it is impossible to establish from this particular study the degree to which this was a result of a fathering deficit in the maintenance of emotional attachments across distances. Further research with a more purposeful sampling strategy would therefore be useful, as would research that captured fathers' as well as children's accounts.

In being able to bring their children to live with them in the United Kingdom, as well as being free to cross borders in order to exchange visits, care was potentially more mobile and circular among these Polish fathers than might be the case among other nationalities in other migration scenarios. However, the precise arrangements made by Polish fathers and their families were diverse and dynamic, especially across the life course, serving to highlight the interplay between structures and agency in configuring migrant men's father-care arrangements. Moreover, what might be considered *counter*-circulatory forces were revealed, which also acted to mediate the circulation of care. These included the fathers' positioning as migrants in the UK labour market, and in particular their access to time and money. They also included, however, more individualised factors, such as the stage in the family life cycle and specifically the age of children as it was relevant to their education, as well as the quality of personal relationships. Thus, paralleling Kilkey and Merla's (2013) argument in relation to the choices transnational families have around their care arrangements, there is also a need to acknowledge the 'situatedness' of caregiving and the ensuing constraints on its circulation (see also Chapter 5, this volume).

## NOTES

1. I am grateful to Asuncion Fresnoza-Flot, Loretta Baldassar and Laura Merla for their helpful comments on an earlier draft of this chapter.
2. The study was funded by the Economic and Social Research Council (Grant RES-000–22–2590). Grant holders were Majella Kilkey and Diane Perrons, and the research officer was Ania Plomien (see Kilkey et al. 2013a for full details). I would like to acknowledge the contribution of Diane Perrons and Ania Plomien to the project while noting that they are not responsible for the arguments in this chapter.
3. See Hondagneu-Sotelo and Avila (1997) on recruitment of temporary (male) agricultural workers from Mexico by the United States under the Bracero Program (1942), which officially precluded family reunion; McDowell (2009) on the Baltic Cygnet scheme, a female-worker recruitment programme operating in Britain in the immediate post-World War II period, which was restricted to those without dependants; and Castles (2006) on the post-World War II 'temporary' guestworker systems in a number of European states, which made no provisions for dependants, whether the workers were male, female or married couples. As Castles notes, however, while the European guestworker systems formally sought to minimise family reunion, in practice it occurred and constituted one of the main sources of migration to Europe when the guestworker schemes ended (Böhning and Maillat 1974). Similarly, in the United States, 'temporary' Mexican agricultural workers eventually settled there, bringing family members from Mexico when the programme was ended and new rights were granted under the 1965 Immigration Act (Ramirez and Hondagneu-Sotelo 2009).
4. Cantú's (2009) research on men's migration experiences through the lens of sexuality provides a further example of research challenging the economistic paradigm of work on men and migration.
5. It is important to acknowledge, however, that not all migrations provide opportunities for male breadwinning.
6. I am not suggesting here that fathers' accounts should be privileged over children's. Rather, it is important to access both.
7. This is likely to be an underestimate because, as with all population surveys, the Labour Force Survey underrepresents migrants, especially recent migrants.
8. A short-hand term that refers to the eight Central and Eastern European countries that joined the EU in 2004.
9. It was often difficult, however, to establish from interviewees precise information on their employment status. The Trades Unions Congress in Britain (2008, 181–182) highlights a 'vast scale' of 'bogus self-employment' in the UK construction industry—workers 'classified as self-employed but in reality are dependent workers who do not have the independence and autonomy over their work that characterise genuine self-employment' and are without entitlement to basic employment rights.

Part D

# The Mobilities of Care as a Resource Within and Beyond Transnational Families

# 10 Care Circulation in Transnational Families

## Social and Cultural Capitals in Italian and Caribbean Migrant Communities in Britain

*Tracey Reynolds and Elisabetta Zontini*

## INTRODUCTION

Our chapter draws on our research of Italian and Caribbean migrant communities in Britain in order to investigate the interplay between care circulation (Part A, this volume) and social and cultural capitals in transnational family relationships. Our analysis highlights theories of cultural and social capital to show how care circulated in transnational families can be interpreted as a cultural and social resource. We begin our discussion showing how specific practices of circulated care among transnational families are linked to particular understandings of cultural identity. Within the context of social capital, we approach our understanding of care circulation as both an obligation and a resource—something that flows multidirectionally across countries and generations and also helps to maintain bridging and bonding networks across geographical and generational divides. Transnational care flows also provide individuals and family networks with cultural resources, which help strengthen their sense of belonging to their local, ethnic, diasporic and transnational communities. Thus, in the second part of our discussion, we adopt a Bourdieusian framework of cultural capital to examine the role that cultural capital plays in shaping the circulation of care amongst migrant families and their children (i.e., the second generation). In particular, we highlight ways in which the circulation of care establishes cultural capital and social mobility amongst particular migrant communities. We similarly assess how migrant and minority ethnic groups might be able to utilise their cultural capital as part of circulating care transnationally.

This chapter is based on our ongoing research of Caribbean and Italian families and communities based in Britain. The origins of the research stemmed from our work within the Families and Social Capital Research Group at London South Bank University in the United Kingdom. The group's work focused on the dynamics of family change and processes of social capital, paying particular attention to identities and values, trust and reciprocity and caring for and about. Our broad perspective on understanding transnational families led us to examine the lived experiences of family members scattered across national boundaries and the issues this raised about such matters as migration, identities, communities, resources and relationships in the contemporary world. The Caribbean project investigated processes of identity formation among Caribbean diasporic youth looking at how these young people utilise social capital resources within their family relationships and community networks. The material was collected through thirty in-depth interviews with second- and third-generation Caribbean young people and fifty kinship/family members in the United Kingdom and the Caribbean across all age groups. The Italian project explored various aspects of family life and social capital. These included the functioning of mutual and reciprocal relations related to care, the role of rituals and the formation of transnational identities. The material was collected through participant observation and fifty in-depth qualitative interviews in a number of sites in both the United Kingdom and Italy. Italians from the three main migration waves to the United Kingdom (pre-war, post-war and recent student and professional migrants) were interviewed, including first-generation migrants and their offspring. This research has developed into new projects that focus more specifically on specific stages of the life course, such as youth (Reynolds 2010a) and old age (Zontini 2012).

## CONTEXTUALISING CARE AMONGST MIGRANT COMMUNITIES

Baldassar and Merla's invitation to examine migrants' caring relationships, practices and exchanges through the lens of care circulation encouraged a re-reading of our original data. A key finding of our previous research was that care operates as a crucial social capital resource circulating within transnational families networks (Reynolds and Zontini 2007; Zontini and Reynolds 2007; Goulbourne et al. 2010). Yet to what extent can these care exchanges be said to represent a cultural resource in the lives of Caribbean and Italian families? The term 'cultural capital' is a way of conceptualising the tangible and intangible assets, benefits and resources that transnational families gain by investing and capitalising on cultural values, identity and norms that emerge within their family networks, and upon which they draw in circulating care as part of their everyday lives.

We understand care circulation as the 'reciprocal, multidirectional and asymmetrical exchange of care that fluctuates over the life-course within transnational family networks subject to the political, economic, cultural and social contexts of both sending and receiving societies' (Introduction, this volume) and as the everyday attempts of migrants to socially and emotionally bridge distance and reestablish proximity (Chapter 3, this volume). The interplay between care circulation as something that simultaneously occurs normally in geographically dispersed families and a process that is based on differentiated power relations, where it does not flow smoothly and evenly, is a theme we continue to return to throughout our analysis. Following Bonizzoni and Boccagni (Chapter 3, this volume), we pay particular attention to the diverse and often asymmetric ways in which care flows through distances, taking into account issues of gender, generation, class and geographical location.

Care circulation implies more than just the sending and receiving societies but pertains more widely across the transnational social field of our respondents, which might include more than two countries. By exploring a number of intra- and intergenerational relationships that get articulated across family life courses, our analysis moves away from a narrow focus on care that privileges exchanges between parents (especially mothers) and their children. The lens of care circulation and our discussion of cultural capital, and its relationship to social capital, draws attention to the way in which these inter- and intragenerational care exchanges are interpreted, offered, negotiated and accessed by migrants inhabiting a transnational social field. Migrants' participation in transnational caring exchanges also brings into focus the importance of family and social networks in shaping how they understand and experience ethnicity, cultural identity and belonging (Reynolds and Zontini 2006). Our previous research illuminates examples of how care circulation operates in practice. For instance, we observed that family members located in different countries are providers and recipients of care irrespective of their social and economic status. These care exchanges flow in a reciprocal and multidirectional manner. Family care circulates within generations and nations, but it also crosses these dimensions (Reynolds and Zontini 2007; Zontini and Reynolds 2007; see also Baldassar 2007b; Merla 2011, 2012a, 2012b).

The rich body of literature on the feminist ethics of care has also influenced our understanding of care circulation among Italian and Caribbean transnational families. In line with other feminist scholars, we differentiated between two forms of care exchange: caring about and caring for (Ackers and Stalford 2004; Finch and Groves 1983; Fisher and Tronto 1990). *Caring about* encompasses contact and emotional support and refers to emotional functions connected with sociability, advice, comfort and self-validation (Di Leonardo 1992). Examples of *caring about* activities we observed include providing small favours and money loans, communication by telephone, letters, e-mails, visits to give advice, support or just merely 'checking in'; participation in family decision making; and financing the purchase of care. *Caring for* refers to concrete, 'hands-on' caregiving on a personal level (Ackers and Stalford 2004; Finch and Groves 1983). Examples of caring for activities we noted included 'kin-keeping', domestic help such as childcare and financial assistance such as remittances; organising regular family meals (e.g., with married children and their families); family celebrations (such as birthdays, Christmas and Easter dinners);

regular visits 'home' (i.e., to the Caribbean and Italy); hosting kin in the United Kingdom; and gift-giving. It was noted in both of our studies that family members devote considerable time and energies to this despite the geographical distance.

The reciprocal caring exchanges operating between family members at transnational, intergenerational and intragenerational levels reveal the moral discourses informing their behaviour towards kin (Reynolds and Zontini 2006, 2007; see also Merla 2010). Individuals usually have a need to negotiate their caring relationships within these moral guidelines and according to particular contexts (Finch and Mason 1993; Williams 2004). Among the Caribbean and Italian migrants interviewed, we found that strong moral obligation and expectation towards care existed towards family members living in different nation-states. This moral obligation enabled the maintenance of caring roles and responsibilities across geographical borders. In many ways, this supports the earlier debates on transnationalism that interpreted migrants' need to keep up links and networks with their country of origin as a sign of their marginalisation and precarious position in their countries of settlement (Glick Schiller et al. 1992).

Aside from using the feminist ethics of care to differentiate forms of care provision, this care literature has been vital to us in moving our understanding of care beyond conventional models that characterise care as being one-directional and originating from a single source, flowing from a caregiver (the 'haves') to a care receiver (the 'haves not') (Ackers and Stalford 2004; Sevenhuijsen 2000). We reject a dependency model of care, which focuses exclusively on those dependent and in need of financial and personal assistance, such as, for example, children, young people, the elderly and those individuals experiencing ill health and socioeconomic disadvantage. Instead, the notion of care circulation allows us to view care as representing an ongoing human activity that places individuals in relations of interdependence with each other throughout their life course (Noddings 2003; Ruddick 1989; Tronto 1993; Sevenhuijsen 1998). We also saw the individuals involved in these transnational care exchanges as relational and interdependent rather than as the autonomous and free-floating subjects as suggested by individualisation theories that demarcate families as increasingly fragmented, fractured and dispersed (see Beck 1992; Beck and Beck-Gernsheim 2002; Irwin 1999; McRae 1997).

There is little evidence, furthermore, to suggest that family members are less involved in caring relationships as a result of growing individualism. Indeed, while individualism is a dominant aspect of Caribbean society and greater autonomy exists for individuals to choose their lifestyles, family forms and living arrangements, connections and responsibilities to family members are maintained (Goulbourne 2002; Reynolds 2004). One could argue that their relative success in sustaining their family connections and providing collective and individual responsibility for care within this individualised framework is because the individualised self is understood as relational to others within their networks. In contrast, in Italian and Southern European families, despite increased diversity in living arrangements, the individual is still understood as interconnected and interwoven into the family (Finch 1989b; Ginsborg 2003). Italian families in recent times have been going through structural changes, including the decline of the extended family households. While extended households are no longer as common in Southern Europe as they were, family members continue to live close to one another, maintaining important economic and emotional links (Vaiou1996; Zontini 2004b). Yet despite the apparent cultural differences concerning the ways in which this relationship between the individual and the family is articulated—Caribbean as relational and Italians as interconnected—we found commonalities in the way in which individuals from both ethnic groups are embedded in webs of personal relationships and care provision, which represented an important social capital resource for connecting and relating to other kinship members.

## SOCIAL CAPITAL AND CARE CIRCULATION

As indicated above, migrants inhabit a transnational social field, and consequently the way in which transnational families circulate care takes places within this field. This reference to the term 'social field' is especially influenced by the work of Pierre Bourdieu and his idea that society comprises a plurality of social fields. Bourdieu's claim is that the position and possibilities of the various actors and individuals in any field are determined by the various forms and proportion of capital they possess within each social field. Capital (social, cultural, economic, symbolic) here refers to the variety of resources, tangible and intangible, available to individuals that lead to the development and extension of 'habitus' and give access to power and influence. Bourdieu's notions of social field, capital and habitus allow us to conceptualise how different types of cultural identity and values are formed and come to influence how we understand and act in the world (Connelly 1998). Bourdieu's (1986) writing on social capital addresses the formation and durability of ties and networks, and it acknowledges that the value of individuals' ties depends on the number of connections they can mobilise and the quantity of capital possessed by each connection. His discussion of the interplay between social and cultural capitals emphasises the way in which cultural capital gives access to what is seen as actual or potential social assets and resources within particular communities (Barron 2011). It is also used to explain entrenched forms of societal inequality, particularly how this interplay between the two forms of capitals give rise to the reproduction of social class divisions and social class hierarchy in society and, under appropriate conditions, is transmitted from one generation to the next (Lareau and Weininger 2003).

Writing around the same period on social capital, the American sociologists James Coleman (1990) and Robert Putnam (1993) became highly influential in this study area. In our previous work, we reviewed at length some of the main debates by Coleman and Putnam (see Evergeti and Zontini 2006; Goulbourne et al. 2010; Zontini 2004b, 2006, 2010; Reynolds 2004, 2006, 2010a), and so what follows is a brief overview of this work. For Coleman, social capital is generated in the family. He stresses the importance of closure of social networks for the creation and maintenance of social capital, which in his view allows the emergence of norms and increases the level of trust among the members of the network. Social capital is therefore embedded in family and community relations because it creates an expectation of obligations and mutually beneficial relationships that are based on a normative expectation of mutual obligation and reciprocity for its members (Edwards et al. 2003; Barron 2011). What distinguishes Putnam's position from that of Coleman is that, whereas the latter is interested in social capital for the generation of human capital, Putnam's interest lies in the impact of social capital for democracy and economic prosperity. For Putnam, social capital is a public good that is generated in the community and not in specific families. In his definition, social capital refers to 'features of social organizations, such as networks, norms and trust, which facilitate action and co-operation for mutual benefit' (Putnam et al. 1993, 35). Social capital is differentiated according to its capacity for 'bridging' (relationships and networks of trust and reciprocity between different groups and communities; outward looking) or 'bonding' (relationships and networks of trust and reciprocity that reinforce bonds and connections within groups; inward looking).

Studies drawing on social capital in relation to transnational families highlight that similar networks of trust and reciprocity and civic participation are not constrained by geographic boundaries and can cross geographical neighbourhoods and nation-states (see also Levitt 2001; Bryceson and Vuerola 2002b; Goulbourne and Solomos 2003; Reynolds 2006; Anthias 2007; Ryan et al. 2008; Zontini 2010; Baldassar et al. 2007; Merla 2012b). These studies of migrant families embedded within transnational social fields provide various examples of the diverse forms of social capital generated across ethnic and migrant groups. Perhaps the most significant aspect of such studies is that they bring to the fore the qualitative and temporal experience of migrants in relation to social capital, as well as highlighting racial-ethnic, gender and class power relations in the construction and use of social networks, which in the past have received insufficient attention.

By and large, many of the studies on transnational families demonstrate positive social capital and positive care circulation between family members (see Goulbourne et al. 2010; Merla 2011, 2012a). However, it is also important to highlight some of the more negative implications of social capital, which present a challenge to the assumption that transnational families live in harmony and only participate in pleasurable exchanges of care. Negative emotions are connected with care exchanges, which include anxiety, hurt, feelings of disrespect and guilt (see Merla 2010; Baldassar 2007b). Many of the negative feelings that were reported to us by participants originated, on the one hand, from families struggling to cling to particular family practices and expectations and, on the other hand, from the mismatch between the ideal family and the reality of everyday family life. The issue of the gender division of labour was a source of tensions and conflict within families, which also exacerbated underlying intergenerational conflicts. Some second-generation women resented the particular gender division of care work that they associated with Italian families and resented their parents' defence of these practices. Young women felt that their families' protection and support was often a double-edge sword as those giving support wanted to influence the choices of those receiving it and that support was linked to obligations and adherence to shared norms and values (see De Tona 2011). Some of our interviewees discovered through their experiences that departing from such expectations would result in a decline in support. These strong and often tense relationships of dependence especially between mothers and daughters occurred both locally and transnationally (Goulbourne et al. 2010; Zontini 2010).

Most of our interviewees also struggled to reconcile the ideal Italian family with the reality of their everyday family life. This centred in particular around unmet expectations that resulted when family members had different and in some cases conflicting expectations of their duties and when families failed to achieve the highly valued togetherness despite the *sacrifici* undertook to this end. This happened, for instance, when migrants' offspring chose to move elsewhere for work or study or when families realised that return migration was not going to occur. Linked to this, we identified the feeling of guilt, which accompanied the experiences of several of our interviewees. For first-generation migrants, it was associated with having left the home of origin and therefore not being able to be near and caring for ageing parents, for their offspring the guilt arose from having failed their parents in their expectations that in old age they would be looked after at home. For Caribbean families, much of the alienation came from the pressures to conform to group norms and live up to cultural expectations of a Caribbean identity. Relationships with family and friends contributed to shape the processes of ethnic identity formation and interviewees' fear of being excluded and alienated if they did not conformed to what they perceived as culturally accepted practices (see Goulbourne et al. 2010). Pressures to conform to particular family or cultural practices, the unequal distribution of care work across the transnational social field, especially by gender, and the unequal power dynamics generated by care circulation were found in the experiences of both groups studied and should be taken into account alongside more positive interpretations of transnational families.

What is clear from our study of transnational families, using Caribbean and Italian migrants as our case studies, is that individuals are enmeshed in interpersonal networks, which constitute (positive and negative) points of connections in the way that they circulate care as part of their everyday lives. Yet the question of how these care exchanges are experienced as cultural assets that may be valued in the family, ethnic community or wider society is a relatively under-researched area. The choices and decisions individuals make in life are influenced by 'habitus' and the existing social networks to which they have access. According to Bourdieu, an individual's 'habitus' is a structured set of values and ways of thinking that is built up over time, usually from the family, through socialisation of culture and traditions. Cultural symbols become markers of distinction, both signalling and constituting individuals' position in the social structure (Field 2008).

## CARE CIRCULATION AS CULTURAL RESOURCES

Bourdieu's work on cultural capital has been most widely applied to the debates around schooling and education. However, the application of this concept has been expanded on and updated to include diverse social fields, such as migration and migrant communities in recent years. In our analysis, we adopt a Bourdieusian notion of cultural capital to examine the care exchanges of migrant and ethnic minority communities in two ways. First, we highlight the perpetual inequality experienced by some migrant and minority ethnic groups in terms of the resources they have to access and provide care at formal and informal levels. For instance, our individual studies addressing social care amongst migrant elders suggest that there is systematic inequality in care circulation at the level of formalised state care provision. As a result, they tend to prefer accessing care resources provided by family and ethnic-specific community associations or networks in far greater numbers than white UK elders. We also suggest that a key factor in why these elderly migrants experience inequality of access to more formal institutionalised care is that, compared to white UK elders from a middle-class background, they are not so imbued with the appropriate social connections, embodied cultural capital or 'habitus' that encourage them to more confidently access care within this field (Reynolds 2012b; Zontini Forthcoming).

In the following section, we apply Bourdieu's ideas concerning cultural capital to highlight issues of the cultural identity amongst migrants and the relational mores, norms, values and ties they draw on to circulate care. This concept has particular resonance with researchers in the field of migration studies. For instance, Vertovec (2009, 67) talks of *bifocal habitus* and *transnational habitus* as a particular dual frame of reference through which migrants constantly compare their situation in the 'home' country with that of the 'host one'. Similarly, Weenink (2008) also refers to the term 'cosmopolitan habitus' in his study exploring how parents construct and perceive cultural capital for their children attending internationalised educational settings. Research by Erel (2010, 644) exploring cultural capital amongst Turkish and Kurdish migrant women in Britain and Germany focuses on the notion of *converting cultural capital* to highlight processes of adapting and applying the meanings, knowledge, customs, achievements and outlooks that migrant families bring to new environments in order to enhance individuals' mobility in particular social settings. These and other studies (e.g., Weine et al. 2004) investigating migrant communities and cultural capital offer an important corrective to the taken-for-granted assumption that migrant and minority ethnic communities are lacking in cultural capital.

Applying a care circulation framework to our research findings points to the existence of cultural capital within Caribbean and Italian families. We recognise that the cultural capital valued in these families and migrant groups may have little value in wider society and among the white UK majority because how cultural capital is valued depends on the social field it is located within. Yet our research suggests that individual family networks are in possession of cultural capital because they are able to generate, mobilise and access resources, tangible and intangible, to successfully bridge the cultural barriers of host and migrant communities and achieve success and inter- and intragenerational social mobility. In our analysis of Caribbean and Italian families, we are not interested in simply measuring or differentiating levels of cultural capital across these ethnic groups. Rather, using the lens of care circulation, we focus our understanding on how care resources circulated and developed within the social capital networks of transnational families and community (re)produce cultural capital amongst these migrants. We then attempt to shed light on the various ways in which those individuals in possession of cultural capital are able to better circulate care resources within their networks, further increasing the social assets and social capital of group members.

With this objective in mind, we observed that cultural signifiers—the obvious markers being food, language, regional and ethnic pride—represent an essential part of the emotional process of 'caring about' and the emotional functions connected with sociability, comfort, self-validation and belonging. Cultural signifiers, which are legitimatised by group members and individuals, are converted into cultural capital as a result of the care circulated amongst family members. In the Italian context, a legitimised cultural signifier would be the ideal of the 'normative Italian family' and the cultural values associated with this: co-operative, solidarised, interdependent and reciprocal units (Baldassar and Gabaccia 2011). The ideal of the 'normative Italian family' can be utilised as an ethnic resource to pool labour. For instance, if we look historically at the Italians of first- and second-migration waves, during the pre-war and 1945 post-war period, with limited access to higher educational qualifications, we could see that some enjoyed a certain degree of economic success in the catering trade. Italian migrants were able to open ethnic stores, restaurants, coffee shops and ice-cream bars (Zontini 2004b). This was largely achieved because of the cohesion of their families. As Palmer (1977, 251) explains, 'their production is only made possible by the mobilisation of family labour, with everyone working long hours'. These Italians were successful in trading on their ethnicity, not only by selling 'ethnic' products but also by turning specific family values into economic success (Colpi 1991). Such cultural values of the 'normative Italian family' as being co-operative, solidarised, interdependent and reciprocal units, utilised as an ethnic resource to pool labour, arguably contributed to the social mobility and economic capital of some Italian individuals and family networks, enabling some to enjoy a 'bi-focal' habitus, although social mobility for the ethnic group as a whole was restricted.

The Rossi family exemplifies this well. Mr Rossi migrated in the late 1950s to become a factory worker in a town in central England. He later was joined by his wife, who also became employed in the textile industry. They had three children. The couple was working in alternate shifts in order to be able to look after the children and work full time so as to maximise savings. They hardly spent any money except for the annual trip to Italy back to their village of origin. All of their children enjoyed travelling to Italy, and contrary to other so-called second-generation youth, they learned Italian well and grew up bilingual. Five years ago, Tommaso, Mr. Rossi's youngest son, opened his Italian café. He was able to do so thanks to the capital donated by his parents who gave him part of their life savings. He also modelled the business on the cafes he saw in Italy during his frequent trips. Some of the products he sells arrive directly from Italy through some of his friends and relatives there. Tommaso and his siblings regularly visit Italy, particularly around the time of the village festival. They have acquired a 'bi-focal habitus' that allow them to navigate different national fields and acquire new useful resources, such as language skills and knowledge about what is fashionable in terms of food and drink in contemporary Italy. With his earnings, he is now able to give something back to his parents. At the time of the last interview, he was planning a surprise trip to Italy with his parents. He wanted to take them on a vacation to Rome since he felt that they never travelled much beyond their village of origin.

Another example is that of the knife grinders from Northern Italy. Their migration histories go back more than one hundred years when they started to carry out their itinerant work as far as the United Kingdom and the United States. Initially, women stayed behind looking after children and elderly people. Eventually they settled abroad, with women continuing to perform caring work, this time in the countries of immigration, where they cooked and hosted the recently arrived villagers as well as their own families. While abroad they kept strong kin and village ties with each other in the diaspora as well as with the village back in Italy. In the United Kingdom, they passed on this specialised artisanal skill down the generations while modernising their activities. Some of those interviewed today have achieved upward social mobility and now own highly mechanised workshops that serve top hotels and restaurants throughout London.

It could be similarly argued that the offspring of Caribbean migrants (second and third generation) to a far lesser extent have been able to utilise the strong ethnic-specific bonding ties, most closely associated with the black neighbourhood and related notions of ethnic belonging, identity and affinity to carve out ethnic-specific employment opportunities and social enterprise initiatives within these locales. Following on from Caribbean mass migration to Britain during the post- World War II period and settlement across several towns and cities, including London, Birmingham and Manchester, the term 'black neighbourhoods' was coined to reflect the way in which these urban spaces acted as critical sites of struggle and resistance for black community members responding to racial discriminatory practices (Goulbourne 1989).[1] Community bonds in such neighbourhoods created opportunities for the development of day-to-day strategies and networks of survival and self-reliance. An essential survival strategy included establishing a vast array of ethnic-specific public service and community sectors in order to serve the community and provide a range of welfare care services for the most vulnerable of its community members. These include black supplementary schools, black housing associations and black mental health organisations amongst others (Reynolds 2012a). Many individuals employed in such organisations speak of being influenced by a strong desire to provide care and public service for their community and sharing a cultural affinity with group members. However, we also suggest that individuals participating in such Caribbean (or black) community services have been able to translate collectivised notions of affinity and 'caring about' community members into individual opportunities for social mobility and career progression.

Such is the case of Kim and Maureen Vincent, two sisters of first-generation Caribbean migrants, who left Barbados in the early 1960s and settled in Kennington, South London. Kim and Marie strategically utilised their bridging and bonding social capital networks of the black welfare-based community organisations they worked in to rapidly progress the career ladder and secure senior/middle management posts, which otherwise would not have been so readily available to them in mainstream welfare services providing care. Kim is the managing director of one of the larger black housing associations in London, and Marie is a manager of a day centre that provides a range of services catering for children, young people, parents and the elderly residents located within a 'black neighbourhood' with longstanding patterns of Caribbean settlement and that is poorly resourced with high indices of poverty and deprivation. Both sisters have utilised their professional networks in the United Kingdom to set up a charitable youth organisation in Barbados, which is their parents' country of residence and where they still continue to have strong family connections. Marie, in particular, regularly visits 'home' to undertake charitable and fundraising activities for this organisation. One of the consequences of this work is that they have been able to establish contacts with, and patronage from, wealthy and influential members of industry and popular culture in the United States, Canada and Britain.

The strategic utilisation of language and intercultural skills represents a further example of how affinity to ethnic and cultural identity may be translated into a form of cultural capital for second- and third-generation migrants. Richard Alba's (2005) study on boundary processes amongst immigrant groups is especially pertinent here because it highlights how language draws a 'bright'[2] ethnic boundary between the majority and migrant populations. While being bilingual in certain 'minority' or homeland languages reinforces difference and distance between the migrants and majority populations, those second- and third-generation migrants who are able to speak fluently in high-prestige European languages (French, German and Spanish) can regard this ability to do so as a cultural asset, facilitating their integration into mainstream culture. We further suggest, however, that young people with proficiency in 'minority' languages have utilised this as a cultural resource within the profession of social care. A few of our second- and third-generation migrants who were bilingual in English and their native tongue or other languages discussed how they have strategically employed and manipulated these linguistic skills in order to secure employment opportunities and get on in society. These migrants' language and intercultural skills provided translating and interpreting employment opportunities within care and public services agencies (e.g., departments within the National Health Service, local authority social service departments and the police force) that regularly deal with individuals from migrant communities with limited proficiency in the English language.

The following case study of Guliana, a second-generation Italian, offers us some insight into the way in which migrants who maintain strong kinship networks within their homeland are able to utilise their bilingual language skills in order to create employment opportunities for themselves. Giuliana, who was born in the United Kingdom and is in her mid-forties, maintained strong networks in the village where both her parents came from, and she has visited this Italian village throughout her life. Giuliana is employed by a local county council as a welfare rights officer. This post was funded by the Italian government to provide advice and services to Italian nationals in the United Kingdom. In this role, Giuliana is able to successfully utilise both her knowledge of the UK welfare system and her bilingual skills. A further benefit, which can be viewed as a cultural asset, is that Giuliana is from the same community (in terms of parents' village of origin) in which she is serving. This is particularly important because many of the elderly Italian service users are distrustful of public officials. However, they feel safe to talk to Guliana because they know her and her family background. These Italian elders access informal advice from Giuliana about formalised and institutionalised state welfare care provision. As a result of Giuliana's ability to bridge these two worlds, and the way in which she is able to utilise her bilingual skills and knowledge of the homeland to establish rapport and trust relationships with the Italian community members, she was recently appointed as the new chairperson of the Association of Elderly Italians. This voluntary role is afforded high status within the community she serves.

Arguably, having multi/bilingual skills is important in a globalised and transnational world. Migrant parents or kin who provide their children with these language skills could be said to be undertaking an important 'caring for' task. Our analysis suggests that migrant individuals who are bi/multilingual are able to translate this into a cultural capital resource because, in contrast to non-foreign language English-speaking people, they can seek out employment opportunities where speaking a second language is an essential requirement of the job. The next example of Adrienne, a second-generation Caribbean with parents originating from Guyana and Martinique who is fluent in French, provides an example of how she has used her bilingual skills for career enhancement and social mobility. Adrienne is a senior analyst in a major international bank. Adrienne is one of only a few women who have reached this relatively senior position and the only individual from a minority ethnic background. Adrienne directly attributes her career progression and success to her language skills. She comments:

> We deal with a lot of international clients and what gives me an edge over my team-mates is that I can speak French fluently, not the French that they teach in the classroom but the real native French. My mum raised us to speak French [. . .] I can't remember learning to speak French, it is just something I do, like speaking English. I didn't realise it could work to my advantage [. . .] it has worked out that way. [. . .] In this industry we meet a lot of international clients and lots of them feel more comfortable discussing business in French. The clients will ask for me because sharing the language it easier to establish a good relationship with them. I've built a pretty impressive business portfolio having a second language [. . .] in this industry its becoming pretty mandatory that you have a second language if you want to build your client base and progress up the company ladder.

Our third example similarly builds on the theme of parents' developing bilingual skills in their children with the intention of creating better life opportunities for them. Marcella is a second-generation migrant of Italian origin with two sons. During the interview, Marcella described how her children benefitted from the language skills that they learned as part of their transnational family life. Although her sons were born in Italy, they came to live in the United Kingdom as children with their mother after Marcella and her husband divorced. Despite the acrimonious relationship with the ex-husband that followed the divorce, Marcella still continued to regularly take her children to visit their father and his family in Italy throughout their childhood. As a result, her children have grown up to be bilingual in Italian and English. Today, both of her children are studying languages at one of the most prestigious universities in the United Kingdom, which she credits to them gaining these important language skills as children.

With the examples we present above, we do not mean to suggest that migrants only acquire cultural capital in their country of residence. Many migrants are already in possession of cultural capital that originated in their homeland. However, this is transformed and negotiated as a consequence of migration and settlement in the United Kingdom, and this negotiation process shapes their care flows. In relation to 'caring for' tasks and practices, we found complex negotiations occurring in families and Italian and Caribbean local community organisations concerning kinship responsibilities for caring. Often these negotiations are both explicit and implicit and involve a range of interconnected factors including professional or educational status within the family/community, social class, age, gender and so on. In both family and community, we observed the existence of 'key players' who control the access and level of care provision for its members. In terms of family, we identified that those with high-income professional backgrounds and also those with expertise or currently working in the social care sector were able to acquire additional levels of care resources for family members. In such instances, these individuals' cultural capital, alongside economic capital, enabled them to provide 'caring for' resources, such as domestic assistance, where required. Sometimes it was simply a matter of having the economic capital to purchase care provision. However, in most instances, individuals' cultural capital meant that they had 'insider knowledge' about services and a 'habitus' that gave them confidence to not only access particular forms of care networks but also to tap into a wide array of institutional care provisions and communicate with the related health and social care professionals. Jennifer, a second-generation Caribbean who is a day-centre manager at a community care organisation providing services for African Caribbean older people, comments:

> The Government is moving more towards individualised and personalised care agendas which in theory should give elders and their carers more say in the care services received. I have been trained in person support planning and I use these person-centred planning tools when working together with an older person attending the centre. I have the networks and partnerships with statutory and voluntary organisations so that if I don't know something I know who to go to, to find out this information pretty quickly but lots of people would not have the first clue about where to begin planning for their care in later life.

In some cases, accessing particular forms of care was extended to care provision for family members in the homeland. This was particularly the case in caring for sick or elderly parents or significant kin members who were left back home following migration or who had returned back home after living many years in Britain to live out their final years. Generally speaking, we observed that the greater level of social and cultural capital individuals possessed, the greater level of care was obtained for their sick or elderly parents or kin.

With regard to care provision taking place within ethnic-specific community associations, we observed that hierarchal structures existed. At the top of the structure were group-appointed representatives, viewed as having cultural capital, within the particular group that acted as 'cultural mediators' and 'cultural gatekeepers'. These representatives provided an important function in terms of establishing bridging with social care professionals and inter-ethnic networks to generate further resources for the group. However, in this role, they also controlled the group members' access to care resources, as the following case study suggests.

Mr. Giacometti is the president of a centre for elderly Italians. In this role, he is responsible for organising the activities of the centre, keeping accounts of the membership fees and liaising with external organisations such as the local authority. The centre is important for those who attend its weekly meetings. However, it is also a place where subtle exclusions operate based on hierarchies of gender, status and respectability. The space there is gendered and also hierarchical. Men and women sit at different tables. Men play cards, and the women are divided into those who play bingo and those who sit at the periphery of the group and chat. There is a separate table where the male committee members and the chairperson sit talking about 'important' issues to do with the running of the group. Women do not know anything about what the committee discusses and decides because there are no women on it. Some elders felt excluded from the inner circles that develop at the group and stopped attending. They also resented the gossip and the social control. On the whole, however, they are positive places for the elders that attend them, giving them a sense of purpose and community (Zontini 2012).

Increasingly, however, new media are impacting on established power dynamics and inter/intrageneral family and community relations. Many of our younger (second- and third-generation) participants were increasingly utilising these new technologies as cultural assets in their 'caring about' activities with kin members. For example, they would regularly use new media—such as Skype, instant messaging, social networking sites and other Internet- and mobile phone–based platforms—to keep in touch and to maintain the emotional and intimate connections with family members living across distances and nation-states. In this role, younger migrants are transforming practices of intimacy across distance and encouraging the development of lateral kin relationships (e.g., among cousins) that otherwise might have been lost. By drawing on digital technologies in their 'caring about' and 'caring for' exchanges, younger migrants were increasingly bypassing the traditional kin-keeping role of the older generation. Directing care exchanges through new media by controlling the flow of information between families created for young migrants a potential source of cultural capital (see also Baldassar 2010a; Baldassar 2011). In our related work exploring second-generation 'return' migration among Caribbean and Italian young adults, we similarly noted that digital technologies represented an important return migration strategy, in terms of influencing the decision to (re)migrate and putting practical plans in place to facilitate the 'return' to the homeland (e.g., using Skype, instant messaging and e-mails to search for employment opportunities, conduct job interviews and project manage the building/purchasing of property) (Reynolds 2010b; Goulbourne et al. 2010).

The growing body of research investigating the role of new media and digital technologies on transnational kinship ties certainly supports our data. Heather Horst and Daniel Miller (2006) identify that migrant young people are at the forefront of the use of new technologies in terms of creating new meanings for how people live transnationally and how family members in different nation-states keep in touch. New media change transnational movements from the actual to the virtual and change how people imagine and belong to their home and host countries (Miller 2011), with diasporic youth utilising a range of new media to maintain symbolic relationships within a particular locality, as well as intergenerational and 'caring about' exchanges (Reynolds and Zontini 2006). This point is most eloquently expressed in Madianou and Miller's (2012) study of Filipino mothers separated from their children. These authors argue that parenting relationships, and the way in which care is circulated between them, are dependent on the media itself, especially for mothers who spend many years separated from their children. Yet the mothers' and children's opinions differed regarding the use of technology. Whereas mothers felt that new media allowed them to carry out their mothering role and caring tasks, the children in contrast were more skeptical, feeling in some instances that mothers were becoming overinvolved using this media to control them from afar. Based on this evidence, one can arguably suggest that care circulated between transnational kin members is transformed because of the new media, but crucially this technology also sustains these relationships and, as such, represents a valuable cultural resource in mediating care flows within transnational kinship networks.

## CONCLUSION

In our chapter we attempt to investigate the interplay between social and cultural capitals in the circulation of care in transnational family relationships.

For us this is a new and relatively unexplored area of analysis because our previous work has primarily focused on social capital produced and resulting from the transnational kinship ties of migrant families. In our discussion, we move away from the general consensus concerning cultural capital and migrant communities, which tends to position migrant communities as being in deficit in cultural capital or undertaking a 'rucksack approach' (Erel 2010), whereby individual migrants arrive with cultural resources that either fit or do not fit in their country of destination. Through the lens of care circulation and drawing principally on case studies of Caribbean and Italian migrants and their transnational family networks, we start to map out a framework for examining the complex interplay of gender, ethnicity, language, generation, socioeconomic status and migration status in determining the level and form of social and cultural capitals that are generated, accessed and mobilised by individuals within transnational care flows.

What our analysis does confirm is that the care circulated represents an important social and cultural resource for transnational families, mediating their relationships, reproducing kinship ties and generating for them cultural identity and a sense of belonging to families and communities spanning different generations and nation-states. The care circulated and (re)produced in caring for and caring about transnational families creates cultural capital and social mobility for individual family members to varying degrees, but we show that this is very much contingent on their ethnicity, gender, migration history and language skills, among other factors. We also highlight how individuals' cultural capital is utilised, through the transnational care circulated, to benefit and generate additional resources for their kin and ethnic group members. Finally, we identify that new media and digital technologies have created significant changes in the way in which care is circulated among family members, not only in terms of who controls the flows and direction of these care exchanges but also the nature by which hierarchy and structure are established and maintained in transnational family relationships.

## NOTES

1. For example, in the South London neighbourhood of Brixton, which is arguably viewed as the historical 'capital of Black Britain', the large concentration of a Black Caribbean population facilitated political organising and protest.
2. Alba's (2005) discussion of the nature of the ethnic boundary experienced by immigrant groups in the United States and European nations draws a distinction between 'bright' and 'blurred' boundaries. The former is unambiguous (e.g., citizenship). Individuals know exactly what side of the boundaries they are on, and the issue of exclusion/inclusion is sharply brought into focus. The latter, in contrast, is a much more temporal, porous and ambiguous location (e.g., religion and language), whereby cultural elements of the immigrant groups are incorporated into the majority culture.

# 11 'Boomerang Remittances' and the Circulation of Care

## A Study of Indian Transnational Families in Australia

*Supriya Singh and Anuja Cabraal*

## INTRODUCTION

An estimated 215 million people across the globe migrated in 2010 (Swing 2010). As people move, nuclear and extended families splinter across national borders. In Australia, roughly half of Australia's population is migrant or the Australian-born child of a migrant (Hugo 2012a) and so in some measure belong to a transnational family. However, transnational families are studied most often within the frameworks of migration rather than family studies. This is partly because in the West, as Bryceson and Vuorela (2002a, 28) note, 'there has been a tendency to make the family synonymous with the household. . . . This conflation . . . would woefully fail to capture the composition and structure of transnational families'. The focus on the couple in the West, rather than the family, also contributes to this neglect of the transnational family (Singh 1997).

In this chapter, we use the term 'transnational family' broadly to include the family members who have migrated and those who have been left behind (Baldassar, Baldock and Wilding 2007). Although these transnational families are separated by distance and national borders, as Bryceson and Vuorela (2002a, 3) note, they 'hold together and create something that can be seen as a feeling of collective welfare and unity, namely "familyhood", even across national borders'. Most often, the transnational family has been studied as if it were in two parts—in the countries of origin and destination. With 'twice or thrice migrants' (Bhachu 1995), that is, people whose family and personal histories include more than one migration, the transnational family can stretch across several national boundaries.

Although migration creates transnational families, these families share much with families in general and families separated by distance in particular. There is the same need for negotiation and reciprocity (Finch 2007). The transnational family differs from families separated by distance, in that the transnational family has to overcome distance as well as different state regimes related to passports, workforce regulations, residence, education and health care (Kilkey and Merla 2013; Chapter 5, this volume). The transnational family, as with all other kinds of families, has a developmental cycle, which changes with life stage (Yeoh, Huang and Lam 2005). Family practices over life stage and generation display a sense of being part of the family. As Finch (2007, 67) says,

> Display is the process by which individuals, and groups of individuals, convey to each other and to relevant audiences that . . . their actions do constitute 'doing family things' and thereby confirm that these relationships are 'family' relationships.

In transnational families, in the absence of face-to-face interaction, the need to display care is greater. Work by Baldassar (2007a) and Baldassar, Baldock and Wilding (2007) has brought frameworks of two-way care to the forefront of the study of the transnational family. Drawing on comparative studies of care in transnational families, Baldassar (2008a, 271) argues

> that all family caregiving is mediated by a dialectic comprising the capacity (ability, opportunity), the culturally informed sense of obligation and the negotiated family commitments of individual members to provide care within specific family networks . . . these practices are largely organised by the structures of kinship and community, in particular the sense of obligation to engage in reciprocal care exchanges.

These frameworks concentrate on the care that 'circulates' (Part A, this volume) between transnational families, rather than the 'global care chains' that typically involve a female migrant domestic worker being paid to look after children of the employer's family while her children are cared for by older children or the extended family (Yeates 2005a).

## INDIAN TRANSNATIONAL FAMILIES IN AUSTRALIA

In this chapter, we report on research about three groups of Indian migrants in Australia—first-generation migrants who arrived between the 1970s and 1990s, the second generation who were born in Australia or migrated before they were 12 years old and Indian students who came to study in 2005 or later with a view to migration. We compare and contrast the different ways they display care in the transnational family, with a particular focus on remittances.

Our research draws on eighty-six open-ended interviews with people from the Indian diaspora in Australia conducted between May 2005 and March 2010. The study began with interviews with eighteen first-generation migrants between 2005 and 2010. Most were professionals, representing a mix of direct migrants from India and 'twice or thrice migrants' who had migrated from India to Malaysia, Singapore, Kenya, Fiji or the United Kingdom, and then to Australia. There were an equal number of men and women and varied across religions.

We then explored migration experiences amongst twenty second-generation Indian Australians between 2009 and 2010, focusing on issues of identity and belonging. All of them were university students or professionals. There were thirteen women and seven men, mostly single, eighteen to thirty-nine years old. We also interviewed Indian international students and community leaders between 2009 and 2010, when there were incidents of racist violence towards Indian students in Melbourne (Singh 2011a). Our students, as with the Indian students in Melbourne, were predominantly from Punjab, between eighteen and twenty-nine years old, male, middle class and from regional cities, towns and villages. They were Sikh, Hindu and Christian. There was a lack of Muslim representation. We asked students about their continuing connections with family and their migration experience in Australia with a particular focus on racism. Community leaders were mainly drawn from Sikh, Hindu, Christian and Muslim organisations and were asked about the kind of support they offered to Indian students. The approach to the research was that of grounded theory. The interviews were analysed with the help of N8, a program for the analysis of qualitative data.

In this chapter, we compare these three groups in the Indian diaspora in Australia, showing that the perception and experience of the circulation of care differs with migration experience. The first generation felt the caring went mostly one way from Australia to their transnational families, through remittances, telephone calls and visits. In contrast, the Indian students experienced money and care as primarily flowing from India to Australia. In time, money and care also went back to India. The second generation stood apart as their immediate family resided in Australia. Most had little connection with their extended family in India. In the few cases where there was a meaningful relationship, the relationship had to be reciprocal for it to exist at all.

## REMITTANCES AS A MEDIUM OF CARE

We have found it useful to use Fisher and Tronto's (1990) distinction between 'caring about', 'taking care', 'caregiving' and 'care receiving' to distinguish different dimensions of care in our empirical study of care in the transnational family. They say 'Caring about involves paying attention to our world in such a way that we focus on continuity, maintenance, and repair. Taking care of involves responding to these aspects—taking responsibility for activities that keep our world going' (Fisher and Tronto 1990, 40). Fisher and Tronto (1990, 40) distinguish the first two from 'caregiving' and 'care receiving', which involve 'the concrete tasks, the hands-on work of maintenance and repair' and responses by the person who receives care. Although these four dimensions of caring are connected, they do not always constitute an orderly process. In the transnational family, as

Zechner (2008, 41) points out 'caring about' and 'taking care' dominate as they can happen over distance. Caregiving and receiving require 'physical contact or simultaneous presence with the caree'. What a focus on the circulation of care brings to this discussion is attention to the patterns and flows of caregiving over the family life cycle and migration process.

Remittances, that is, money sent home by migrant workers, are one of the important ways that migrants show they 'care about' and 'take care of' the families they left behind. In the Indian family, money is a medium of care and relationship. Money is ritually gifted at births, marriages and deaths to symbolise relationship. Money circulates between parents and adult children. The family is an important boundary of domestic money, with information about money shared often between fathers and sons, between brothers and at times even among extended kin. Money is an important way for parents to express care for their children and for children to express their filial piety. In the Indian patrilineal family, sending money home is the mark of being a 'good' son. Receiving money from children is testimony to being a good parent with filial children. Sending money home becomes one of the important ways of displaying family relationships (Singh 1997; Singh and Bhandari 2012 ).

Anglo-Celtic middle-income families in Australia differ from the Indian patrilineal family, for the couple rather than the family is the domestic financial unit. Information about money is private to the couple, rather than being shared across generations between father and son, or between husband, wife and adult children. Money in the Anglo-Celtic middle-income family usually flows one way from grandparents and parents to grandchildren and adult children. Children express their care for their parents and grandparents through actions such as cleaning the gutters or taking the parents out shopping or banking. Parents and grandparents also emphasise their independence, not wanting to place a financial burden on their children. These values operate within the context of a social welfare system (Singh 1997).

The literature on remittances as a medium of caring and support for transnational families is geographically diverse. Some of the most important literature deals with the links between the United States, Latin America and the Caribbean, placing remittances as part of a wider give and take within the transnational family and community (see Horst 2006; Mahler 2001, 2007; Mahler and Pessar 2006; Pessar and Mahler 2003; Viruell-Fuentes 2006). In her book *The Purchase of Intimacy*, Zelizer (2005a, 222) argues that money is a medium of care, support and filial relationship across countries:

> Remittances . . . maintain long-distance household ties between the emigrants and people back home. We can therefore better understand conflict and bargaining within households by looking directly at these immigrant transactions. More visibly than husband-wife struggles,

> remittances involve a whole set of third parties—children, grandparents, siblings, and others. What is more, they transform households at both origin and destination.

Remittances give the senders a sense of continued belonging to a family and displays this belonging to the whole family. At the same time, remittances set up reciprocal obligations of care from the recipient. Reciprocal flows of money and care characterise 'trust networks' (Tilly 2007). Ryan's (2004) study of Irish women who migrated to England in the 1930s and sent money home illustrates some of the detailed negotiation of money and care that takes place—the care flowing both ways, but the money and financial support going only from England to Ireland. Ryan (2004, 362) says the women:

> sent money home, they paid for younger family members to join them, they found jobs for siblings, cousins and neighbours and provided accommodation for as many as they could fit into their flats or houses. . . . Several women also mentioned that they sent their children to Ireland for school holidays thus availing of grandparents as a free child minding service. Although remittances, gifts and parcels usually flowed from the migrants back to family members in Ireland, the fact that families back home also provided practical assistance indicates the potential for mutual support that familial networks could provide across national boundaries.

## BOOMERANG REMITTANCES

The literature on remittances, with its emphasis on migrant workers sending money to the source country, revolves around a one-way flow from migrant to the family and community in the home country. When the World Bank enumerates inwards and outwards remittances, that is, remittances flowing into and out of a country, it includes three categories: workers' remittances, compensation of employees and migrants' transfers (Ratha, Mohapatra and Silwal, 2011). There is no enumeration of money that may flow from the stay-behind migrants' families in the homeland to the migrants in the host country. We are calling this flow of money 'boomerang remittances'.

Even narrowly defined, remittances are one of the largest international flows of funds. Remittances that go through formal money transfer channels to developing countries in 2012 are estimated at US$374 billion. India and China are the two largest recipients, with India receiving US$64 billion in 2011 and China receiving US$62 billion. Remittances, including those to high-income countries, are expected to reach US$615 billion by 2014 (Ratha and Silwal 2012).

For individual countries, remittances can be greater than foreign direct investment (Mohapatra et al. 2010). The total value of remittances is even greater as informal remittances are estimated to be at least 50 percent of recorded remittances (Development Prospects Group 2007). In Asia, they could be anywhere between 15 and 80 percent of the true value of remittances (Buencamino and Gorbunov 2002). The International Organization for Migration (IOM) estimates that in 2009, recorded remittances 'were nearly three times the amount of official aid and almost as large as direct foreign investment flows to developing countries' (Swing, 2010, 2).

Boomerang remittances have become important in Australia, as international students and their families contributed A$19.1 billion to Australia as a whole in 2009–2010 (Australian Education International [AEI] 2011a). Using Birrell and Smith's (2010) more conservative figures, an international student contributed A$28,691 per year rather than the ABS assumption of A$49,654. Birrell and Smith's estimate is close to that of Access Economics Pty Limited (2009) for 2007–2008. Access Economics Pty Limited (2009, i) estimates that 'Each international student (including their friend and family visitors) contributes an average of A$28,921 in value added to the Australian economy and generates 0.29 in full-time equivalent (FTE) workers'. Given that 619,119 international students enrolled in Australia at the end of December 2010 (Australian Education International [AEI] 2011b), even on 2007 estimates, they represent a contribution of A$17.9 billion and generated 179,544 FTE jobs. This figure does not include the money that flows from the origin country after the student has received permanent residence for possible investment in housing and small business.

## INTERNATIONAL INDIAN STUDENTS: PAYING TO STUDY AND MIGRATE

International Indian students are the first large group of Indian migrants who have had to pay to migrate. They are a new kind of migrant group, created by a policy linking international education and migration in 2001. This is the first young migrant group that is paying for an Australian education as a possible pathway to migration. This need to pay first has meant they are conscious of their transnational family's financial and emotional support. This support has strengthened their feelings of filial obligation in the present and in the future, as they seek ways of ensuring care for their parents in Australia. Their migration experience sets them apart in other ways from the earlier wave of professionals who migrated from India in the 1970s to 1990s. Indian students are young, often male and mostly single. For many, this is their first experience of living without family. Unlike the earlier migrants who could access welfare support, these students are wholly dependent on their families and their own abilities to earn money in Australia (Singh and Cabraal 2010).

The migration of Indian students is a two-step process. They pay for their education and living expenses in order to qualify for the possibility of migration. Migration is the main impetus for study in Australia. Eighteen of the thirty-five international students and spouses we studied already had a bachelor's degree or above. For the twenty-four students from regional cities, small towns and villages, one push factor was the difficulty of getting a job that could afford a middle-class life for the family. Others migrated because they saw it as an opportunity to move themselves and their families out of deprivation. Among our participants, only three said that they came to Australia for education. One decided to apply for permanent residence and stay, whereas the second plans to go back to India to join his family business. The third student's plans are still to be finalised.

## RECEIVING MONEY FROM INDIA

Family support with or without loans was crucial for financing study and living expenses. Parents were at the centre of this financial support, although in one case, it was the father's younger brother in the United States who financed his nephew's study in Australia. We also heard in casual conversation with Indian students how the extended family contributed to money that had to be shown in the bank account for the granting of an Australian visa. Only one of the thirty-five students financed himself through his savings from working in Europe.

Education in Australia was an expensive investment decision for families, as the expenses ranged from A$20,000 to A$30,000 a year per person. For one family that migrated—the woman who was studying, her husband and their one and a half year old daughter—the expenses came to about A$80,000 over two years. In this case, it was the husband's parents and elder brother, together with the couple's savings, that made up the sum. Thirteen of the thirty-five students were financed with bank loans, in addition to family support. Another seven students did not say whether they took out loans.

At times there were additional costs, such as a second-hand car so the student could get regular work. Parents also visited to help their children, particularly to look after the grandchildren. Families that were relatively well off also helped their children to buy homes and set up businesses once they got permanent residence. Two of the students we interviewed who had been in Melbourne for five years had homes. This support was hinted at rather than elaborated. One of the students later said, 'The money that goes to India after the children start working is in the hundreds. But the money that comes for homes and businesses is in the thousands'.

Although our participants came nearly evenly from the upper middle and middle classes, many of the students were aware their families had to struggle to meet these costs. We heard one case where the student's father mortgaged his home to get a loan. Most of the students we interviewed tried hard not to draw on their loans to prevent the 12 percent interest from accruing. When they did draw on the loans for living expenses, particularly at the beginning of their stay, they tried to send money home to pay for the interest as soon as they could. Five persons at different stages of their studies were already repaying loans. This was not always easy, particularly for those with little English and no prior work experience. They tolerated exploitation because they had to pay the rent and knew their parents had done what they could (Singh 2011a).

The students who knew their families were in need tried to send money home regularly or at least when asked. Jay (all the names of our participants are pseudonyms) in his mid to late twenties, the one student who financed himself, had a well-paid job in Melbourne because of his international work experience. He tried to send A$200 to A$300 a month to his parents. For Jay, this family practice continues from his time in India and Europe when he used to send 20 to 30 percent of his salary to his parents.

The students we studied usually sent money to their parents. But for Tirath in his late twenties, who now has permanent residence and a job, the money is sent home to his stepmother-in-law. His story is one of betrayal over inheritance by his sister in India after his parents' death. So he feels that when his parents died, he lost them and his only sibling, together with the rest of his extended family. His family is now his wife and his affinal family. He also explains that his wife was the only earning member of her family before she left India. And now they are also his only transnational family.

## FEELING 'CARED ABOUT' AND 'CARED FOR'

Hearing the stories of the students, the overwhelming theme is their gratitude to their families for their financial and emotional support. Students are at the receiving end of care. They were 'cared about' and 'cared for'. The early months and even the first year for the students is usually the most difficult because this is often the first time they have been without family. One student admitted he cried most of the first year. The mobile phone is a life line for support from parents.

Students also received caregiving, as parents flew to Australia to support their children and grandchildren. Ekta, in her late twenties, found herself trapped in a hastily arranged marriage that led to financial and domestic abuse. She had a daughter by the time she decided to walk out on the marriage. Although her sister had joined her shortly before she decided to leave, Ekta talked of how her mother flew to Melbourne to look after them. She still cannot speak of that period in her life without tears.

For our two married couples with children, the grandparents in India were the primary carers for at least some of the time. Knowing the pressures that would be on them from study and work, both couples left their children with the husband's parents in India. In one way the arrangement was a continuation because both couples had lived in a patrilineal joint family before they migrated. Indu and Inder, both thirty years old, were one of these two couples. They come from an upper middle-class family in Gujarat. Unlike the other stories we heard, both Indu and Inder had highly paid jobs. They decided to migrate for a better quality of life, as they hardly saw each other because of the severity of work. By the time they decided to migrate, their daughter was one year old. They left their daughter with Inder's parents because Indu was enrolled in a graduate degree and Inder hoped to work full time. It did not work out as planned. Indu said it was a rude shock to go from living in a joint family with eleven family members to a family where 'we were just two. We left our daughter as well, so we were missing home and India'. Indu missed her daughter sorely. She went back after four months and brought her daughter back. Now one grandparent or the other comes to look after the granddaughter for three to six months at a stretch.

Uncertainties about getting a professional job in Australia, and about the policy framework relating to family reunion, lead to students thinking of mobility rather than settlement. With an Australian education, they have a global passport, in that their qualifications are more easily recognised in other countries. Yet it is difficult for students to plan how they in turn will care for their parents when the time comes. Hence, for many the decision to settle in Australia depends partly on their parents being able to come to Australia. This rests on the ability of the student to pay nearly A$40,000 per parent to fast track the application, and also on the parents' willingness to come. When the student is the only child or the only son, this aspect becomes a central point in the decision to settle. When Charandeep, age thirty-one and the only living son of a retired policeman, gained permanent residence, he began to think of a family reunion. He began to save money for a house in Canada because in Canada family reunion is said to be less onerous. However, a promising job in his field in Australia led to his decision to stay in Australia. After many delays, his parents have finally visited him in Melbourne. He is now putting in their papers for permanent residence so that he can care for his parents.

In their stories, the students we spoke with relate how their experience in Australia has led to a greater desire for independence and a recognition of the dignity of work. There is also a greater awareness in the way they recognise their parents' difficulties when they receive care. There is a reluctance to ask for more than necessary. For some, such as Gobind and Gita, this is a big change from their dependence on their parents when they were in India.

## GOBIND AND GITA: RECEIVING CARE AND CAREGIVING

Gita in her late twenties and Gobind in his early thirties got married six years ago. It was an arranged marriage. Both belong to upper middle-class families in a regional city in Punjab. Gobind's parents are both senior government servants (recently retired), and Gita's father is a businessman. They lived with Gobind's parents, who looked after all the expenses. Gita has a master's in Hindi and Gobind has a master's in defence studies and a B.Ed. Neither of them could get a regular job.

When they had twin daughters four years ago, Gobind began looking for a job that would support his family. He tried education, but permanent teaching jobs in government schools are frozen in Punjab. Teaching jobs in the private sector offer Rs 5,000 a month compared with the Rs 12,000 in government schools. He then tried for a job with a call centre and marketing. None of these jobs would offer a middle-class life. After two years searching for a job, he seriously began thinking of migrating. Gobind's father finally agreed, but his mother did not want them to go. 'She was very emotional', Gita says.

Gita was able to get a 6.5 score on her IELTS, and they received a visa for her to study community welfare. They knew that it was going to be a struggle, for Gita's brother in Melbourne continues to drive a taxi, as he cannot get a job in information technology, which is his area of study. They came with A$2000 in hand in 2008. Gobind's parents have paid their fees and for a while also helped with living expenses. They also helped Gobind buy a second-hand car. Gobind points out his parents have been paying for all of this from their retirement fund.

When they told their story, leaving their children in India with Gobind's parents was an unspoken sorrow. Gita went to India once when her father died but has not been back since then. Gobind works as a casual factory worker at A$18 an hour. He was only able to get this work after he got a car. In a good week, he works for five days, but this is not consistent. He now goes through a recruitment agency and works wherever the agency sends him. He has not found out whether his B.Ed. is accepted in Australia. He has also not used his considerable expertise in cricket to network, except to teach a few children in the neighbourhood, fearing injury and loss of working days.

Gita has been unable to get a job. She says the employers want Australian experience. She can get call centre work, but they don't offer part-time work. One of Gita's friends works in aged care, but the course costs A$1200. Gobind says they have asked his parents for the fees, for the car. They can't ask for another $1200. He says, 'They send money in lakhs and it translates only to thousands here'.

They have been able to support themselves, not in the way they had hoped, but they are now able to pay their way. Gobind says in India he had grown up with a 'silver spoon'. He had no idea how much things cost. Gobind says, 'My parents would give me as much money as I wanted when I was studying. . . . I would spend in a day what I earn here in a week. Before, I did not think about it. I thought it was my parents' duty'. He says,

> We now have the confidence that we can survive on our own without family, kin or friends. We have to solve our problems together, between

> the two of us. Before, the two of us would talk to each other, but not too much. If she had a problem, she would discuss it with her mother or my mother.

Gita says, 'Now we only have each other'.

Gobind has not told his parents that he does manual work in a factory. They will be distressed, he says. 'In India I used to get up at 6am to play cricket. Here I wake up at 5am to go to work'. But they were coming to visit soon after the interview and bringing the children to Melbourne once Gita finished her course in a few months. Gobind says they will have to know when they come here. But they will then be able to see it is honest, acceptable work in Australia.

## SHIFTING PERCEPTIONS OF CARE—THE FIRST- AND SECOND-GENERATION EXPERIENCE

Indians—predominantly lone males—first arrived in Australia in the first half of the nineteenth century to work as labourers, camel drivers and hawkers (Voigt-Graf 2003). They later worked in cane and banana fields. They saw themselves as sojourners and only brought their families to Australia in the 1960s (Dusenbery 2001). It was only in the 1970s, after the dismantling of the white Australia policy that Indian professionals arrived in larger numbers as nuclear families. For the most part, they gained work in their areas of expertise.

The first generation of Indian migrants we studied displayed and maintained caring for the transnational family through regular telephone calls, e-mail, visits home and presence at celebrations and commemorations. Sending money home was an important way of expressing caring for and about the family. In contrast to the Indian students' unfailing sense of gratitude in *receiving* money and care, for the first generation, the emotions around *giving* money and care are more complex. They are sometimes troubled because they perceive that communication, caring and money are going primarily one way from Australia to the home country in the transnational family. This perceived imbalance signals a lack of 'caring about' the migrant offshoot of the transnational family by the stay-behind kin.

Among some of our first-generation participants, there was a perception that the dollar sent was not the dollar received. Because an Australian dollar can be worth thirty to fifty Indian rupees, this diverts attention from the migrants' costs of settlement and the tax regime. The family in the home country does not sufficiently value the kinds of negotiations that have to take place in balancing the interests of the nuclear family in Australia and the natal family in the home country. Money sent home is pitted against the day-to-day physical 'caregiving' provided by other family members, usually siblings in the home country. In some cases, these tensions over care and money flow into issues of inheritance, one of the most significant expressions of belonging in the family (see also Baldassar et al. 2007; Olwig 2002; Zelizer 2005a).

## MULTIGENERATIONAL CARE

Unlike the Indian students, the first generation of Indian migrants has been through different life stages—nurturing their family in Australia, the passing away of parents and inheritance, children's marriages and grandchildren. The 'twice migrants' in this group also have a multigenerational perspective on shifting perceptions of care. As Levitt (Levitt 2002, 139) says, 'Transnational activities do not remain constant across the life cycle. Instead, they ebb and flow at different stages'.

The first-generation migrants we interviewed spoke of their efforts to ensure they did as much of the physical caregiving as possible in two directions—their parents or grandparents in the homeland, on the one hand, and their children's families—in Australia or elsewhere—on the other. We have two cases where the migrant children have provided separate houses for their parents in Australia. We also have three families where the father came to stay with his son or daughter's family in Australia.

Anita and Anand's story best shows how care becomes multigenerational spanning more than one country. Anita and Anand migrated from India to Australia in 1973 with their baby daughter. When Anita's mother fell ill, Anita and her daughter went for long periods to look after her. After her mother died, Anita brought her father to live with them in Australia, as there was no effective family left in India. Both Anita and Anand also spend a few months at a time, turn by turn, in the United States to help their eldest daughter with child care. For Anita and Anand, the transnational family now spans India, Australia and the United States, with Australia at the centre.

## CARE AND SECOND-GENERATION INDIANS

The second-generation Indians stand apart on issues of care from the first-generation migrants and the Indian students. The second-generation experience of family revolves around their nuclear families in Australia.

Rumbaut (2002, 89) observed in a decade-long longitudinal study of 1.5 and second-generation young adults from Mexico, the Philippines, Vietnam, China and a host of other Latin American and Asian countries, transnational attachments are 'always under 10 percent'. Rumbaut (2002, 91) notes that, 'unlike their parents . . . there appears to be no "tingling" sensation, no phantom pain, over a homeland that was never lost to them in the first place'. There is also none of the first generation's angst over imbalance of care because there are no unfulfilled expectations.

In our study, the second generation saw the nuclear family as 'family'. They expressed a sense of mutual obligation and care but have not as yet had to follow through on physical care or financial contributions. In one case, the son offered, but the offer was refused. With Anita and Anand, the idea that the daughter in the United States may send them money was met with a shudder of disapproval.

Most of the time, the connection with the extended family outside Australia is through visits to grandparents, attending weddings and communicating with cousins intermittently via the telephone but now more often through Facebook or e-mail groups. However, the connection does not always mean closeness. For transnational family relationships to exist amongst the second generation, the care has to be circular and seen to be reciprocal.

Four of the twenty second-generation Indians we interviewed did speak of the loss of the extended family left behind. These four had come to Australia when they were one to twelve years old and either had memories of closeness and being with cousins or, in one case, had an aunt look after them as a baby so felt a sense of gratitude. Over time, this sense of loss lessened as cousins moved away, grandparents or significant members of the parental generation died and/or more of the extended family moved to Australia.

The second-generation and Indian students belong to the same age group but have little in common with each other. Only five of the thirty-five Indian students we interviewed had some peripheral contact with the second generation. Most of the Indian students were focussed on supporting themselves and often paying off their loans. A few also supported their parents during this time. They were struggling in a way they felt put them apart from the second generation. The second-generation Indians interviewed felt some empathy for the difficulties faced by the Indian students. They also felt that the differences in worldview, particularly gender relationships, were a barrier in developing relationships.

## CONCLUSION

Reciprocal care is as important in transnational families as in families within national borders. When families flow across national borders, caring has to be more consciously planned and displayed, as it cannot rely on the everyday face-to-face relationships. As our study shows, caring is influenced by the group's migration experience, life stage and generational changes. Caring in a transnational family can ground both ends of the family in an aura of comfort and love. At the same time, as with all families, there is the possibility of conflict around care, particularly where money and inheritance are involved.

In Australia, in the last decade, there has been an important change within the Indian diaspora in that remittances now flow two ways. The concept of the circulation of care as introduced by Baldassar and Merla in this volume makes this change visible. The older concept of the one-way flow of remittances from migrants to their kin back home was true for the first-generation migrants, most of whom were professionals who migrated with their families between the 1970s and 1990s. In contrast, our research found that with the international student migrants, money moves both ways—from host to source country and also from source to host country. The flow of money now mimics the circularity of care.

This two-way flow of money and care pre-supposes migration from the aspirational middle and upper middle classes in middle-income countries, where access to money and foreign exchange is relatively free. It also marks a generational shift from settlement to what Baas (2010) calls an 'imagined mobility'. With Indian students, there is a feeling that they are entitled to a good education and a duty of care because they have paid to study. With an Australian education, they have improved prospects for mobility to other countries if they so choose.

'Boomerang remittances' draw attention to the need to chart the two-way flow of family and market money across national borders. At present, the conceptual separation between market activities such as trade and investment, on the one hand, and the flow of family money, on the other, prevents a holistic picture of money flows between the two countries. A broader framing of money flows will draw attention to the combined flow of the personal money of family remittances, the community nature of diaspora philanthropy and the migrant dimensions of foreign direct investment.

As Figure 11.1 shows, there is a circular flow of family remittances and investment. Community philanthropy at times goes both to the origin and host countries, although at times the funds are channelled to the origin country through institutions in the host country (Singh 2011b).

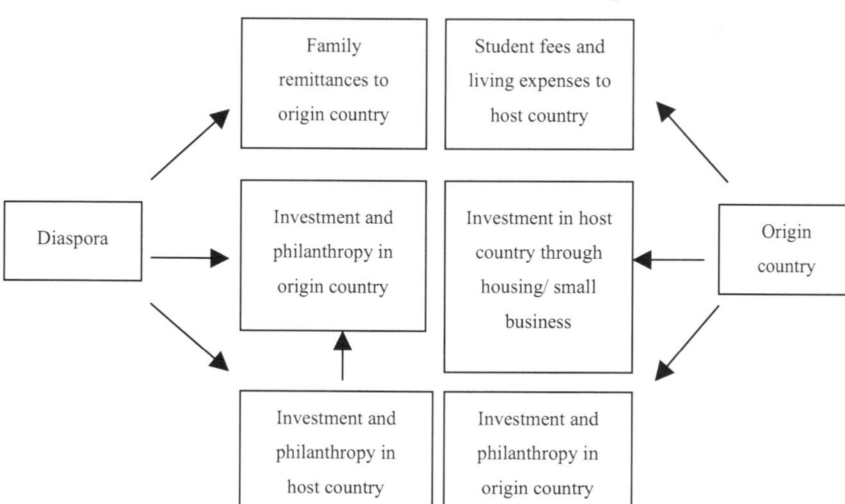


*Figure 11.1* Two-way flow of migration money.

As William Lacy Swing (2010, 3), the director general of the IOM, says,

> A new narrative is needed—one based on factual accounts of migrant contributions to society and the global economy. This can be achieved through trade, investment and development linkages, including the role of migrants as a channel for development finance in the form of remittances, the transfer of skills and ideas, and the establishment of commercial and cultural networks.

This new narrative can influence policy and perceptions about the value of migration and also reframe public debates about the virtues of assimilation as opposed to transnational ties. It needs to be recognised that transnational ties are an important part of personal and national well-being as well as family strength. Multiculturalism is not only an important cultural policy, but is one with far-reaching economic consequences at a time when labour mobility coincides with the need for a younger skilled labour force in high- and medium-income countries. With the international Indian students, migration is linked with mobility. Their choices of settlement depend on how they can further individual and family prosperity while providing the caring that keeps families strong and together. Hence, policy settings, such as those of family reunion, need to facilitate caregiving in transnational families if a country wants to keep its skilled migrant workers.

## ACKNOWLEDGMENTS

We would like to thank the Global Cities Research Institute, RMIT University, for funding this research.

# 12 Middle-Class Transnational Caregiving
## The Circulation of Care Between Family and Extended Kin Networks in the Global North

*Loretta Baldassar and Raelene Wilding*

## INTRODUCTION

As has been discussed throughout this book, attention to 'global' family care has been dominated by accounts of the disruption of family caregiving relations. The primary example documents the flow of mothers away from their own children in the global south in order to offer care for the children and families of the global north, thereby earning higher incomes but at the expense of the maternal care of their own children (e.g., Hochschild 2000; Parreñas 2005a). These are important insights into contemporary experiences of mobility and care in an unequal world. However, in this chapter, we point to an alternative experience of global family care, one in which the members of the global north do not necessarily benefit from the low-cost labour of the global south, and in which migrants and their kin move across national borders in order to provide informal, unpaid care to each other, rather than provide paid care to the families of wealthier others. It is our intention to use these examples to demonstrate that there are additional forms of global care to the care chain scenarios and that these circuits of care sometimes intersect with, and sometimes run parallel to, the global care chains identified by other scholars.

Our argument is based on a qualitative study of transnational families.[1] We interviewed migrants in Perth, Western Australia, and their ageing parents living in Italy, Ireland, the Netherlands, Singapore, New Zealand and Iran (see Baldassar, Baldock and Wilding 2007), exploring their exchange of financial, emotional, practical, personal and accommodation support as well as their migration, visiting and caregiving histories. What follows is based on a subset of that larger sample, comprised of those who might be defined as the Australian 'middle class' by virtue of their professional occupations, higher education status and capacity to access significant economic, social and cultural resources. We identify this group as the relatively privileged elites in the global system of mobility, particularly when compared with the precarious situations of the refugee sample and their family members in transit in Iran, but also when compared with the working-class labour migrants who arrived in Australia in the 1970s and earlier. Our aim is to theorise the experiences of middle-class transnational families in Australia as part of the diversity of global care circuits.

There are at least two ways in which the contexts of the global care practices of these families are distinct from those presented in the discussions of global care chains, both of which are linked to Australia's specific history of immigration and labour relations. The Australian immigration program has, since the 1970s, increasingly focused on importing skilled migrants (Castles & Miller 2009; Hawthorne 2005). These migrants are less interested in moving for economic reasons, being in a position to migrate in search of a better lifestyle (Khoo, Hugo and McDonald 2011; Abel 2013). In this respect, they represent a different set of experiences to economic migrants. At the same time, the relative wealth of the middle classes in Australia is not associated with the capacity to easily employ labour to assist with their own caregiving tasks and responsibilities—the other end of the care chain. Australia's emphasis on permanent rather than temporary migration means that it does not have a history of facilitating large-scale temporary immigration of low-paid domestic or care workers to provide child care or eldercare. Simultaneously, the protection of wages and regulation of work conditions means that the majority of the middle classes in Australia cannot afford to employ live-in domestic servants or full-time nannies. Instead, Australia relies heavily on child-care centres and informal care arrangements provided from within the family, usually by women (Fine 1999; AIHW 2003). Thus, the classic global care chain examples are not descriptive of the caregiving practices in which either Australians or migrants in Australia participate.

The families we discuss below are also influenced by Australian migration policy, which tends to produce families in which migrants live with their children but are separated from ageing parents (Baldassar, Baldock and Wilding 2007). Aged migration to Australia is not an option for most families because of the stringent criteria and small caps applied to this stream.[2] In addition, most families acknowledge the difficulties associated with migrating in later life, especially if it involves moving to a country where the language is different. Australian migrant families are thus geographically distanced from yet another potential source of caregiving support and obligation—grandparents. However, in what follows, we demonstrate that the assumption that distance prevents the circulation of care within family networks is problematic. Just as Khoo et al. (2011) have described a process of 'brain circulation' as characterising skilled migration, the skilled migrants we describe are also engaged in 'care circulation'. They are actively providing and receiving care across time and space in irregular, asymmetrical and yet persistent ways. In the four stories that follow, we identify some of the patterns and dimensions of this global care circulation.

## GENERALISED ASYMMETRICAL RECIPROCITY: THE EXTENSION OF EVERYDAY FAMILY CARE INTO GLOBAL FAMILY CARE

Clare[3] has lived her whole life in Ireland. She has twelve adult children dispersed across the world with their partners and children. Two of them live in her home, three more live in the same town, three are in Ireland but at a distance, three are in Australia and one is in Asia. As she talks about their lives, it is clear that they are in constant communication. 'We are a very close family', she says. The exchange of care is such a normalised part of everyday life for Clare that she finds it difficult to respond to questions about who does what for whom. Rather, the forms and directions of care become clear when she is encouraged to simply describe her family. When listing where they all live, the description is automatically interspersed with stories about the forms of support that each family member contributes to and benefits from. Within Ireland, this exchange of support is particularly intense. For example, the entire family congregated in Dublin within a day to provide emotional support for a daughter-in-law and son who unexpectedly lost their newborn baby; an uncle used his training as a teacher to provide additional tuition for a nephew with dyslexia; Clare travels across the country to care for grandchildren when their parents have to travel for work or to provide company during a pregnancy; grandchildren walk or bus to Clare's home to be cared for until their parents finish work; a son collects her at least three times a year to join his family for a seaside holiday; all of the children pass through regularly and drop in to check on Clare or drive her to nearby towns for shopping, appointments and meetings with friends; one son who lives only a couple of miles away checks in at least twice a week as well as calling every day; and the exchange of telephone calls across the family network is regular—even interrupting our interview a couple of times as children called to check if 'the visitor from Australia' had arrived.

It might be expected that the children living in Australia would feel particularly absent and alienated from the family given the limits that distance places on their ability to participate in this intimate familial environment of ongoing circulation of care and support. Indeed, the sense of being surrounded by family is perhaps what they miss most about living away. Clare explained that she sent videos of family events to her daughter Karen for this reason,

> This is what Karen says she misses most, is that, just being around family all the time, and that's why she enjoyed the video that I sent, you

> know, it was just ah, she felt she was in the middle of it, you know, . . . Just the kids out in the yard playing, and people dropping in and stopping for tea, and everyone just together.

It becomes apparent through the stories that both Clare in Ireland and her daughter Karen in Australia tell about their family that the circulation of care is not so much disrupted by long-distance migration as it is transformed. In part, this appears to be the result of Clare's willingness to travel. She laughed as she commented. 'People joke when they meet me in the street, they ask me whether I'm coming or going'. But it is also in part the legacy of being a close family. The types of support exchanged between Australia and Ireland is diverse, reciprocal and continuous. For example, on the day of our interview, Clare commented that she was going to call her daughter in Australia to see whether she could find a particular craft book that her own library was unable to locate.

Rather than Clare seeing her family as being disrupted by migration, it appears instead to have been expanded. Her own siblings had dispersed across the world, prompting her to travel in order to visit them from early adulthood. When two of her own daughters went to England for work, she said, 'We'd think nothing of dropping over . . . to see them, all the time. . . . We'd go over to one and then go down to see the other, you know, and they themselves would go down to each other, you know, from Liverpool to London and that'. When one of her daughters decided to move to Australia so that her husband could pursue new employment opportunities, Clare reflected, 'It's not like years ago when people went away you'd never see them again, you know, but the world has got very small'. At the same time, she recognised that moving to Australia 'was a large step, for sure', and so Clare travelled out to spend time with her daughter to help her adjust. In part, her trip was prompted by reports from a friend who visited Australia on holiday: 'When he came home he said "she's not happy", and ah, then I said "well I'll go out".' Airfares were expensive at the time, and money was short, but the money to pay for this trip was contributed by another of her daughters, who offered her share of an inheritance from a grandparent.

Later trips to Australia were characterised by a continuation of the circulation of care that is a feature of Clare's family life. For example, Clare would look after the children while Karen was working, Karen would find groups who shared Clare's interests and drive her to craft sessions and outings. However, the biggest advantage of the regular trips Clare made to Australia was that,

> because I've been there, when Karen talks to me I know who she's talking about [and] exactly where that was, and this is the thing . . . she's always telling me all the news about all her friends and I know who she's talking about. I think that's what Karen loves now, because it's

> harder for people who aren't close like and nobody knows what you're talking about, you know, so getting to know the place.

Getting to know the place, and the people in Karen's life, is an important part of the emotional support and care that Clare contributes through her visits. In a similar way, Karen and her husband made a commitment to visit Ireland in order to make sure that their extended families had an opportunity to get to know their children. As Karen explained, 'We never could afford to go, but if you waited until you could afford to do anything, you'd never do anything, so you have to go with the plan first and then afford it, do you know what I mean? . . . [Mum] just wanted to see me and wanted to see the children . . . [and] the cousins could see them as well, I think that's the reason'. The contact between cousins is maintained via the Internet, establishing the foundations for another generation of the exchange of family support.

One of the advantages of a large family is that it appears people are always available to provide care and support, without any one person being overly burdened. Karen explained, 'There's so many of them that, if I thought she was sitting . . . in a house in Ireland all on her own, you know, but I've never known it any other way . . . the fact that they're all there and they're looking after her, I don't have to worry'. At the same time, any concerns Clare might have about her children in Australia are alleviated by the fact that they all live in Perth within a fifteen-minute drive of each other, and they use this proximity to share child care and exchange other forms of everyday support on an ongoing basis.

## CIRCULATION OF FAMILY: INTERSECTIONS OF LIFE CYCLE AND FAMILY CARE

Anita was born and grew up in Italy, where she completed a university degree specialising in English. While she was working in her first teaching job in an English school nearby her hometown, she met and fell in love with a visiting teacher, Albert, from Australia. They decided to marry and move to Australia so they could both pursue postgraduate degrees. They both felt that this kind of degree from an Australian university was more prestigious than something similar in Italy. Anita's parents were excited by the opportunities the marriage and move to Australia represented, but they were also devastated by the thought that they would be separated from their daughter. They consoled themselves, saying it was only to be for a short time. To try to make up for moving away, Anita and Albert decided to have two weddings, one in Italy and one in Australia, so that no family member missed out. A few family members and friends attended both weddings, including Anita's sister who travelled to Australia for the Perth wedding and Albert's sister who travelled to Italy.

Anita successfully obtained her postgraduate qualification, but her marriage to Albert ended in divorce. Anita painstakingly hid the demise of her marriage from her parents because she knew they would worry and fret about her. Her father was not in good health, and she feared the additional stress would further weaken him. Anita's sister provided constant support by making regular phone calls and even sending motivational music compilations. Eventually, Anita broke the news to her parents during a visit home. They were keen for Anita to return to live in Italy, where they could be closer to her. Anita, however, had found an excellent job in Australia and decided to settle there. This decision was not well supported by her parents as they felt being single she should not go. Eventually, Anita met and married another Australian man, Matthew, and had three children. Once again, Anita held a wedding in both countries, but by this time, air travel was cheaper, and both sets of parents attended both weddings. Anita and her family enjoy annual trips home to visit their extended families and to have summer holidays. Recently, Matthew was offered an excellent job in Italy through Anita's family's network of friends. This provided them with the opportunity to live in Italy for two years. They enjoyed this experience very much, and their three children became fluent in Italian and got to know their grandparents, aunts, uncles and cousins very well.

Anita and Matthew continue to visit Italy with their children each year and also host regular visits from their family in Australia. Anita's parents contribute financially to the cost of their trips home by gifting money to them for birthdays and Christmas. Anita's parents also assisted with the purchase of their house in Australia, and they plan to contribute to the children's private school fees, partly as a way of making up for not being able to provide the level of child care they are able to offer their local grandchildren. When Anita's father was ill, she applied to go part-time at the school where she worked and negotiated some extended unpaid leave during the teaching breaks. Anita used this time to make an additional trip home each year to provide personal 'hands-on' care to her father and to give her mother and sister a break. When her father was clearly close to death, Anita did not think twice about immediately flying home to be by his bedside.

Despite the relative ease of transnational caregiving in Anita's family, certain difficulties were still often mentioned. Anita's mother, Franca, took her grandmother duties very seriously and suffered deeply at the thought that she was not able to care for and share her love with her Australian grandchildren to the same extent as with her local grandchildren. There was no mention that the money she gifted for their trips to Italy could have been spent on something else. Similarly, Franca and Matthew would only occasionally mention that their obligation to visit Italy as often as possible limited them from doing other things. When pressed, both independently saw the issue as a mute point: 'We just couldn't . . . and that's just the way it is'.

## THE FLYING GRANDMOTHER: CULTURALLY SPECIFIC FAMILY CARE IN TRANSNATIONAL CONTEXT

Christine was the first to acknowledge that she was a 'favourite' daughter. When she failed to get the points necessary to attend university in her home country, Singapore, her father provided her with full financial support to complete a degree in Australia. This provision of finance for her overseas education was the beginning of a long story of transnational care. Christine's mother, Evelyn, explained, 'Every year we sent her a lump sum of money, including fees, lodging, food, whatever is needed for her we send it to her. And we visit her maybe once or twice a year . . . we are happy with our contact with one another'.

In the final year of her degree, Christine met Peter, a student from New Zealand, the man she later married. When the relationship was revealed to her parents a year after it had begun, her mother immediately travelled out to Australia. As Christine explained,

> Dad sent his bodyguard over, which is my mother, to suss [check] out the relationship. She was deliberately hard on me to see Peter's reaction. . . . I suppose she liked what she saw, because if it didn't work out the way she wanted it . . . she would have been able to drag me back to Singapore (laughs). She had the power. I would not be happy, but I'd go kicking and screaming. . . . Then Dad came because Mum must have given him favourable reports.

This close observation was just one of the ways in which Christine's parents demonstrated their significant and ongoing care for their daughter, a theme that permeated her description of their long-distance relationship.

After marrying, Christine and Peter settled in Perth, maintaining contact with their distant kin through regular visits and frequent telephone calls. Christine would call her mother at least once a week and often twice a day. Her mother laughed as she said, 'Now she has a family of her own, and she rings more often than before! . . . I don't normally call her unless I have something special to talk to her. Sometimes . . . she calls twice [a day]. That's how we contact each other'. Christine also visited Singapore at least once a year, taking her children with her after they were born. During times of crisis, the visits were extended into longer periods of time. As Evelyn explained, 'Christine stayed with me for one month after my husband died. When she left, I felt a bit lonely, but she keeps on calling me practically every day'. At other times, the annual visits were combined with holidays to other parts of Asia. She took both the children with her to Singapore en route to a family holiday in Thailand. The intensity of the family connections of support and care became particularly evident when Christine's children were born. For the first birth, her mother travelled out to stay for a month to provide hands-on support. Yet, Christine explained, 'I wished she stayed a little bit longer, but never mind . . . she received a lot of flack [criticism] from . . . my grandma and her relatives for having so short a stay with me. . . . But she stayed a little longer because she was "encouraged" to do so with the second one'. Each of these visits was characterised by substantial support. As Christine explained, 'Oh, she did everything. She was priceless. I loved her. And Peter really, really got to see her and was most grateful for her existence, basically . . . my mother was admirable. She cooked dinner, she did the housework. She did the children. She did me. She did us'. Her mother's contributions even extended to managing the marital relationship: 'Peter and I had a couple of blow-ups, which really saddened my mum. But she tried to sort us out without being too interfering. Well, a lot of people would think it's interference, but I think Peter and I were most grateful for her intervention actually'.

For Evelyn, the regular visits to Australia were a natural and expected response to the transnational circumstances. Indeed, she places the visits and phone calls within a broader context of members of the family network, doing what is necessary to provide the expected care and support to other family members. She explained that one of her sisters lived in Sydney, and 'so she comes back practically every year to see my mother. And I did that too, to my daughter. I used to visit her . . . maybe . . . three times [a year] when my husband was alive. But now maybe I cut short and less the visit, maybe once or twice a year'. Evelyn feels some pressure to visit even more often:

> '[Christine] keeps asking me to go back and look after her children and stay with her. But I don't like . . . to stay there long. And also, I have a pension here. I cannot go to other countries for more than three months . . . but I also don't like to leave my family [in Singapore] for long period of time. I have my son, my grandchildren here, my mother and brothers and sisters. I feel more comfortable here'.

What is particularly remarkable about Evelyn's commitment to travelling to care for her grandchildren is that she dislikes travel, 'although I love children, I never like travelling. I never like travelling'. Despite her aversion to travel, she undertakes visits on a regular basis in order to fulfil what she sees as her grandmothering duties.

## ROUTINISED FAMILY CONTACT: STRETCHING THE OBLIGATIONS ACROSS DISTANCE

John and Caitlin had never intended to migrate to Australia from New Zealand. They set off on a round-the-world trip, worked in Singapore, Hong Kong and Thailand, and many years later found themselves buying a house in Perth. Caitlin explained, 'I think at that stage, that was the "go overseas adventure", and we had every intention of going back'. They acknowledged that their families in New Zealand were probably surprised and even disappointed that they had not returned to New Zealand after all, but this was an unspoken disappointment and not worth mentioning out loud. Indeed, there was still a sense that the return to New Zealand could actually happen at any moment. They had made several trips back 'home' for weddings and funerals and simply to catch up with the family, and they felt that their contact with family was probably the same as it would have been if they had moved back because their families lived in rural New Zealand while their work required them to live in the city. John explained, 'We've probably maintained almost as much face-to-face contact now as we did when we were actually living in New Zealand. The distance is different, but'.

At first their visits to the family were opportunistic and erratic, complemented by similarly opportunistic visits from their family to Perth. A visit between New Zealand and Australia occurred at least once every two years and sometimes as often as twice in one year, usually coinciding with a trip to Europe or Asia or a funeral, wedding or significant birthday. However, more recently, they had noticed that their parents were ageing. As Caitlin explained, 'My mum couldn't travel anymore, and I think that was when it hit us that they were getting older, and we kind of made a decision then to go back at least every second year'.

Caitlin and John didn't feel that their parents needed any specific care from them; rather, the visits were simply a means of maintaining their connection with their families. As Caitlin explained, 'Yes, I felt a need to see [my mother]—not so much probably because I was worried about her . . . but I just like to catch up with her, and because . . . both sets of parents . . . they're virtually around the corner from each other so visiting one was like visiting everybody'. The desire to spend time with family did not mean that such visits were easy. They were characterised by the same fractious relationships and moments of joy that feature in most family interactions. As Caitlin explained,

> Frankly, going back was quite arduous—that's not overstating it because you felt a certain amount of obligation to catch up with all sorts of people and then spend 'x' amount of time with one set of parents and 'x' amount with the other set of parents and if you didn't get the proportions right, that caused problems so it was always quite full of—a certain amount of tension.

The family closeness extended to taking for granted that they would be available to their parents and siblings in a moment of crisis. For Caitlin, this meant resigning from her job when her parents needed her to return to her hometown at short notice:

> Basically, I just said that this is what I've got to do. I didn't really have any doubts about—or question in my mind that it was the right thing

> to do or the right time to go or whatever. . . . And so I resigned and went when my dad was ill and he subsequently passed away and then the same with Mum, when I found out how ill she was, I just rang my employer and I said look, I'm sorry, I want to be with her until she's well, and they said fine, just go and take care of it. [With Dad being ill], I gave up my job. I think I was away for three months.

For John and Caitlin, 'hopping over' to New Zealand on a regular basis and supplementing this with additional 'crisis visits' was simply a way of 'doing family'.[4] Importantly, they suggested that there were no significant costs to this. They had access to money to pay for the travel, and there was no need to organise visas. For Caitlin, even her job was disposable, reflecting her easy access to employment in her field in Perth. While there was a significant distance to travel to get from one place to another, their fields of work would require them to travel in order to maintain their family relations in any case, being urban professionals from rural family backgrounds.

## CARE CIRCULATION FROM THE AUSTRALIAN MIDDLE-CLASS MIGRANT PERSPECTIVE

That middle-class and privileged families are relatively absent in the transnational migration literature is an interesting point and worthy of reflection (Conradson and Latham 2005). Miller (2010, 84) goes so far as to argue that 'the middle class of suburbia, [is] a class so universally derided by theorists that no one had bothered to theorise them properly'. Perhaps there is an assumption that these families are less important for analysis because their relative wealth, compared with poorer families, ensures their needs are met. After all, the wealthy families, particularly women, of the north participate in the care chains as the beneficiaries of the unequal power relations. The care chains literature tends to define these women as using their significant purchasing power to obtain the care support they need to allow them to pursue paid employment and professional careers at the expense of the family care requirements of the female domestic workers they employ (Ehrenreich and Hochschild 2003b). This representation of women 'in the north' is arguably overly simplistic, in particular with regard to women in southern Europe, where access to non-family care is unequal across the social strata (Saraceno 2010, 40). Women in these countries commonly employ domestic workers to care for their ageing family members, but they are often themselves un- or underemployed and carry significant care burdens looking after children or grandchildren of their own (Campani 2012; Costa 2013). The relatively small cost of domestic migrant labour is often paid for out of limited government subsidies and the pensions of the elderly, pensions that do not meet the costs of institutional care in those countries (Naldini and Saraceno 2008).

Ironically, Australian women, while relatively wealthy and with considerable access to educational, health and employment resources, do not participate in global care chains because they cannot afford the high wages and conditions of care workers in their country; even if they could, there is no significant pool of such labour to access.[5] Even general house cleaning is usually contracted through small or private businesses and is often too expensive for most Australians. The practice of employing live-in domestics is largely absent and considered unusual or even objectionable by most Australians. There is, however, an increasing interest in hosting students in exchange for nanny and au pair duties (Morokvasic 2004). It has been argued that the international student and working-holiday visa regimes may contribute informally as a de-facto temporary worker scheme (see Chapter 11, this volume). Even so, these entrants are generally relatively wealthy and from First World countries, including increasing numbers of young graduates from Europe (Khoo et al. 2011).[6] While not engaged in chains of care that involve the commodification of care labour in return for improved career advancements, women in both southern Europe and Australia are still very much involved in circuits of care and mobility.

Our data locate the circuits of transnational care across the so-called global north, that is, between migrants residing in First World countries. This analysis of the middle classes sits somewhat uneasily within the limitations of theories and conceptualisations of the care chain framework (Kofman 2012) because the exchange of care tends to circulate through extended kin relations within the same family and, as such, is informal rather than commodified. The practices of care in these families are certainly global in reach, stretching from Australia to Europe, Singapore and New Zealand and back again, but the movement of this care might be better described as flowing sideways (rather than upwards or downwards) through care circuits that link individuals of more equal economic and power relations. This is not to suggest that the families are not sites of unequal power relations. Indeed, our research has documented the uneven gendered and age relations, for example, that inform the various decisions made about who provides what to whom (Baldassar, Baldock and Wilding 2007; see also Finch and Mason 1993). However, these inequalities are of a different order to those outlined in discussions of global care chains, which position women in terms of both local gender inequalities and unequal international political economies. Our analysis shows that members of the extended global north family networks contribute to the transnational circulation of care for their members; while these kin are mostly similarly placed in the economic and class structure of home and host countries, the types of care they contribute to the transnational context are distributed and distinguished along the lines of gender, age and skill. The model of this exchange is thus one of generalised asymmetrical reciprocity, accomplished through the ongoing synchronous and asynchronous communications and visits that characterise the uneven circular flows of care for and about each other (Wilding 2007; Baldassar 2008).

In identifying this sample of migrants in Australia as 'privileged', we do not mean to suggest that they are particularly wealthy elites. This sample would identify themselves as 'normal' or 'average' in the Australian context. They have sufficient incomes to purchase airfares for travel on a regular basis and access the communication technologies that have become so central to transnational engagement.[7] Their 'privilege' is also based on another resource, largely taken for granted by Australians, that they readily access and which is of particular importance in a mobile world: the capacity to legitimately cross borders with ease by accessing visas and passports.[8] In the Australian context, the easiest border-crossing of non-citizens is available to those with New Zealand passports, who are able to freely enter Australia to work, study or holiday without needing additional visas. Yet Australia also has a long history of seeking to ensure that those migrants who are eligible for permanent residency acquire Australian citizenship as quickly as possible, also evident in the decision to allow dual citizenship, encouraged for immigrants since 1986 and available for Australian emigrants since 2002. Most of the people whose transnational families we describe above have accessed this entitlement, supporting their capacity to be members of transnational families. Perhaps more importantly, and unlike the refugee sample we describe in the larger study (Baldassar, Baldock and Wilding 2007), their family members are also able to travel in and out of Australia relatively easily on short-term visas.[9] For those not on the list of preferred countries of origin, applying for a tourist visa (subclass 676) or sponsored family visitor visa (subclass 679) requires passing health, character, financial and age requirements in addition to paying a fee. Meeting these requirements is particularly difficult for those from countries or regions identified on the Department of Immigration's 'high risk' list as unstable and as sources of asylum seekers and humanitarian refugees. However, for those coming from places such as Italy, Ireland, Singapore and the Netherlands, access for up to six months at a time is easily organised either online or through a travel agent. Obtaining these visas is often automatic with the purchase of an airline ticket through a travel agent.

Partly because such visa arrangements make visits possible and relatively easy, distance in these middle-class families is to some extent 'normalised'. Family members can and do maintain contact and thus continually generate the feeling of being a well-connected family. In many ways, the experience of belonging to family and exchanging caregiving for the transnational kin is not so different from more local kin; they are considered very much a part of the family network. Many people in our study commented that they probably see their family members as often as they would if they had never migrated. This is particularly relevant to countries such as Australia, where distances between places can be enormous. But it is also pertinent to people who live in smaller countries because it is not so much the geographical distance that limits mobility, as the time and resources, including money and visas, required to bridge that distance. While the frequency and form of care provision and reception may be different, this is not necessarily seen as a deficit. Rather, transnational caregiving is often characterised by family members as special, extended and quality time. Just how much contact and what form of care might be considered desirable and sufficient depends on the different families, their members and their histories and patterns of obligation and support (Finch and Mason 1990). Similarly, Olwig (Chapter 6, this volume) argues that it is not the distance between people but the quality of their relationships that matter most.

Desirable circulations of care are also informed by culturally specific notions about the obligation to care as well as the structurally determined availability of resources and familial expectations of how those resources might be distributed. Thus, the flying grandmother in the Chinese-Singaporean family is expected to and chooses to take care of her daughter and grandchildren for extended periods of time, whereas the Italian grandparents manage their obligations and desires to care by providing financial support to cover the costs of their children's visits home, as well as by assisting with the purchase of a house and contributing to the fees of private school education. Thus, when the cultural norms of proximate families prove to be impossible to maintain, alternatives are identified and pursued. The New Zealand family was perhaps the most insistent that the distance was actually insignificant to their family relations, pointing to the fact that if they lived in New Zealand, they would be likely to see their parents as frequently as they do from Australia. What is interesting in this example is the ways in which geographic distance is possibly being measured just as much through cultural similarity as through kilometers or miles. The boundaries and distance separating New Zealand and Australia are perceived as insignificant in part because they do not require the negotiation of a different language or different cultural expectations of family relations. Although Singapore is closer than New Zealand in terms of air travel, the differences between Singapore and Perth contribute to a sense of visits across these borders being more significant and thus 'larger'.

Despite this variance in the perceptions or experiences of distance, in all of these families, there appears to be an emphasis on doing as much as one can and working at keeping up the contact and thereby maintaining family connections. These priorities are evident in the decisions of the Irish family to travel across borders for regular visits in order to ensure that the Irish grandmother knows the community of her daughters, and the Australian-born children know and have relationships with their aunties, uncles and cousins in Ireland. Indeed, the importance of physical co-presence in sustaining the Irish family is clear and overrides the perceived challenges of doing so across long distances, as is evident in the decision of one sibling to provide her mother with the airfare to visit another sibling in Australia. This case is a compelling illustration of the generalised asymmetrically reciprocal exchange of care (Introduction, this volume) in transnational families, in that care is not measured and exchanged in a two-way equivalent swap but shared between members of the family, given as and when needed by who is best able to provide at that particular time.

The Italian migrant's decision to repeat her wedding in two countries is an important symbol of the willingness and capacity to remain equally connected to kin both here and there and is reinforced by the decision of both her parents and parents-in-law to attend both weddings. Even for a relatively privileged family, these are significant investments of time and money in what might otherwise easily be dismissed as unnecessary repetitions of family events. Indeed, in an era of increasing communication opportunities, it is striking that co-presence is privileged over the possibility of experiencing the wedding through photographs, video and/or Skype. While such resources are clearly available to these families, the visit is emphasised in the decisions they make about how to sustain relationships and express mutual support and care. In this respect, it becomes clear that access to money, passports, visas and time to travel ensures that transnational families are able to make choices from among a range of options regarding how they will sustain family ties across time and space. It also underlines the privileged place of embodied co-presence over virtual forms. As noted in Chapter 1 (this volume), the greater the intensity of transnational virtual communication, the greater the sense of obligation to visit, particularly in the case of the middle classes who have access to the resources to fulfill these obligations (see also Wilding 2006).

An important feature of these families is that the movement of one person tends to provoke the movement of another, such that the visits between Singapore and Australia, between Italy and Australia, between New Zealand and Australia and between Ireland and Australia are part of a broader cycle of exchange throughout the family. They are not always evenly matched, and there is a tendency for the migrant to return more frequently than for any specific family member to visit them. However, within the broader family network, the flow of individuals in both directions ensures that the social field is active and activated. Yet this is not necessarily new to the twenty-first century or specific to the relatively affluent social classes. Evidence indicates that this circulation of people across space and time has always been relevant to understanding the lives of migrants (Agunias 2006). Labour migration flows are often characterised by migration chains in which the movement of family members triggers and facilitates the movement of other kin and associates. What has transformed is the compression of the time period within which such circulation occurs. Whereas a relatively privileged Italian migrant of the 1950s or an Irish migrant of the 1800s might have made only a couple of return visits during their lifetime and exchanged letters at three-month intervals, today's travel and communication opportunities have intensified such exchanges so that they can visit annually or more and communicate constantly if desired (Baldassar 2011).

Similar to the patterns of travel and communication, the circulation of care and support are also arguably intensified by distance. While there is ample evidence of the circulation of resources within local family networks across the life cycle according to need and capacity, less attention has been paid to this circulation across distance over the life course. Indeed, the protection of this feature of family life, the 'generational contract' (see Introduction, this volume), is arguably the underlying goal of the constant communication and travel being conducted by both parent and adult child following migration. As we have argued elsewhere (Baldassar, Baldock and Wilding 2007), each visit, telephone call or offer of financial support is not only an event in itself, but also a promise that there will be more to come—that the family remains a source of love, care and support, albeit also of tension and contest. Thus, each moment of the circulation of resources is a reinforcement of the social field that both generates and requires the further circulation of resources.

## CONCLUSIONS

Overall, these case studies suggest that families can be maintained as 'close' with ongoing caregiving exchange to adequately meet the needs of kin from a distance. Perhaps what is exceptional about the middle-class transnational families' experiences presented in this chapter compared to the less privileged families that populate each of the other chapters in this volume—and understandably and appropriately dominate in the transnational family literature—is the ability of the middle-class family members to feel they have more or less adequately met their obligation to provide care and that their needs for care are more or less adequately met. This is particularly evident in the case studies we selected. The experiences of these four relatively privileged transnational families allow us to illustrate two broader points. First, they enable us to demonstrate that the management of distance and absence in some families—particularly those with the advantages of relative wealth and access to visas—is experienced as part of broader familial practices of the circulation of care. Second, the capacity to be mobile, reliant on access to a variety of resources, enables such middle-class transnational families to be perceived by their members as both fairly commonplace, ordinary ways of practising familyhood, and as providing satisfactory and adequate flows of care and support that are associated with positive experiences of extended family relationships.

It is not our intention to use the positive stories represented in these case studies to encourage an uncritical acceptance of the transnational family form as equivalent to the local or proximate family. There are other examples in our middle-class sample of family members who, despite enjoying relative wealth and capacity to travel, engage in transnational communication and so on, still feel that their family obligations of care are not well met. For example, one Italian mother simply insists that she would be happier and healthier if her only daughter, living in Australia, were permanently living close by in Italy. She feels this way despite the fact that she is able to afford a live-in domestic who adequately attends to her every physical need and despite her daughter ringing daily and visiting each year for four to six weeks. Her daughter, consequently, feels a constant sense of guilt for not meeting her mother's expectations, despite doing all she can to provide as much care as possible from a distance (Baldassar, Wilding and Baldock 2007). Despite the evidence that families with resources and willingness to maintain relations of support across space and time will do so and can manage effectively, there is also evidence in our sample of ways in which distance can be used to defend against unwanted family obligations or interference. The most obvious example here is that of Anita, who demonstrates that distance makes it easy to keep up appearances by hiding her failing marriage from her parents. This kind of charade is usually only temporary, given the sheer amount of contact and people's ability to suspect something is amiss through the sound of one's voice on the phone and, in particular, the eventual visits that take place. Distance does result in feelings of loss, longing and sadness that are not easily resolved and may only be temporarily reduced by the practices and processes of transnational communication. This said, these sentiments are also the experience of proximate families. Distance can encourage visits and moments of contact that are extra special and out of the ordinary, thereby resulting in profound and deep connections. Distance can also allow contacts to become weaker and more perfunctory. Yet it must be acknowledged that such problematic family relations are also a frequent feature of proximate family relations, not being unique to transnational family forms. Indeed, it might be suggested that such examples are an illustration of the continuation of complex family forms across distance and national borders and the circulation of family care.

The experience of transnational family life is affecting a growing number as well as 'types' of families. North–north flows are increasingly relevant, particularly in the current global economic crisis, which has led to a resurgence in emigration from European countries such as Italy and Spain and Ireland with some of it towards Australia, most of it young graduates and professionals (Flavell et al. 2007). There are also new 'north–south' flows as young graduates leave Europe for Latin America (Solimano 2009).[10] Thus, there is a growing need to better understand the transnational lives of these relative elites, some of whom are not particularly wealthy themselves, although they are likely to have families in the homeland who can support them (see Chapters 10 and 11, this volume), but are rich in social and cultural capital that provide good opportunity and life chances. By outlining some of the specific family networks, strategies and experiences that characterise the global family care processes of middle-class migrants in Australia, and placing these in the context of the specific migration histories and policies of Australia, we offer an important additional dimension to the care chain perspective. Global care is not always or only a unilinear displacement of care in return for money. It is often also the product and practice of reciprocal and circular, if asymmetrical, flows of care within the family networks that are transformed by migration into transnational family forms.

## NOTES

1. The research reported in this chapter was supported by the *Transnational Families* Project conducted by Loretta Baldassar, Cora Baldock and Raelene Wilding and funded by the Australian Research Council (ARC) from 2000 to 2004. It also draws on two other ARC-funded Linkage projects: *Italian Lives* conducted from 2005 to 2009 and coordinated by Baldassar and *Australian diasporas and brain gain*, conducted from 2009 to 2011, on which Baldassar was a chief investigator.
2. For example, the Aged Parent subclass 804 visa remained capped at 550 places in 2012–2013; see www.immi.gov.au
3. All of the participants in this chapter and the family members they discuss have been given pseudonyms to protect their anonymity.
4. See Baldassar, Baldock and Wilding 2007, Chapter 6, for an overview of types of visits.
5. Australia is noteworthy for its long history of carefully controlled and monitored immigration programing. Temporary worker visas have only recently been introduced in Australia, including the popular working holiday visa, which permits people ages eighteen to thirty years to remain in Australia for one year.
6. In addition, due to the strict regulations governing Australian professional practice, it has been argued that many humanitarian and refugee entrants, a large number of whom are professionals in their homelands, end up in working-class employment in Australia (Constable et al. 2004; Colic-Peisker and Tilbury 2006)
7. See Baldassar, Baldock and Wilding 2007, Chapter 5, on transnational communication and the use of new technologies.
8. This relative freedom of physical movement over borders is also reflected in the movement of other kinds of goods and services, many of which are linked to the nation's care of its citizens. For example, Australians can receive pension payments while living overseas, subject to various criteria.
9. Currently, visitors with a European Union (EU) passport are able to apply free of charge for an 'eVisitor' visa that allows them to enter Australia for up to three months for short-term tourism or business purposes. The 'Electronic Travel Authority' is available for those with a passport from one of thirty-four nominated countries or territories (including Singapore as well as EU countries) for a small fee through a travel agent, and it also permits up to three months' stay in Australia. Once in Australia, these visas can be extended for up to six months.
10. 'Exodus of Workers from Continent Reverses Old Patterns', *Wall Street Journal*, 14 January 2012. http://online.wsj.com/article/SB10001424052970203550304577137174048327642.html

# References

Abbott, Pamela, and Claire Wallace. 2000. *An Introduction to Sociology. Feminist Perspectives.* London and New York: Routledge.
Abel, Emily K., and Margaret K. Nelson. 1990. "Circles of Care: An Introductory Essay." In *Circles of Care: Work and Identity in Women's Lives*, edited by Emily Abel and Margaret Nelson, 4–34. Albany: State University of New York Press.
Abel, Gillian. Forthcoming 2013. *British Transnationals Through the Lens of Consumption: A Critique of Labour and Lifestyle Migration Approaches in the Case of "Middling" Migrants in Western Australia.* PhD thesis, University of Western Australia.
Abrego, Leisy. 2009. "Economic Well-Being in Salvadoran Transnational Families: How Gender Affects Remittance Practices." *Journal of Marriage and Family* 71 (4): 1070–1085.
Access Economics Pty Limited. 2009. *The Australian Education Sector and the Economic Contribution of International Students.* Australian Council for Private Education and Training.
Ackers, Louise. 2004. "Citizenship, Migration and the Valuation of Care in the European Union." *Journal of Ethnic and Migration Studies* 30 (2): 373–396.
Ackers, Louise, and Peter Dwyer. 2002. *Senior Citizenship? Retirement, Migration and Welfare in the European Union.* Bristol: Policy Press.
Ackers, Louise H., and Helen E. Stalford. 2004. *A Community for Children? Children, Citizenship and Internal Migration in the EU.* Aldershot: Ashgate.
Adey, Peter. 2010. *Mobility.* London: Routledge.
Agunias, Dovelyn Rannveig. 2006. *From a Zero-Sum to a Win-Win Scenario? Literature Review on Circular Migration.* Washington, DC: Migration Policy Institute.
Ahmed, Sara, Claudia Castaneda, Anne-Marie Fortier, and Mimi Sheller. Eds. 2003. *Uprootings/Regroundings: Questions of Home and Migration.* Oxford: Berg.
AIHW. 2003. *Australia's Welfare 2003.* Canberra: Australian Institute of Health and Welfare. AIHW Cat. No. AUS 41.
Åkesson, Lisa, Jørgen Carling, and Heike Drothbohm. 2012. "Mobility, Moralities and Motherhood: Navigating the Contingencies of Cape Verdean Lives." *Journal of Ethnic and Migration Studies* 38 (2): 237–260.
Alba, Richard. 2005. "Bright vs. Blurred Boundaries: Second-Generation Assimilation and Exclusion in France, Germany and the United States." *Ethnic and Racial Studies* 28 (1): 20–49.
Alba, Richard and Mary Waters. Eds, 2011 *The Next Generation: Immigrant Youth in a Comparative Perspective.* New York: New York University Press
Alber, Erdmute. 2003. "Grandparents as Foster Parents. Changes in Caregiving Relationships Between Grandparents and Grandchildren among the Baatombu in Northern Benin." *Anthropos* 98 (2): 445–460.

Al-Ali, Nadje. 2002. "Loss of Status or New Opportunities? Gender Relations and Transnational Ties Among Bosnian Refugees." In *The Transnational Family: New European Frontiers and Global Networks*, edited by Deborah Bryceson and Ulla Vuorela, 83–102. New York: Berg.

Alicea, Marixsa. 1997. "'A Chambered Nautilus': The Contradictory Nature of Puerto Rican Women's Role in the Social Construction of a Transnational Community." *Gender & Society* 11 (5): 597–626.

Ambrosini, Maurizio. 2011. "Undocumented Migrants and Invisible Welfare: Survival Practices in the Domestic Environment." *Migration Letters* 8 (1): 34–42.

Ames, Morgan G., Janet Go, Joseph "Jofish" Kaye, and Mirjana Spasojevic. 2010. *Making Love in the Network Closet: The Benefits and Work of Family*. Videochat, at Savannah, Georgia.

Amit, Vered. 2007. "Globalization Through 'Weak Ties': A Study of Transnational Networks Among Mobile Professionals." In *Going First Class? New Approaches to Privileged Travel and Movement*, edited by Vered Amit, 53–71. New York and Oxford: Berghahn Books.

Anca Gheaus, Anca. 2011. "Care Drain: Who Should Provide for the Children Left Behind?" *Critical Review of International social and Political Philosophy*: 1–23.

Andall, Jacqueline. 1999. "Cape Verdean Women on the Move: 'Immigration Shopping' in Italy and Europe." *Modern Italy* 4 (2): 241.

Anderson, Bridget. 2000. *Doing the Dirty Work? The Global Politics of Domestic Labour*. London and New York: Zed Books.

Anthias, Floya. 2007. "Ethnic Ties: Social Capital and the Question of Mobilisability." *Sociological Review* 55 (4): 788–805.

Appadurai, Arjun. 1996. *Modernity at Large*. Minneapolis: University of Minnesota Press.

———. 1991. "Global Ethnoscapes: Notes and Queries for a Transnational Anthropology." In *Recapturing Anthropology*, edited by Richard Fox, 191–210. Santa Fe, NM: School of American Research Press.

———. 1990. "Disjuncture and Difference in the Global Cultural Economy." *Public Culture* 2 (2): 1–24.

Archer, Margaret. 2006. "Persons and Ultimate Concerns: Who We Are Is What We Care About." In *Conceptualization of the Person in Social Sciences*, edited by Edmond Malinvaud and Mary Ann Glendon, 261–283. Rome: Vatican City Press.

———. 2000. *Being Human*. Cambridge: Cambridge University Press.

Arendell, Terry. 2000. "Conceiving and Investigating Motherhood: The Decade's Scholarship." *Journal of Marriage and Family* 62 (4): 1192–1207.

Ariza, Marina. 2005. "Juventud, Migración y Curso de Vida. Sentidos y Vivencias de la Migración Entre los Jóvenes Urbanos Mexicanos." In *Jóvenes y niños. Un enfoque sociodemográfico*, edited by Mier-y-Terán Marta and Cecilia Rabell, 39–70. Mexico City: Instituto de Investigaciones Sociales, UNAM, FLACSO, Porrúa Editores and Cámara de Diputados.

Ariza, Marina and Orlandina de Oliveira. 2007. "Familias, Pobreza y Desigualdad Social en Latino América: una Mirada Comparativa." *Estudios demográficos y urbanos* 22 (1): 9–42.

———. 2001. "Contrasting Scenarios: Non-Residential Family Formation Patterns in the Caribbean and Europe." *International Review of Sociology* 11 (1): 47–61.

———. 1999. "Formación y Dinámica Familiar: Diferencias entre México, Centroamérica y el Caribe." In *México Diverso y Desigual: Enfoques Sociodemográficos*, edited by Beatriz Figueroa, 161–176. México: Sociedad Mexicana de Demografía y El Colegio de México.

Ariza, Marina and Alejandro Portes. 2007. "La Migración Internacional de Mexicanos: Escenarios y Desafíos de Cara al Nuevo Siglo." In *El País Transnacional. Migración Mexicana y Cambio Social a través de la Frontera*, edited by Marina Ariza and Alejandro Portes, 11–44. México: UNAM, Instituto de Investigaciones Sociales.

Ariza, Marina, Mercedes González de la Rocha, and Orlandina de Oliveira. 1994. "Características, Estrategias y Dinámicas Familiares en México, América Central y el Caribe." Informe final. *Population Quality of Live Independent Comission.*

Asis, Maruja, Shirlena Huang, and Brenda Yeoh. 2004. "When the Light of the Home Is Abroad: Unskilled Female Migration and the Filipino Family." *Singapore Journal of Tropical Geography* 25 (2): 198–215.

Asis, Maruja, and Fabio Baggio. 2003. "The Other Face of Migration: Children and Families Left Behind." Paper presented at the Eighth International Metropolis Conference, Vienna, Austria, September 15–19.

Attias-Donfut, Claudine. 2000. « Rapports de Générations. Transferts Intrafamiliaux et Dynamique Macrosociale. » *Revue française de sociologie*: 643–684.

Attias-Donfut, Claudine, Nicole Lapierre, and Martine Segalen. 2002. *Le Nouvel Esprit de Famille.* Paris: Odile Jacob.

Australian Education International (AEI). 2011a. "Export Income to Australia from Education Services in 2009–10." Accessed May 12, 2011. https://aei.gov.au/AEI/PublicationsAndResearch/Snapshots/Default.htm

———. 2011b. "International Student Data." Accessed May 8, 2012. https://www.aei.gov.au/research/International-Student-Data/Pages/InternationalStudentData2011.aspx#2

Avila, Ernestine. 2008. *Transnational Motherhood and Fatherhood: Gendered Challenges and Coping.* PhD diss., University of Southern California. Accessed August 22, 2011. http://digitallibrary.usc.edu/assetserver/controller/item/etd-Avila-20080715.pdf

Baas, Michiel. 2010. *Imagined Mobility: Migration and Transnationalism among Indian Students in Australia.* London: Anthem Press.

Bacigalupe, Gonzalo, and Maria Camara. 2012. "Transnational Families and Social Technologies: Reassessing Immigration Psychology." *Journal of Ethnic and Migration Studies*: 1–14.

Baldassar, Loretta. 2011. "Italian Migrants in Australia and Their Relationship to Italy: Return Visits, Transnational Caregiving and the Second Generation." *Journal of Mediterranean Studies* 20 (2): 255–282.

———. 2010a. "Transnational Families, Care-Giving and the Inter-generational Contract." Paper presented at the ERSC seminar Transnational and the Second-Generation, University of Nottingham, England, September 24.

———. 2010b. "Ce "Sentiment de Culpabilité": Réflexion sur la Relation entre Emotions et Motivation dans les Migrations et le Soin Transnational." *Recherches Sociologiques et Anthropologiques* 1: 55–76.

———. 2008a. "Debating Culture Across Distance: Transnational Families and the Obligation to Care." In *The Family in Question: Immigrant and Ethnic Minorities in Multicultural Europe*, edited by Ralph Grillo, 269–291. Amsterdam: Amsterdam University Press.

———. 2008b. "Missing Kin and Longing to Be Together: Emotions and the Construction of Co-presence in Transnational Relationships." *Journal of Intercultural Studies* 29: 247–266.

———. 2007a. "Transnational Families and Aged Care: The Mobility of Care and the Migrancy of Ageing." *Journal of Ethnic and Migration Studies* 33: 275–297.

———. 2007b. "Transnational Families and the Provision of Moral and Emotional Support: The Relationship Between Truth and Distance." *Identities* 14: 385–409.

———. 2007c. "L'Aide Transnationale au sein des Familles d'Immigrés Qualifiés Etablis en Australie: une Comparaison entre les Immigrés Italiens et les Réfugiés Afghans." *Enfances, Familles, Générations*. Accessed August 20, 2011. http://www.erudit.org/revue/efg/2007/v/n6/016485ar.html?vue=integral.

———. 2001. *Visits Home: Migration Experiences Between Italy and Australia*. Melbourne: Melbourne University Publishing.

Baldassar, Loretta, and Cora Baldock. 2000. "Linking Migration and Family Studies: Transnational Migrants and the Care of Ageing Parents." In *Theoretical and Methodological Issues in Migration Research. Interdisciplinary and International Perspectives*, edited by Biko Agozino, 61–89. Aldershot: Ashgate.

Baldassar, Loretta, Cora V. Baldock, and Raelene Wilding. 2007. *Families Caring Across Borders: Migration, Ageing and Transnational Caregiving*. London: Palgrave Macmillan.

Baldassar, Loretta, and Donna R. Gabaccia. Eds. 2011. *Intimacy and Italian Migration: Gender and Domestic Lives in a Mobile World*. New York: Fordham University Press.

Baldassar,, Loretta and Joanne Pyke. Forthcoming. "The Role of Intra-Diaspora Knowledge Transfer and 'New' Italian Migration". *International Migration Journal*

Baldassar, Loretta, Joanne Pyke, and Danny Ben-Moshe. 2012. *The Italian Diaspora in Australia: Current and Potential Links to the Homeland*. Report of an Australian Research Council linkage project, Centre for Citizenship and Globalisation, Deakin University.

Baldassar, Loretta, Raelene Wilding, and Cora Baldock. 2007. "Long-Distance Care-Giving, Transnational Families and the Provision of Aged Care." In *Family Caregiving for Older Disabled People: Relational and Institutional Issues*, edited by Isabella Paoletti, 201–228. New York: Nova Science.

Baldassar, Loretta, and Ros Pesman. 2005. *From Paesani to Global Italians: Veneto Migrants in Australia*. Crawley: University of Western Australia Press.

Baldock, Cora V. 2000. "Migrants and Their Parents: Caregiving from a Distance." *Journal of Family Issues* 21: 205–224.

Baldwin-Edwards, Martin, and Albert Kraler. 2009. *REGINE—Regularisations in Europe*. Amsterdam: Pallas Publications, European Commission and Amsterdam University Press.

Banfi, Ludovica, and Paolo Boccagni. 2011. "Transnational Family Life and Female Migration in Italy: One or Multiple Patterns?" In *Gender, Generations and the Family in International Migration*, edited by Albert Kraler, Eleonore Kofman, Martin Kohli and and Camille Schmoll, 285–310. Amsterdam: Amsterdam University Press.

Barron, Ian. 2011. "The Shadows of Difference: Ethnicity and Young Children's Friendship." *Journal of Race, Ethnicity and Education* 14 (5): 655–674.

Barrow, Christine. 2010. *Caribbean Childhoods "Outside", "Adopted" or "Left Behind"*. Kingston: Ian Randle Publishers.

Basch, Linda Green, Nina Glick Schiller, and Cristina Szanton Blanc. 1994. *Nations Unbound. Transnational Projects, Postcolonial Predicaments, and Deterritorialized Nation-States*. New York: Routledge.

Basok, Tanya. 2000. "Migration of Mexican Seasonal Farm Workers to Canada and Development: Obstacles to Productive Investment." *International Migration Review* 34 (1): 79–97.

Battaglini, Alex, Sylvie Gravel, Carole Poulin, Michel Fournier, and Jean-Marc Brodeur. 2002. "Migration et Paternité ou Réinventer la Paternité." *Nouvelles Pratiques Sociales* 15: 165–179. Accessed June 12, 2007. http://www.erudit.org/revue/nps/2002/v15/n1/008267ar.html.

Bauböck, Rainer, and Thomas Faist. 2010. *Diaspora and Transnationalism: Concepts, Theories and Methods*. Amsterdam: Amsterdam University Press.

Bauer, Elaine, and Paul Thompson. 2006. *Jamaican Hands Across the Atlantic*. Kingston: Ian Randle Publishers.

———. 2004. " 'She's Always the Person with a Very Global Vision': The Gender Dynamics of Migration, Narrative Interpretation and the Case of Jamaican Transnational Families." *Gender & Society* 16 (2): 334–375.

Bauman, Zygmunt. 1998. *Globalization: The Human Consequences*. Cambridge: Polity.

Beasley, Chris, and Carol Bacchi. 2007. "Envisaging a New Politics for an Ethical Future: Beyond Trust, Care and Generosity—Towards an Ethic of 'Social Flesh'." *Feminist Theory* 8 (3): 279–298.

Beck, Ulrich. 1992. *Risk Society: Towards a New Modernity*. London: Sage.

Beck, Ulrich, and Elisabeth Beck-Gernsheim. 2002. *Individualization*. London: Sage.

Beck, Ulrich and Natan Sznaider. 2010. "New Cosmopolitanism in the Social Sciences." In *The Routledge International Handbook of Globalization Studies*, edited by Bryan S. Turner, 635–652. Abingdon and New York: Routledge.

———. 2006. "Unpacking Cosmopolitanism for the Social Sciences: A Research Agenda." *The British Journal of Sociology* 57 (1): 1–23.

Benavides, Blanca Mirna, Xenia Ortíz, Claudia Marina Silva, and Lilian Vega. 2004. "Pueden las Remesas Comprar el Futuro? Estudio Realizado en el Cantón San José La Labor, Municipio de San Sebastián, El Salvador." In *Desarrollo Económico Local en Centro América. Estudios de Comunidades Globalizadas*, edited by Guillermo Lathrop and Juan Pablo Pérez Saínz, 139–180. San José, Costa Rica: Flacso.

Bengtson, Vern, and W. Andrew Achenbaum. 1993. *The Changing Contract Across Generations*. Hawthorne: Aldine De Gruyter.

Ben-Moshe, Danny, and Joanne Pyke. 2012. *Diasporas in Australia: Current and Potential Links with the Homeland*. Summary report of an Australian Research Council Linkage project into the Italian, Macedonian, Tongan and Vietnamese diasporas, Centre for Citizenship and Globalisation, Deakin University.

Bernardes, Jon. 1999. "We Must Not Define 'The Family'!" *Marriage and Family Review* 28 (3): 21–41.

———. 1986. "Multidimensional Developmental Pathways: A Proposal to Facilitate the Conceptualisation of 'Family Diversity'." *The Sociological Review* 34 (3): 590–610.

Bernardi, Laura. 2011. "A Mixed-Methods Social Networks Study Design for Research on Transnational Families." *Journal of Marriage and Family* 73: 788–803.

Bernhard, Judith K., Patricia Landolt, and Luin Goldring. 2009. "Transnationalizing Families: Canadian Immigration Policy and the Spatial Fragmentation of Care-Giving Among Latin American Newcomers." *International Migration* 47 (2): 3–31.

———. 2008. "Transnationalizing Families: Canadian Immigration Policy and the Spatial Fragmentation of Care-giving among Latin American Newcomers." *Early Childhood Education Publications and Research*. Paper 8. http://digitalcommons.ryerson.ca/ece/8

Bhachu, Parminder. 1995. "New Cultural Forms and Transnational South Asian Women: Culture, Class, and Consumption Among British South Asian Women in the Diaspora." In *Nation and Migration: The Politics of Space in the South Asian Diaspora*, edited by Peter Van der Veer, 222–244. Philadelphia: University of Pennsylvania Press.

Birrell, Bob, and T. Fred Smith. 2010. "Export Earnings from the Overseas Student Industry: How Much?" *Australian Universities' Review* 52 (1): 4–12.

Blackman, Tim. 2000. "Defining Responsibility for Care: Approaches to the Care of Older People in Six European Countries." *International Journal of Social Welfare* 9 (3): 181–190.

Blackman, Tim, Sally Brodhurst, and Janet Convery. 2001. *Social Care and Social Exclusion: A Comparative Study of Older People's Care in Europe*. London: Palgrave Macmillan.

Bledsoe, Caroline. 1990. "'No Success Without Struggle.' Social Mobility and Hardship for Foster Children in Sierra Leone." *Man* 25 (1): 70–88.

Bledsoe, Caroline, and Papa Sow. 2008. "Family Reunification Ideals and the Practice of Transnational Reproductive Life Among Africans in Europe." MPIDR Working Paper WP 2008–001. Rostock: Max Planck Institute for Demographic Research.

Bloch Françoise, and Monique Buisson. 1994. "La Circulation du Don entre Générations, ou Comment Reçoit-On?" *Communications* 59: 55–72.

Boccagni, Paolo. 2013. Forthcoming. "Migration and the Family Transformations It 'Leaves Behind': A Critical View from Ecuador". *The Latin Americanist.*

———. 2012a. "Practising Motherhood at a Distance: Retention and Loss in Ecuadorian Transnational Families." *Journal of Ethnic and Migration Studies* 38 (2): 261–277.

———. 2012b. "Rethinking Transnational Studies: Transnational Ties and the Transnationalism of Everyday Life." *European Journal of Social Theory* 15 (1): 117–132.

———. 2011. "Migrants' Social Protection as a Transnational Process: Public Policies and Emigrant Initiative in the Case of Ecuador." *International Journal of Social Welfare* 20 (3): 318–325.

Boden, Deirdre, and Harvey Molotch. 1994. "The Compulsion to Proximity." In *Nowhere: Space, Time and Modernity*, edited by Roger Friedland and Deirdre Boden, 257–286. Berkeley: University of California Press.

Böhning, W. R., and Dennis Maillat. 1974. *The Effects of the Employment of Foreign Workers*. Paris: OECD.

Bolzman Claudio, Myrian Carbajal, and Giuditta Mainardi. Eds. 2007. *La Suisse au Rythme Latino. Dynamiques Migratoires des Latino-Américains*. Geneva: Les Editions IES.

Bolzman, Claudio, and Ibrahima Guissé. 2010. "La Formation des Etudiants: Réalités et Obstacles à la Mobilité Transnationale dans les Rapports Nord-Sud." In *Transnationalités et Développement: Rôles de l'Interculturel*, edited by Altay Manço and Claudio Bolzman, 141–154. Paris: L'Harmattan.

Bolzman, Claudio, Elisabeth Hirsch-Durret, Simon Anderfuhren, Marilène Vuille, and

Jäggi Monique. 2008. "Migration of Parents under Family Reunification Policies. A National Approach to a Transnational Problem. The Case of Switzerland." *Retraite et société* selection; 93–121.

Bonizzoni, Paola. 2013. Undocumented Domestic Workers in Italy: Surviving and Regularizing Strategies". In *Irregular Migrant Domestic Workers in Europe: Who Cares?*, edited by A. Triandafyllidou, 135–160.London: Ashgate.

———. 2012. "Here or There? Shifting Meaning and Practices of Motherhood Across Time and Space." *International Migration*. [article published on-line available at http://onlinelibrary.wiley.com/doi/10.1111/imig.12028/abstract]

———. 2011. "Civic Stratification, Stratified Reproduction and Family Solidarity: Strategies of Latino Families in Milan." In *Gender, Generations and the Family in International Migration*, edited by Albert Kraler, Eleonore Kofman, Martin Kohli and Camille Schmoll, 313–334. Amsterdam: Amsterdam University Press.

———. 2009. "Living Together Again: Families Surviving Italian Immigration Policies." *International Review of Sociology* 19 (1): 83–101.

Bonizzoni, Paola, and Luisa Leonini. Forthcoming. "Shifting Geographical Configurations in Migrant Families: Narratives of Children Reunited with Their Mothers in Italy." *Comparative Population Studies.*

Bonvalet, Catherine, and Jim Ogg. 2006a. *Enquêtes sur l'Entraide Familiale en Europe. Bilan de 9 Collectes.* Paris: Editions de l'INED.

———. 2006b. "Place de l'Entraide dans les Recherches sur la Famille." In *Enquêtes sur l'Entraide Familiale en Europe: Bilan de 9 Collectes*, edited by Catherine Bonvalet and Jim Ogg, 25–52. Paris: Editions de l'INED.

Bonvalet, Catherine, and Laurent Ortalda. 2006. "Enquête 'Proches et Parents,' Ined, France, 1990." In *Enquêtes sur l'Entraide Familiale en Europe: Bilan de 9 Collectes*, edited by Catherine Bonvalet and Jim Ogg, 85–120. Paris: Editions de l'INED.

Bourdieu, Pierre. 1986. "The Forms of Capital." In *Handbook of Theory for Research in the Sociology of Education*, edited by John E. Richardson, 241–258. Westport, CT: Greenwood Press.

Bowie, Fiona. 2004. "Adoption and the Circulation of Children. A Comparative Perspective." In *Cross-Cultural Approaches to Adoption*, edited by Fiona Bowie, 3–20. London: Routledge.

Bowlby, John. 1969. *Attachment and Loss. Vol. I: Attachment.* London: Hogarth.

Boyle, Paul, Thomas J. Cooke, Keith Halfacree, and Darren Smith. 2003. "The Effect of Long-Distance Family Migration and Motherhood on Partnered Women's Labour-Market Activity Rates in Great Britain and the USA." *Environment and Planning A* 35 (12): 2097–2114.

———. 2001. "A Cross-National Comparison of the Impact of Family Migration on Women's Employment Status." *Demography* 38 (2): 201–213.

Bribosia, Emmanuelle, and Andrea Rea. 2002. "Le Débat sur les Nouvelles Migrations en Belgique à la Lumière des Politiques Migratoires Récentes." In *Les Nouvelles Migrations. Un Enjeu Européen*, edited by Emmanuelle Bribosia and Andrea Rea, 233–260. Bruxelles: Complexe.

Bryant, John. 2005. *Children of International Migrants in Indonesia, Thailand, and the Philippines.* Innocenti Working Paper 2005–05, UNICEF Innocenti Research Centre, Florence.

Bryceson, Deborah Fahy, and Ulla Vuorela. 2002a. "Transnational Families in the Twenty First Century." In *The Transnational Family: New European Frontiers and Global Networks*, edited by Deborah Bryceson and Ulla Vuorela, 3–30. New York: Berg.

———. Eds. 2002b. *The Transnational Family. New European Frontiers and Global Networks.* Oxford: Berg.

Buencamino, Leonides, and Sergei Gorbunov. 2002. "Informal Money Transfer Systems: Opportunities and Challenges for Development Finance." Accessed May 5, 2005. http://www.un.org/esa/esa02dp26.pdf

Bullock, Marcus, and Peter Paik. 2009. *Aftermaths: Exile, Migration, and Diaspora Reconsidered.* New Brunswick, NJ: Rutgers University Press.

Bushin, Naomi. 2009. "Researching Family Migration Decision-Making: A Children-in-Families Approach." *Population, Space and Place* 15 (5): 429–443.

Byron, Margaret. 2005. "Expanding Narratives of Emigration and Return." In *Caribbean Narratives of Belonging. Fields of Relations, Sites of Identity*, edited by Jean Besson and Karen F. Olwig, 206–221. Oxford: Macmillan Education.

———. 1999. "The Caribbean-born Population in 1990s Britain: Who Will Return?" *Journal of Ethnic and Migration Studies* 25 (2): 285–301.

Caestecker, Frank. 2006. "Histoire de la Migration aux XIX° et XX° siècles (1830–2000)." In *Penser l'Immigration et l'Intégration Autrement. Une Initiative Belge*

*Inter-Universitaire*, edited by Bichara Khader, Marco Martiniello, Andrea Rea and Christiane Timmermans, 13–28. Bruxelles: Bruylant.
Caglar, Ayse. 2001. "Constraining Metaphors and the Transnationalisation of Spaces." *Journal of Ethnic and Migration Studies* 27 (4): 601–613.
Caicedo, Maritza. 2010. "Integración Económica y Desigualdad: Tres Generaciones de Mexicanos en Estados Unidos." *Revista Mexicana de Sociología* 72 (2): 255–282.
Calavita, Kitty. 2006. "Contradicciones Estructurales en la Política de Inmigración: los Casos de la Europa del Sur y de los Estados Unidos." *REIS. Revista Española de Investigaciones Sociológicas* 116: 185–212.
———. 1989. "The Contradictions of Immigration Lawmaking: The Immigration Reform and Control Act of 1986." *Law & Policy* 11 (1): 17–47.
Campani, Giovanna. 2012. 'Migrant Women and Gender Gap: Experiences in Southern Europe'. Paper presented at the *Land of Strangers Conference*, University of Padova, October 12–13.
Cantú, Lionel. 2009. *The Sexuality of Migration: Border Crossings and Mexican Immigrant Men*. Edited by Nancy A. Naples, and Salvador Vidal-Ortiz. New York: New York University Press.
Cao, Xiang, Abigail Sellen, A. J. Bernheim Brush, David Kirk, Darren Edge, and Xianghua Ding. 2010. *Understanding Family Communication Across Time Zones, at Savannah, Georgia, USA*. Accessed November 11, 2012, http://research.microsoft.com/en-us/people/daedge/p155-cao.pdf.
Caradec, Vincent. 1996. "Les Formes de la Vie Conjugale des 'Jeunes' Couples 'Agés'." *Population* (French Edition) 51(4/5): 897–927.
Carling, Jørgen, Cecilia Menjivar, and Leah Schmalzbauer. 2012. "Central Themes in the Study of Transnational Parenthood." *Journal of Ethnic and Migration Studies* 38 (2): 191–217.
Carsten, Janet. 2000. "Introduction: Cultures of Relatedness." In *Cultures of Relatedness. New Approaches to the Study of Kinship*, edited by Janet Carsten, 1–36. Cambridge: Cambridge University Press.
Castells, Manuel. 1996. *The Rise of the Network Society*. Cambridge, MA: Blackwell.
Castles, Stephen. 2006. "Guestworkers in Europe: A Resurrection?" *International Migration Review* 40: 741–766.
———. 2004. "The Factors That Make and Unmake Migration Policies." *International Migration Review* 38 (3): 852–854.
Castles, Stephen, and Mark J. Miller. 2009. *The Age of Migration*. 4th ed. Houndmills: Palgrave Macmillan.
CeSPI-FIERI. 2007. "Madri Migranti. Le Migrazioni di Cura dalla Romania e dall'Ucraina in Italia: Percorsi e Impatto sui Paesi di Origine." CeSPI Working Paper No. 34.
Chadeau, Ann, and Annie Fouquet. 1981. "Peut-On Mesurer le Travail Domestique?" *Economie et Statistique* 136: 29–42.
Chamberlain, Mary. 1998. *Caribbean Migration: Globalised Identities*. London and New York: Routledge.
Chavkin, Wendy, and JaneMaree Maher. 2010. *The Globalization of Motherhood. Deconstructions and Reconstructions of Biology and Care. Routledge Research in Comparative Politics*. Abingdon and New York: Routledge.
Cheal, David. 2002. *Sociology of Family Life*. Basingstoke: Palgrave.
Cieraad, Irene. 2006. *At Home: An Anthropology of Domestic Space*. Syracuse, NY: Syracuse University Press.
Clark Rebecca, Jennifer E. Glick, and Regina Bures. 2009. "Immigrant Families Over the Life Course: Research Directions and Needs." *Journal of Family Issues* 30 (6): 852–872.

Coe, Cati. 2008. "The Structuring of Feeling in Ghanain Transnational Families." *City & Society* 20 (2): 222–250.

Coenen-Huther, Josette, Jean Kellerhals, and Malik von Allmen. 1994. *Les Réseaux de Solidarité dans la Famille*. Lausanne: Editions Réalités sociales.

Cohen. Rina. 2000. " 'Mom Is a Stranger': The Negative Impact of Immigration Policies on the Family Life of Filipina Domestic Workers." *Canadian Ethnic Studies* 32 (3): 76–86.

Cohen, Robin. 1997. *Global Diasporas: An Introduction*. Seattle: University of Washington Press.

———. 1987. *The New Helots: Migrants in the International Division of Labour*. Research in Ethnic Relations Series. Aldershot, Averby: Gower Publishing Group.

Cole, Michael, and Shiela Cole. 2001. *The Development of Children*. New York: W H. Freeman and Company.

Colectivo IOE. 2002. *Política Migratoria en España en el Marco Europeo*. Madrid: Mimeo.

Coleman, James S. 1990. *Foundations of Social Theory*. London: Harvard University Press.

Colen, Shellee. 1989a. " 'Like a Mother to Them': Stratified Reproduction and West Indian Childcare Workers and Employers in New York." In *Conceiving the New World Order: The Global Politics of Reproduction*, edited by Faye Ginsburg and Rayna Rapp, 78–102. Berkeley: University of California Press.

———. 1989b. " 'Just a Little Respect': West Indian Domestic Workers in New York City." In *Muchachas No More. Household Workers in Latin America and the Caribbean*, edited by Elsa M. Chaney and Mary Garcia Castro, 171–194. Philadelphia: Temple University Press.

Coles, Anne. 2008. "Making Multiple Migrations: The Life of British Diplomatic Families Overseas." In *Gender and Family among Transnational Professionals*, edited by Anne Coles and Anne-Meike Fechter, 125–148. New York and London: Routledge.

Coles, Anne, and Anne-Meike Fetcher. Eds. 2008. *Gender and Family among Transnational Professionals*. New York and London: Routledge

Colic-Peisker, Val, and Farida Tilbury. 2006. "Employment Niches for Recent Refugees: Segmented Labour Market in Twenty-first Century Australia." *Journal of Refugee Studies* 19 (2): 203–229.

Colpi, Terri. 1991. *The Italian Factor: The Italian Community in Great Britain*. London: Mainstream.

Connell, Raewyn. 1987. *Gender and Power*. Stanford, CA: Stanford University Press.

Connelly, Paul. 1998. *Racism, Gender Identities and Young Children: Social Relations in a Multi-Ethnic, Inner-City Primary School*. London: Routledge.

Conradson, David, and Alan Latham. 2005. "Transnational Urbanism: Attending to Everyday Practices and Mobilities." *Journal of Ethnic and Migration Studies* 31 (2): 227–233.

Constable, Nicole. 1999. "At Home but Not at Home: Filipina Narratives of Ambivalent Returns." *Cultural Anthropology* 14 (2): 203–228.

Constable, Janis, Regine Wagner, Merilyn Childs, and Antoinetta Natoli. 2004. *Doctors Become Taxidrivers: Recognizing Skills—Not Easy as It Sounds*. New South Wales, Sydney: Office of Employment Equity and Diversity, Premier's Department, www.eeo.nsw.gov.au.

Conway, Dennis, and Robert B. Potter. Eds. 2009. *Return Migration of the Next Generations: 21st Century Transnational Mobility*. Farnham, England; Burlington, VT: Ashgate.

Cornelius, Wayne A. 2001. "Death at the Border: Efficacy and Unintended Consequences of US Immigration Control." Working Paper, Center for Comparative Immigration Studies, UC San Diego.

Cortés, Rosalia. 2007. *Children and Women Left Behind in Labour Sending Countries. Global Report on Migration and Children.* Accessed 30 April 2013, http://www.unicef.org/socialpolicy/index_46205.html

Costa, Giuliana. 2013. "Long-Term Care Italian Policies: A Case of Inertial Institutional Change." In *Reforms in Long-Term Care Policies in Europe*, edited by C. Ranci and E. Pavolini. New York: Springer Science.

Cowling, Wendy. 1990. *On Being Tongan: Responses to Concepts of Tradition.* Unpublished doctoral thesis, Macquarie University.

Cresson, Geneviève, and Nicole Gadrey. 2004. "Entre Famille et Métier: le Travail du Care." *Nouvelles Questions Féministes* 23 (3): 26–41.

Damamme, Aurélie, and Patricia Paperman. 2009. "Temps du Care et Organisation Sociale du Travail en Famille." *Temporalités 9.* Accessed November 18, 2012. http://temporalites.revues.org/1036

Datta, Kavita, Cathy McIlwaine, Joanna Herbet, Yara Evans, Jon May, and Jane Wills. 2009. "Men on the Move: Narratives of Migration and Work Among Low-paid Migrant Men in London." *Social and Cultural Geography* 10: 853–873.

D'Aubeterre, María Eugenia. 2000. "Mujeres y Espacio Transnacional: Maniobras Para Renegociar el Vinculo Conyugal." In *Migración y Relaciones de Género en México*, edited by Dalia Barrera Bassols and Cristina Oehmichen Bazán, 63–85. Mexico: GIMTRAP. IIA/UNA.

Dei Ottati, Gabi. Forthcoming. "Transnational Fast Fashion Industrial District: An Analysis of the Chinese Businesses in Prato." Draft paper 18 November 2012, to be published in *Cambridge Journal of Economics.*

Delphy, Christine. 1998. *L'Ennemi Principal I.* Economie Politique du Patriarcat. Paris: Syllepse.

De Tona, Carla. 2011. "Mothering Contradictory Diasporas: Negotiation of Motherhood Traditional Roles among Italian Women in Ireland." In *Intimacy and Italian Migration: Gender and Domestic Lives in a Mobile World*, edited by Loretta Baldassar and Donna Gabaccia, 101–112. New York: Fordham University Press.

D'Emilio, Anna Lucia, Berenice Cordero, Bertrand Bainvel, Christian Skoog, Debora Comini, Jean Gough, Monica Dias, Rhea Saab, and Theresa Kilbane. 2007. *The Impact of International Migration: Children Left Behind in Selected Countries of Latin America and the Caribbean.* New York: Unicef.

Development Prospects Group. 2007. "Migration and Development Brief 2." Accessed August 21, 2007. http://web.worldbank.org/WBSITE/EXTERNAL/NEWS/0,,contentMDK:21124587~pagePK:64257043~piPK:437376~theSitePK:4607,00.html

Díaz Gorfinkel, Magdalena. 2009. "Política de Inmigración y la Población Inmigrante en España y la Unión Europea." *Revista de Derecho de la Unión Europea* 17 (2): 69–84.

Di Leonardo, Micaela. 1992. "The Female World of Cards and Holidays: Women, Families and the Work of Kinship." In *Rethinking the Family: Some Feminist Questions*, edited by Barrie Thorne and Marilyn Yalom, 246–261. Boston: Northern University Press.

———. 1984. *The Varieties of Ethnic Experience: Kinship, Class and Gender among California Italian-Americans.* New York: Cornell University Press.

Domingo, Andreu I Valls, and Rosana Beatriz Martínez. 2006. "La Población Latinoamericana Censada en España en el Año 2001: un Retrato Sociodemográfico." *Notas de Población* 81: 99–127.

Donati, Pierpaolo. 2012. *Relational Sociology: A New Paradigm for the Social Sciences (Ontological Explorations).* Abindgon and New York: Routledge.

Doucet, Andrea. 2006. *Do Men mother? Fathering, Care and Domestic Responsibility*. Toronto: University of Toronto Press.
Doucet, Andrea, and Laura Merla. 2007. "Stay-at-Home Fathering. A Strategy for Balancing Work and Home in Canadian and Belgian Families." *Community, Work and Family* 10: 455–473.
Douglass, Mike. 2006. "Global Householding in Pacific Asia." *International Development Planning Review* 28 (4): 421–445.
Doyle J. and M. Nathan. 2001. *Wherever Next: Work in a Mobile World*. London: The Industrial Society
Dreby, Joanna. 2010. *Divided by Borders: Mexican Migrants and Their Children*. Berkeley: University of California Press.
———. 2008. "Gender and Transnational Gossip." *Qualitative Sociology* 32: 33–52.
———. 2007. "Children and Power in Mexican Transnational Families." *Journal of Marriage and Family* 69 (4): 1050–1064.
———. 2006. "Honor and Virtue: Mexican Parenting in the Transnational Context." *Gender & Society* 20: 32–59.
Dreby, Joanna, and Timothy Adkins. 2010. "Inequalities in Transnational Families." *Sociology Compass* 4: 673–689.
Drinkwater, Stephen, John Eade, and Michal Garapich. 2009. "Poles Apart? EU Enlargement and the Labour Market Outcomes of Immigrants in the United Kingdom." *International Migration* 47: 161–190.
Duncombe, Jean, and Dennis Marsden. 1998. " 'Stepford Wives' and 'Hollow Men'?: Doing Emotion Work, Doing Gender and 'Authenticity' in Intimate Heterosexual Relationships." In *Emotions in Social Life: Critical Themes and Contemporary Issues*, edited by Gilian Bendelow and Simon Johnsson Williams, 209–224. London: Routledge.
———. 1993. "Love and Intimacy: The Gender Division of Emotion and 'Emotion Work'." *Sociology* 27 (2): 221–241.
Dusenbery, Verne A. 2001. "Punjabi Sikh Positionings in Australia." In *A Punjabi Sikh Community in Australia: From Indian Sojourners to Australian Citizens*, edited by Rashmere Bhatti and Verne A. Dusenbery, 242–251. A Centenary of Federation Project supported by the Commonwealth and presented by Woolgoolga Neighbourhood Centre Inc.
ECMI-CBCP/AOS-Manila, SMC and OWWA. 2004. *Hearts Apart: Migration in the Eyes of Filipino Children*. Manila: Episcopal Commission for the Pastoral Care of Migrant and Itinerant People-CBCP/Apostleship of the Sea-Manila, Scalabrini Migration Center and Overseas Workers Welfare Administration.
Edwards, Rosalind, Jane Franklin, and Janet Holland. 2003. "Families and Social Capital: Exploring the Issues." Families and Social Capital ESRC Research Group Working Paper 1. London: South Bank University.
Ehrenreich, Barbara, and Arlie R. Hochschild. Eds. 2003a. *Global Woman: Nannies, Maids and Sex Workers in the New Economy*. London: Granta Books.
Ehrenreich, Barbara, and Arlie R. Hochschild. 2003b. "Introduction." In *Global Woman: Nannies, Maids and Sex Workers in the New Economy*, edited by Barbara Ehrenreich and Arlie R. Hochschild, 1–13. London: Granta Books.
Elliott, Anthony, and John Urry. 2010. *Mobile Lives*. London: Routledge.
Elrick, Tim, and Emilia Brinkmeier. 2009. "Changing Patterns of Polish Labour Migration after the UK's Opening of the Labour Market? Insights from Rural Case-Studies in the Opolskie and Świętokrzyskie Voivodships." In *Polish Migration to the UK in the 'New' European Union After 2004*, edited by Kathy Burrell, 49–66. Farnham: Ashgate.

ENDESA. 2008. *Encuesta Demográfica y de Salud 2007*. Santo Domingo: Centro de Estudios Sociales y Demográficos/Macro International Inc.
Engster, Daniel. 2004. "Care Ethics and Natural Law Theory: Toward an Institutional Political Theory of Caring." *The Journal of Politics* 66 (1): 113–135.
Ennuyer, Bernard. 2001. "Ces Vieux que l'On dit 'Dépendants'." In *Vivre au Grand Age. Angoisses et Ambivalences de la Dépendance*, edited by Joëlle Chabert and Bertrand Richard, 9–65. Paris: Autrement.
Epstein, A. L. 1978. *Ethos and Identity: Three Studies in Ethnicity*. Chicago: Aldine.
Erel, Umut. Ed. 2012. Special Issue: "Transnational Care in Europe—Changing Formations of Citizenship, Family, and Generation." *Social Politics: International Studies in Gender, State & Society* 19 (1).
———. 2010. "Migrating Cultural Capital: Bourdieu in Migration Studies." *Sociology* 44 (4): 642–660.
———. 2002. "Reconceptualizing Motherhood: Experiences of Migrant Women from Turkey Living in Germany." In *The Transnational Family. New European Frontiers and Global Networks*, edited by Deborah Fahy Bryceson and Ulla Vuorela, 127–146. Oxford: Berg.
Escriva, Angeles. 2005. "Aged Global Care Chains: A Southern-European Contribution to the Field." Paper presented at the International Conference on Migration and Domestic Work in Global Perspective, Wassenaar, the Netherlands, May 26–29.
Escriva, Angeles, and Emmeline Skinner. 2008. "Domestic Work and Transnational Care Chains in Spain." In *Migration and Domestic Work. A European Perspective on a Global Theme*, edited by Helma Lutz, 113–126. Farnham, Burlington: Ashgate.
Esparragoza, Maria Eugenia. 2003. "Guayaquil . . . Italia." In *Classi Meticce. Giovani, Studenti, Insegnanti nelle Scuole delle Migrazioni*, edited by Enrico Fravega and Luca Queirolo Palmas, 86–90. Roma: Carocci.
Esping-Andersen, Gøsta. 1990. *The Three Worlds of Welfare Capitalism*. Cambridge and Oxford: Polity Press.
Eurostat. 2010. *Combating Poverty and Social Exclusion. A Statistical Portrait of the European Union 2010*. Luxembourg: European Commission.
Evans, Peter. 1996. "Government Action, Social Capital and Development: Reviewing the Evidence on Synergy." *World Development* 24 (6): 1119–1132.
Evergeti, Venetia, and Elisabetta Zontini. 2006. "Social Capital, Migration and Transnational Families: Some Critical Reflections." *Ethnic and Racial Studies* 29 (6): 1025–1039.
Evergeti, Venetia, and Louise Ryan. 2011. "Transnational Family Life and Care." In *Gender, Generations and the Family in International Migration*, edited by Albert Kraler, Eleonore Kofman, Martin Kohli and Camille Schmoll, 355–373. Amsterdam: Amsterdam University Press.
Evers, Adelbert, Marja Pilj, and Clare Ungerson. Eds. 1994. *Payments for Care*. Aldershot, UK: Avebury.
Faist, Thomas. 2000. *The Volume and Dynamics of International Migration and Transnational Social Spaces*. New York: Oxford University Press.
Falzon, Mark-Anthony. 2009. *Multi-Sited Ethnography: Theory, Praxis and Locality in Contemporary Research*. Farnham: Ashgate.
Favell, Adrian. 2008. "The New Face of East-West Migration in Europe." *Journal of Ethnic and Migration Studies* 34: 710–716.
Fernández Sánchez, Pablo Antonio. 2002. "El Derecho de Reagrupación Familiar de los Extranjeros." *Derecho y Conocimiento* 1: 375–395.
Field, John. 2008. *Social Capital*. London: Routledge.
Fihel, Agnieszka, and Paweł Kaczmarczyk. 2009. "Migration: A Threat or a Chance? Recent Migration of Poles and Its Impact on the Polish Labour Market." In *Polish*

*Migration to the UK in the 'New' European Union After 2004*, edited by Kathy Burrell, 23–48. Farnham: Ashgate.
Finch, Janet. 2007. "Displaying Families." *Sociology* 41 (1): 65–81.
———. 1989a. *Family Obligations and Social Change*. Cambridge, UK: Polity Press.
———. 1989b. "Kinship and Friendship." In *British Social Attitude. Special International Report*, edited by Roger Jowell, Sharon Witherspoon and Lindsey Brook, 87–104. Aldershot: Gower.
Finch, Janet, and Dulcie Groves. Eds. 1983. *A Labour of Love: Women, Work, and Caring*. London: Routledge.
Finch, Janet, and Jennifer Mason. 1993. *Negotiating Family Responsibilities*. London: Routledge.
———. 1991. "Obligations of Kinship in Contemporary Britain: Is There Normative Agreement?" *The British Journal of Sociology* 42 (3): 345–367.
Finch, Tim, Jill Rutter, Maria Latorre, and Naomi Pollard. 2009. "Shall We Stay or Shall We Go Now? Re-migration Trends Among Britain's Immigrants." London: IPPR. Accessed September 26, 2009. www.ippr.org/publicationsand reports/.
Fine, Michael. 1999. "The Responsibility for Child and Aged Care: Shaping Policies for the Future." SPRC Discussion Paper No. 105, Social Policy Research Centre, Sydney.
Fisher, Berenice, and Joan Tronto. 1990. "Towards a Feminist Theory of Caring." In *Circles of Care: Work and Identity in Women's Lives*, edited by Emily K. Abel and Margaret K. Nelson, 35–62. New York: New York Press.
Fisher, Mike. 1994. "Man-Made Care: Community Care and Older Male Carers." *British Journal of Social Work* 24: 659–680.
Flavell, Adrian, Miriam Feldblum, and Michael Smith. 2007. "The Human Face of Global Mobility: A Research Agenda." *Transaction Social Science and Modern Society* 44 (2): 15–25.
Foner, Nancy. 2001. *Islands in the City: West Indian Migration to New York*. Berkeley and London: University of California Press.
Fresnoza-Flot, Asuncion. 2011. "Le Vécu Masculin de la Migration des Femmes: le Cas des Maris Philippins restés au Pays." *Cahiers du Genre* numéro hors-série: 199–217.
———. 2010. "The Catholic Church in the Lives of Irregular Migrant Filipinas in France: Identity Formation, Empowerment and Social Control." *The Asia Pacific Journal of Anthropology* 11: 345–361.
———. 2009a. *Migration, Genre et Famille Transnationale: l'Exemple des Mères Migrantes Philippines en France*. Lille: Atelier National de Reproduction des Thèses.
———. 2009b. "Migration Status and Transnational Mothering: The Case of Filipino Migrants in France." *Global Networks* 9: 252–270.
Furedi, Frank. 2005. *Politics of Fear: Beyond Left and Right*. London and New York: Continuum.
Gamburd, Michele Ruth. 2000. *The Kitchen Spoon's Handle: Transnationalism and Sri Lanka's Migrant Housemaids*. Ithaca: Cornell University Press.
Garapich, Michal. 2008. "Odyssean Refugees, Migrants and Power: Construction of the 'Other' Within the Polish Community in the United Kingdom." In *Citizenship, Political Engagement and Belonging: Immigrants in Europe and the United States*, edited by Deborah Reed-Danahay and Catherine Brettell, 124–144. New Brunswick: Rutgers University Press.
Gardner, Katy, and Ralph Grillo. 2002. "Transnational Households and Ritual: An Overview." *Global Networks* 2: 179–190.
Gerstel, Naomi, and Sally Gallagher. 2001. "Men's Caregiving: Gender and the Contingent Character of Care." *Gender & Society* 15: 197–217.

Ghana Statistical Service. 2008. *Ghana Demographic and Health Survey*. Accra: Ghana Statistical Service.
Gheaus, Anca. 2011 "Care Drain: Who Should Provide for the Children Left Behind?" *Critical Review of International social and political Philosophy*: 1–23.
Gille, Zsuzsa. 2012. "Global Ethnography 2.0—from Methodological Nationalism to Methodological Materialism." In *Beyond Methodological Nationalism: Research Methodologies for Cross-Border Studies*, edited by Anna Amelina, Devrismel D. Nergiz, Thomas Faist and Nina GlickSchiller, 91–110. London: Routledge.
Ginsborg, Paul. 2003. *Italy and Its Discontents 1980–2001*. London: Penguin Books.
Giralt, Rosa Mas A., and Adrian J. Bailey. 2010. "Transnational Familyhood and the Liquid Life Paths of South Americans in the UK." *Global Networks* 10 (3): 383–400.
Glenn, Evelyn Nakano. 1992. "From Servitude to Service Work: Historical Continuities in the Racial Division of Paid Reproductive Labor." *Signs* 18: 1–43.
Glick, Jennifer E. 2010. "Connecting Complex Processes: A Decade of Research on Immigrant Families." *Journal of Marriage and Family* 72 (3): 498–515.
Glick Schiller, Nina, Linda Basch, and Cristina Szanton-Blanc. 1992. *Towards a Transnational Perspective on Migration*. New York: New York Academy of Sciences.
Glick Schiller, Nina, and George Eugene Fouron. 2001. *George Woke Up Laughing: Long-Distance Nationalism and the Search for Home*. Durham, NC: Duke University Press.
Gmelch, G. 1980 'Return Migration'. *Annual Review of Anthropology* 9:135–159
Godbout, Jacques, and Johanne Charbonneau. 1996. *La Circulation du Don dans la Parenté*. Montréal: INRS-Urbanisation.
Goodman, Robert, Howard Meltzer, and Veira Bailey. 1998. "The Strengths and Difficulties Questionnaire: A Pilot Study on the Validity of the Self-Report Version." *European Child and Adolescent Psychiatry* 7: 125–130.
Goody, Esther N. 1982. *Parenthood and Social Reproduction. Fostering and Occupational Roles in West Africa*. Cambridge: Cambridge University Press.
Goulbourne, Harry. 1989. "The Contribution of West Indian Groups to British Politics." In *Black British Politics in Britain*, edited by Harry Goulbourne, 12–31. London: Avebury.
———. 2002. *Caribbean Transnational Experience*. London: Pluto Press.
Goulbourne, Harry, and John Solomos. 2003. "Families, Ethnicity and Social Capital." *Social Policy and Society* 2 (4): 329–338.
Goulbourne, Harry, Tracey Reynolds, John Solomos, and Elisabetta Zontini. 2010. *Transnational Families: Ethnicities, Identities and Social Capital*. London: Routledge.
Grillo, Ralph. 2010. "Contesting Diversity in Europe: Alternative Regimes and Moral Orders." MMG Working Paper 10 (02).
———. Ed. 2008. *The Family in Question: Immigrant and Ethnic Minorities in Multicultural Europe*. Amsterdam: Amsterdam University Press.
———. 2007. "Betwixt and Between: Trajectories and Projects of Transmigration." *Journal of Ethnic and Migration Studies* 33 (2): 199–217.
Grillo, Ralph, and Valentina Mazzucato. 2008. "Africa-Europe: A Double Engagement." *Journal of Ethnic and Migration Studies* 34 (2): 175–198.
Grundy, Emily. 2005. "Reciprocity in Relationships: Socio-Economic and Health Influences on Intergenerational Exchanges Between Third Age Parents and their Adult Children in Great Britain." *British Journal of Sociology* 56 (2): 233–255.
Gubrium, Jaber F., and James A. Holstein. 1990. *What Is Family?* Houston: Mayfield Publishing Company.

Guzmán, José Miguel. 2002. *Envejecimiento y Desarrollo en América Latina y el Caribe*. Santiago de Chile: CEPAL.

Hafford, Carol. 2010. "Sibling Caretaking in Immigrant Families: Understanding Cultural Practices to Inform Child Welfare Practice and Evaluation." *Evaluation and Program Planning* 33: 294–302.

Hage, Ghassan. 2005. "A Not So Multi-Sited Ethnography of a Not So Imagined Community." *Anthropological Theory* 5 (4): 463–475.

Hardill, Irene. 2004. "Transnational Living and Moving Experiences: Intensified Mobility and Dual-Career Households." *Population, Space and Place* 10 (5): 375–389.

———. 2002. *Gender, Migration and the Dual Career Household*. London and New York: Routledge.

Hardill, Irene, and Sandra MacDonald. 1998. "Choosing to Relocate: An Examination of the Impact of Expatriate Work on Dual-Career Households." *Women's Studies International Forum* 21 (1): 21–29.

Harvey, William. 2008. "Brain Circulation? British and Indian Scientists in Boston, Massachusetts, USA." *Asian Population Studies* 4 (3): 293–309.

Hashim, Iman M. 2005. "Exploring the Linkages Between Children's Independent Migration and Education: Evidence from Ghana." Working Paper T12. Sussex: Sussex Centre for Migration Research.

Hawthorne, Lesleyanne. 2005. " 'Picking Winners': The Recent Transformation of Australia's Skilled Migration Policy." *International Migration Review* 39 (3): 663–696.

Hays, Sharon. 1998. *The Cultural Contradictions of Motherhood*. New Haven, CT: Yale University Press.

Held, David, Anthony David Goldblatt McGrew, and Jonathan Perraton. 1999. *Global Transformations*. Cambridge: Polity.

Herrera, Gioconda. 2010. "Stratified Workers/Stratified Mothers: Migration Policies and Citizenship Among Ecuadorian Immigrant Women." In *The Globalization of Motherhood. Deconstructions and Reconstructions of Biology and Care*, edited by Wendy Chavkin and JaneMaree Maher, 55–76. Abingdon and New York: Routledge.

———. 2008. "Políticas Migratorias y Familias Transnacionales: Migración Ecuatoriana en España y Estados Unidos." In *América Latina Migrante: Estado, Familia, Identidades*, edited by Gioconda Herrera and Jacques Ramírez, 71–88. Quito: Flacso-Ecuador, Ecuador.

Herrera Lima, Fernando. 2001. "Transnational Families: Institutions of Transnational Social Space." In *New Transnational Social Spaces: International Migration and Transnational Companies in the Early Twenty-First Century*, edited by Ludger Pries, 77–93. London: Routledge.

Hibbins, Raymond, and Bob Pease. 2009. "Men and Masculinities on the Move." In *Men. Critical Studies of Masculinities and the Migration Experience*, edited by Mike Donaldson, Raymond Hibbins, Richard Howson and Bob Pease, 1–20. New York: Routledge.

Ho Elsie, and Richard Bedford. 2008. "Asian Transnational Families in New Zealand: Dynamics and Challenges." *International Migration* 46 (4): 41–62.

Hobson, Barbara, and Susanne Fahlén. 2009. "Competing Scenarios for European Fathers: Applying Sen's Capabilities and Agency Framework to Work–Family Balance." *American Academy of Political and Social Science* 624: 214–233.

Hochschild, Arlie Russell. 2005. "Love and Gold." In *Feminist Politics, Activism and Vision: Local and Global Challenges*, edited by Luciana Ricciutelli, Angela Miles and Margaret McFadden, 34–46. Toronto: Zed/Innana Books.

———. 2003. "Love and Gold." In *Global Woman: Nannies, Maids and Sex Workers in the New Economy*, edited by Barbara Ehrenreich and Arlie Russell Hochschild, 15–30. London: Granta Books.

———. 2000. "Global Care Chains and Emotional Surplus Value." In *On the Edge. Living with Global Capitalism*, edited by Will Hutton and Anthony Giddens, 130–146. London: Vintage.

———. 1997. *The Time Bind: When Work Becomes Home and Home Becomes Work*. New York: Metropolitan Books.

Holmes, Mary. 2006. "Love Lives at a Distance: Distance Relationships over the Lifecourse." *Sociological Research Online* 11 (3).

———. 2004. "An Equal Distance? Individualisation, Gender and Intimacy in Distance Relationships." *The Sociological Review* 52 (2): 180–200.

Hondagneu-Sotelo, Pierrette. 2001. *Doméstica. Immigrant Workers Clearing and Caring in the Shadows of Affluence.* Berkeley and Los Angeles: University of California Press.

Hondagneu-Sotelo, Pierrette, and Ernestine Avila. 1997. " 'I'm Here, But I'm There': The Meanings of Latina Transnational Motherhood." *Gender & Society* 11: 548–571.

Horst, Heather. A. 2006. "The Blessings and Burdens of Communication: Cell Phones in Jamaican Transnational Social Fields." *Global Networks* 6 (2): 143–159.

Horst, Heather, and Daniel Miller. 2006. *The Cell Phone: An Anthropology of Communication.* Oxford: Berg.

Horton, Sarah. 2009. "A Mother's Heart Is Weighed Down with Stones: A Phenomenological Approach to the Experience of Transnational Motherhood." *Culture, Medicine and Psychiatry* 33 (1): 21–40.

Huang, Shirlena, Leng Leng Thang, and Mika Toyota. 2012a. "Transnational Mobilities for Care: Rethinking the Dynamics of Care in Asia." *Global Networks* 12 (2): 129–134.

———. Eds. 2012b. "Transnational Mobilities for Care: Rethinking the Dynamics of Care in Asia." *Global Networks* 12 (2).

Hugo, Graeme. Forthcoming. "From Permanent Settlement to Transnationalism—Contemporary Population Movement Between Italy and Australia: Trends and Implications."" *International Migration.*

———. 2012. "Australia's Changing Population and the Future." *Migration Australia* 1: 32–41.

———. 2009. "Returning Youthful Nationals to Australia: Brain Gain or Brain Circulation?" In *Return Migration of the Next Generations: 21st Century Transnational Mobility*, edited by Dennis Conway and Robert Potter, 187–220. Farnham, England; Burlington, VT: Ashgate.

____. 2005. "Migrants in Society: Diversity and Cohesion." A paper prepared for the Policy Analysis and Research Programme of the Global Commission on International Migration.

Illés, Sandor, and Aron Kincses. 2012. "Hungary as Receiving Country for Circulars." *Hungarian Geographical Bulletin* 61 (3): 197–218.

Instituto Nacional de Estadística y Geografía (INEGI). 2011. "Tabuladores Básicos, Censo de Población y Vivienda 2010." Accessed September 2, 2011. http://www3.inegi.org.mx/sistemas/TabuladosBasicos/Default.aspx?c=27303&s=est

———. 2009. "Encuesta Nacional de Dinámica Demográfica: Panorama Sociodemográfico de México: Principales Resultados." México: Instituto Nacional de Estadística y Geografía, Consejo Nacional de Población. "Immigrant Waiting List by Country [on line] Travel State Gov." Accessed August 21, 2011. www.travel.state.gov/pdf/waitingListItem.pdf

Irwin, Sarah. 1999. "Resourcing the Family: Gendered Claims and Obligations and Issues of Explanation." In *The New Family?*, edited by Elizabeth B. Silva and Carol Smart, 31–45. London: Sage.

Isaksen, Lise Widding, Sambasivan Uma Devi, and Arlie Russell Hochschild. 2008. "Global Care Crisis: A Problem of Capital, Care Chain, or Commons?" *American Behavioral Scientist* 52: 405–425.

Isiugo-Abanihe, Uche C. 1985. "Child Fosterage in West Africa." *Population and Development Review* 11 (1): 53–73.

Iuliano, Susanna. 2010. *Vite Italiane: Italian lives in Western Australia*, Crawley (WA): UWA Publishing.

Jenson, Jane. 2003. *Redesigning the "Welfare Mix" for Families: Policy Challenges.* Ottawa: Canadian PolicyResearch Networks

Joseph, Alun E., and Bonnie C. Hallman. 1985. "Over the Hill and Far Away: Distance as a Barrier to the Provision of Assistance to Elderly Relatives." *Social Science and Medicine* 56 (6): 631–639.

Judge, Tejinder K., and Carman Neustaedter. 2010. *Sharing Conversation and Sharing Life.* Video Conferencing in the Home, at Atlanta, Georgia, USA.

Kapur, Devesh. 2001. "Diasporas and Technology Transfer." *Journal of Human Development* 2 (2): 265–286.

Kapur, Devesh, and John McHale. 2005. *Give Us Your Best and Brightest: The Global Hunt for Talent and Its Impact on the Developing World.* Washington, DC: Center for Global Development, Brookings Institution Press.

Kastner, K. 2010. "Moving Relationships: Family Ties of Nigerian Migrants on Their Way to Europe." *African and Black Diaspora: An International Journal* 3 (1): 17–34.

Kearney, Michael. 1995. "The Local and Global: The Anthropology of Globalization and Transnationalism." *Annual Review of Anthropology* 24 (1): 547–565.

Keller, Wolfgang. 2004. "International Technology Diffusion." *Journal of Economic Literature* 42 (3): 752–782.

Kergoat, Danièle. 2000. "Division Sexuelle du Travail et Rapports Sociaux de Sexe." In *Dictionnaire Critique du Féminisme*, edited by Héléna Hirata, Françoise Laborie, Hélène Le Doaré and Danièle Senotier, 35–44. Paris: PUF.

Khoo, Siew-Ean. 2003. "Sponsorship of Relatives for Migration and Immigrant Settlement Intention." *International Migration* 41 (5): 177–199.

Khoo, Siew-Ean, Graeme Hugo, and Peter McDonald. 2011. "Skilled Migration from Europe to Australia." *Population, Space and Place* 17 (5): 550–566.

Kicinger, Anna. 2009. "Beyond the Focus on Europeanisation: Polish Migration Policy 1989–2004." *Journal of Ethnic and Migration Studies* 35: 79–95.

Kilkey, Majella, and Harriet Clarke. 2010. "Disabled Men and Fathering: Opportunities and Constraints." *Community, Work and Family* 13: 127–146.

Kilkey, Majella, and Laura Merla. 2013. Forthcoming. "Transnational Families' Care-Giving Arrangements: Towards a Situated Transnationalism." *Global Networks.*

Kilkey, Majella, Diane Perrons, and Ania Plomien, with Pierrette Hondagneu-Sotelo and Hernan Ramirez. 2013a. *Gender, Migration and Domestic Work: Masculinities, Male Labour and Fathering in the UK and USA.* Basingstoke: Palgrave Macmillan.

Kilkey, Majella, Ania Plomien, and Diane Perrons. 2013b. "Migrant Men's Fathering Practices and Projects in National and Transnational Spaces: Recent Polish Male Migrants to London." *International Migration Review*, Published online.

King, Russell, and Anastasia Christou. Eds. 2012. Special Issue: "Of Home, Belonging and Return: Transnational Links of the Mediterranean-Origin Second Generation." *Journal of Mediterranean Studies* 20 (2).

King, Russel, Warnes, T. and Williams, A. 2000. *Sunset Lives: British Retirement Migration to the Mediterranean.* Oxford: Berg.

Kirk, David, Abigail Sellen, and Xiang Cao. 2010. "Home Video Communication: Mediating 'Closeness'." CSCW no. 2010: 135–144.
Kivisto, Peter. 2001. "Theorizing Transnational Immigration: A Critical Review of Current Efforts." *Ethnic and Racial Studies* 24 (4): 549–577.
Kobayashi, Audrey, and Valerie Preston. 2007. "Transnationalism Through the Life Course: Hong Kong Immigrants in Canada." *Asia Pacific Viewpoint* 48 (2): 151–167.
Kofman, Eleonore. 2012. "Rethinking Care Through Social Reproduction: Articulating Circuits of Migration." *Social Politics: International Studies in Gender, State & Society* 19 (1): 142–162.
———. 2004. "Family-Related Migration: A Critical Review of European Studies." *Journal of Ethnic and Migration Studies* 30 (2): 243–262.
Kofman, Eleonore, and Parvati Raghuram. 2009. *The Implications of Migration for Gender and Care Regimes in the South*. Vol. Programme Paper Number 41. Social Policy and Development, UNRISD.
Kraler, Albert, and Eleonore Kofman. 2009. "Civic Stratification, Gender and Family Migration Policies in Europe." *IMISCOE Policy Brief*: 15.
Kramer, Betty J., and Edward H. Thompson, Jr. 2002. *Men as Caregivers. Theory, Research, and Service Implications*. New York: Springer.
Kurotani, Sawa. 2007. "Middle-Class Japanese Housewives and the Experience of Transnational Mobility." In *Going First Class? New Approaches to Privileged Travel and Movement*, edited by Vered Amit, 15–32. New York and Oxford: Berghahn Books.
Lahaie, Claudia, Jeffrey Hayes, Tinka Piper, and Jody Heymann. 2009. "Work and Family Divided Across Borders: The Impact of Parental Migration on Mexican Children in Transnational Families." *Community, Work & Family* 12: 299–312.
Lamb, Michael E. 2000. "The History of Research on Father Involvement: An Overview." *Marriage & Family Review* 29: 23–42.
Lapeyre, Nathalie, and Nicky Le Feuvre. 2004. "Concilier l'Inconciliable? Le Rapport des Femmes à la Notion de 'Conciliation Travail-Famille' dans les Professions Libérales en France." *Nouvelles Questions Féministes* 23 (3): 42–58.
Lareau, A., and E.B. Weininger. 2003. "Cultural Capital in Educational Research: A Critical Assessment", *Theory and society, 32*(5–6): 567–606.
Laslett, Peter. 1965. *The World We Have Lost*. London: Methuen.
Lash, Scott, and Jonathan Friedman. 1992. *Modernity and Identity*. Oxford: Basil Blackwell.
Lavie, Smadar, and Ted Swedenburg. 1996. *Displacement, Diaspora, and the Geographies of Identity*. Durham & London: Duke University Press.
Lee, Helen. 2003. *Tongans Overseas: Between Two Shores*. Honolulu: University of Hawaii Press.
Le Gall, Josiane. 2009. "Le Lien Familial et la Solidarité à l'Epreuve de la Migration: Le Cas des Musulmanes Libanaises à Montréal." *Les Politiques Sociales* 3–4: 27–44.
———. 2005. "Familles Transnationales: Bilan des Recherches et Nouvelles Perspectives." *Les cahiers du Gres* 5 (1): 29–42.
"Legislación de Extranjeros." 2005. *Boletín Oficial del Estado*. 2ª edición. Madrid: Ministerio de la Presidencia.
Leinaweaver, Jessaca B. 2008. *The Circulation of Children: Kinship, Adoption and Morality in Andean Peru*. Durham, NC: Duke University Press.
———. 2007. "On Moving Children: The Social Implications of Andean Child Circulation." *American Ethnologist* 34 (1): 163–180.
Leira, Arnlaug and Chiara Saraceno. 2006. 'Care: Actors, Relationships, Contexts', *Sosiologi I Dag, Årgang* 36(3):7–34

Levine, Robert. 1976. "Patterns of Personality in Africa." In *Response to Change: Society, Culture and Personality*, edited by George A. DeVos. New York: D. Van Nostrand.

Lévi Strauss, Claude. 1969. *The Elementary Structures of Kinship*. London: Tavistock.

Levin, Irene. 2004. "Living Apart Together: A New Family Form." *Current Sociology* 52 (2): 223–240.

Levitt, Peggy. 2002. "The Ties that Change: Relations to the Ancestral Home over the Life Cycle." In *The Changing Face of Home: The Transnational Lives of the Second Generation*, edited by Peggy Levitt and Mary C. Waters, 123–144. New York: Russell Sage Foundation.

———. 2001. *The Transnational Villagers*. Berkeley: University of California Press.

Levitt, Peggy, and Nina Glick Schiller. 2007. "Conceptualizing Simultaneity. A Transnational Social Field Perspective on Society." In *Rethinking Migration. New Theoretical and Empirical Perspectives*, edited by Alejandro Portes and Josh DeWind, 181–218. New York and Oxford: Berghahn Books.

Levitt, Peggy, and B. Nadya Jaworsky. 2007. "Transnational Migration Studies: Past Developments and Future Trends." *Annual Review of Sociology* 33 (1): 129–156.

Lewis, Jane. 2001. "The Decline of the Male Breadwinner Model: Implications for Work and Care." *Gender, State & Society* Summer: 152–169.

Lin, Ge, and Peter A. Rogerson. 1995. "Elderly Parents and the Geographic Availability of Their Adult Children." *Research on Aging* 17 (3): 303–331.

Lister, Ruth. 1994. "She Has Other Duties. Women, Citizenship and Social Security." In *Social Security and Social Change: New Challenges*, edited by Sally Baldwin and Jane Falkingham. Hemel Hampstead: Harvester Wheatsteaf.

Lodewyckx, Ina, Christiane Timmermans, and Johan Wets. 2011. *Le Regroupement Familial en Belgique: Les Chiffres Derrière le Mythe*. Bruxelles: Fondation Roi Baudouin.

Luster, Tom, Desiree B. Qin, Laura Bates, Deborah J. Johnson, and Meenal Rana. 2008. "The Lost Boys of Sudan: Ambiguous Loss, Search for Family, and Reestablishing Relationships With Family Members." *Family Relations* 57 (4): 444–456.

Lutz, Helma. 2010. "Gender in the Migratory Process." *Journal of Ethnic and Migration Studies* 36: 1647–1663.

Lutz, Helma, and Ewa Palenga-Möllenbeck. 2012. "Care Workers, Care Drain, and Care Chains: Reflections on Care, Migration, and Citizenship." *Social Politics: International Studies in Gender, State & Society* 19 (1): 15–37.

———. 2011. "Care, Gender and Migration: Towards a Theory of Transnational Domestic Work Migration in Europe." *Journal of Contemporary European Studies* 19 (3): 349–364.

MacKinnon, Valerie, and Antonella Nelli. 1996. *Now We Are In Paradise, Everything Is Missing*. Footscray: Victoria University of Technology, Department of Nursing.

Madianou, Mirca, and Daniel Miller. 2012. *Migration and the New Media: Transnational Families and Polymedia*. London: Routledge.

———. 2011. "Mobile Phone Parenting: Reconfiguring Relationships Between Filipina Migrant Mothers and their Left-Behind Children." *New Media & Society* 13: 457–470.

Maguid, Alicia. 2008. "La Emigración Internacional a Través de los Censos en Países de Origen: Evaluación de Resultados y Recomendaciones." *Serie Población y Desarrollo* 86, CEPAL.

Mahler, Sarah J. 2007. "Transnational Migration Comes of Age." In *Sociology of Diaspora*, edited by Ajaya Kumar Sahoo and Brij Maharaj, 194–226. Jaipur: Rawat Publications.

———. 2001. "Transnational Relationships: The Struggle to Communicate Across Borders." *Identities* 7 (4): 583–619.
Mahler, Sarah J., and Patricia R. Pessar. 2006. "Gender Matters: Ethnographers Bring Gender from the Periphery toward the Core of Migration Studies." *International Migration Review* 40 (1): 27–63.
———. 2001. "Gendered Geographies of Power: Analyzing Gender Across Transnational Spaces." *Identities* 7 (4): 441–459.
Manalansan, Martin F. 2006. "Queer Intersections. Sexuality and Gender in Migration Studies." *International Migration Review* 40: 224–249.
Marcus, George E. 1995. "Ethnography in/of the World System: The Emergence of Multi-Sited Ethnography." *Annual Review of Anthropology* 24: 95–117.
Marquet, Jacques. 2009. "Mariages d'Amour et Ruptures pour Désamour." *La Revue du REDIF* 2: 47–52.
Martens, A., and H. Verhoeven. 2006. "Les Minorités Ethniques sur le Marché de l'Emploi en Belgique." In *Penser l'Immigration et l'Intégration Autrement. Une Initiative Belge Inter-Universitaire*, edited by B. Khader, Marco Martiniello, Andrea Rea and C. Timmermans, 271–298. Bruxelles: Bruylant.
Martin, Ruth. 2007. *The Japanese Housewife Overseas: Adapting to Change of Culture and Status*. Kent: Global Oriental.
Martínez Franzoni, Juliana. 2008. *Domesticar la Incertidumbre en América Latina. Mercado Laboral, Política Social y Familias*. San José (Costa Rica): Universidad de Costa Rica.
———. 2005. "Regímenes de Bienestar en América Latina: Consideraciones Generales e Itinerarios Regionales." *Revista Centroamericana de Ciencias Sociales* 2 (2): 41–77.
Mas Giralt, Rosa, and Adrian J. Bailey. 2010. "Transnational Familyhood and the Liquid Life Paths of South Americans in the UK." *Global Networks* 10: 383–400.
Mason, Jennifer. 2004. "Managing Kinship Over Long Distances: The Significance of the Visit." *Social Policy and Society* 3 (4): 421–429.
Maushart, Susan. 2002. *Wifework: What Marriage Really Means for Women*. London: Bloomsbury.
Mauss, Marcel. 1923. "Essai sur le Don: Forme et Raison de l'Echange dans les Sociétés Archaïques." *L'Année Sociologique Nouvelle Série* T.1: 30–186.
Mazzucato, Valentina. 2013. "Transnational Families, Research and Scholarship". In *The Encyclopaedia of Global Human Migration*, edited by Immanuel Ness. Oxford: Blackwell Publishing.
———. 2011. "Reverse Remittances in the Migration—Development Nexus: Two-Way Flows Between Ghana and the Netherlands." *Population Space and Place* 17 (5): 454–468.
Mazzucato, Valentina, and Djamila Schans. 2011. "Transnational Families and the Well-Being of Children: Conceptual and Methodological Challenges." *Journal of Marriage and Family* 73: 704–712.
Mazzucato, Valentina, Bart van den Boom, and Nicholas N. N. Nsowah-Nuamah. 2005. "Origin and Destination of Remittances in Ghana." In *At Home in the World? International Migration and Development in Contemporary Ghana and West Africa*, edited by Takyiwaa Manuh, 139–152. Accra: Sub-Saharan Publishers.
McDowell, Linda. 2009. "Old and New European Economic Migrants: Whiteness and Managed Migration Policies." *Journal of Ethnic and Migration Studies* 35: 19–36.
McKay, Deirdre. 2006. "Translocal Circulation: Place and Subjectivity in an Extended Filipino Community." *The Asia Pacific Journal of Anthropology* 7 (3): 265–278.
McKay, Steve. 2010. " 'So They Remember Me When I'm Gone': Remittances, Fatherhood and Gender Relations of Filipino Migrant Men." In *Transnational*

*Labour Migration, Remittances and the Changing Family in Asia*. Singapore: Asia Research Institute, National University of Singapore.

———. 2007. "Filipino Sea Men: Constructing Masculinities in an Ethnic Labour Niche." *Journal of Ethnic and Migration Studies* 33: 617–633.

McRae, Susan. Ed. 1997. *Changing Britain: Families and Households in the 1990s*. Oxford: Oxford University Press.

Meda, Stefania Giada. 2012. "Famiglie in Transizione: La Migrazione nella Prospettiva Familiare." In *La Famiglia come Intreccio di Relazioni. La Prospettiva Sociologica*, edited by Giovanna Rossi and Donatella Bramanti, 225–253. Milano: Vita e Pensiero.

Merla, Laura. Forthcoming. *Transnational Family Solidarity in Local Contexts*. Routledge, Transnationalism Series.

———. 2012a. "Salvadoran Migrants in Australia: An Analysis of Transnational Families' Capability to Care Across Borders." *International Migration*. Published Online Accessed 29 November 2012. http://onlinelibrary.wiley.com/doi/10.1111/imig.12024/full

———. 2012b. "Salvadoran Transnational Families, Distance and Eldercare: Understanding Transnational Care Practices in Australia and Belgium." In *Migration, Family und Soziale Lage. Beiträge zu Bildung, Gender und Care*, edited by Thomas Geisen, Tobias Studer, and Erol Yildiz, 295–312. Wiesbaden: Springer VS.

———.2011. "Familles Salvadoriennes à l'Epreuve de la Distance: Solidarités Familiales et Soins Intergénérationnels." *Autrepart* 1: 145–162.

———. 2010. "La Gestion des Emotions dans le Cadre du Devoir Filial. Le Cas des Migrants Salvadoriens Vivant en Australie Occidentale." *Recherches Sociologiques et Anthropologiques* 41 (1): 39–58.

Merla, Laura, and Loretta Baldassar. 2011. "Transnational Caregiving Between Australia, Italy and El Salvador: The Impact of Institutions on the Capability to Care at a Distance." In *Gender and Well Being: The Role of Institutions*, edited by Elisabetta Addis, Florence Degavre, Paloma de Villota and John Eriksen, 147–162. London: Ashgate.

———. Eds. 2010a. "Les Dynamiques de Soin Transnationales: Entre Emotions et Considérations Economiques." *Recherches Sociologiques et Anthropologiques* 41.

———. 2010b. "Présentation. Les Dynamiques de Soin Transnationales: Entre Emotions et Considérations Economiques." *Recherches Sociologiques et Anthropologiques* 41 (1): 1–14.

Merla, Laura and Florence Degavre. (2013, Forthcoming) Défamilialisation et politiques de care dans les États sociaux européens. In *Genre, migrations et globalisation de la reproduction sociale. Cahiers genre et développement* N° 9 edited by Christine Verschuur et Christine Catarino, p.105-115. Paris : L'Harmattan

Michel, Andrée. Ed. 1978. *Les Femmes dans la Société Marchande*. Paris: PUF.

Miller, Daniel. 2011. *Tales from Facebook*. Cambridge: Polity.

———. 2010. *Stuff*. Cambridge and Malden: Polity Press.

———. Ed. 2001. *Home Possession: Material Culture Behind Closed Doors*. Oxford: Berg.

Miller, Daniel, and Don Slater. 2000. *The Internet: An Ethnographic Approach*. Oxford: Berg.

Mills, Frank. 1985. *Determinants and Consequences of the Migration Culture of St. Kitts-Nevis*. Washington, DC: Hemispheric Migration Project, Georgetown University and Intergovernmental Committee on Migration.

Mohapatra, Sanket, Dilip Ratha, and Ani Silwal. 2010. *Migration and Development Brief 13*. Accessed March 5, 2011. http://siteresources.worldbank.org/INTPROSPECTS/Resources/334934-1110315015165/MigrationAndDevelopmentBrief13.pdf

Mol, Annemarie. 2008. *The Logic of Care. Health and the Problem of Patient Choice*. London: Routledge.

Moore H. 1988. *Feminism and Anthropology*. Minneapolis: University of Minnesota Press.
Moran-Taylor, Michelle J. 2008. "When Mothers and Fathers Migrate North: Caretakers, Children, and Child Rearing in Guatemala." *Latin American Perspectives* 35: 79–95.
Morawska, Eva. 2001. "Structuring Migration: The Case of Polish Income-Seeking Travellers to the West." *Theory and Society* 30: 47–80.
Morgan, David. 2011a. "Locating 'Family Practices'." *Sociological Research Online* 16 (4): 14.
———. 2011b. *Rethinking Family Practices*. Basingstoke: Palgrave Macmillan.
———. 1996. *Family Connections*. Cambridge: Polity Press.
———. 1975. *Social Theory and the Family*. London: Routledge.
Morokvasic, Mirjana. 2004. " 'Settled in Mobility': Engendering Post-Wall Migration In Europe." *Feminist Review* 77: 7–25.
Morris, Lydia. 2002. *Managing Migration: Civic Stratification and Migrants' Rights*. London: Routledge.
Moulier Boutang, Yann, and Demetrios Papademetriou. 1994. "Sistemas y Políticas Migratorias: Análisis Comparativo de sus Resultados." *Desarrollo* 24: 3–24.
Moulin, Madeleine, Marie-Thérèse Casman, Sylvie Carbonnelle, and Dominique Joly. 2006. *Migrations et Vieillissements. Rapport d'Expertise Commandité par la Fondation Roi Baudouin dans le Cadre de la Mise en Oeuvre de son Programme Justice Sociale*. Bruxelles: Fondation Roi Baudouin.
Mozère, Liane. 2005. "Des Domestiques Philippines à Paris: Entrepreneures d'Elles-Mêmes sur le Marché Transnational de la Domesticité." *Cahiers Genre et Développement*: 155–162.
Mummert, Gail. 2005. "Transnational Parenting in Mexican Migrant Communities: Redefining Fatherhood, Motherhood and Caregiving." Paper presented at the Mexican International Family Strengths Conference, Building Family Relations, Cuernavaca.
Naldini, Manuela, and Chiara Saraceno. 2008. "Social and Family Policies in Italy: Not Totally Frozen but Far from Strucutral Reforms." *Social Policy & Administration* 42 (7): 863–882.
Nedelcu, Mihaela. 2012. "Migrants' New Transnational Habitus: Rethinking Migration Through a Cosmopolitan Lens in the Digital Age." *Journal of Ethnic and Migration Studies* 38 (9): 1339–1356.
Nobles, Jenna. 2011. "Parenting from Abroad: Migration, Nonresident Father Involvement, and Children's Education in Mexico." *Journal of Marriage and Family* 73: 729–746.
Noddings, Nel. 2003, first published in 1984. *Caring: A Feminine Approach to Ethics and Moral Education* (2nd Ed.). California and London: University of California Press.
Notermans, Catrien. 2008. "The Emotional World of Kinship. Children's Experiences of Fosterage in East Cameroon." *Childhood* 15 (3): 355–377.
Nowicka, Magdalena. 2007. "Mobile Locations: Construction of Home in a Group of Mobile Transnational Professionals." *Global Networks* 7 (1): 69–86.
Nydegger, Corinne. 1991. "The Development of Paternal and Filial Maturity." In *Parent-Child Relations Throughout Life*, edited by Karl Pillemer and Kathleen McCarthney, 93–112. Hillsdale, NJ: Lawrence Erlbaum.
OECD. 2012. *Connecting with Emigrants: A Global Profile of Diasporas*. Paris: OECD Publishing.
———. 2007. *Babies and Bosses—Reconciling Work and Family Life: A Synthesis of Findings for OECD countries*. Paris: OECD Publishing.
Olwig, Karen Fog. 2012a. "The Care Chain, Children's Mobility and the Caribbean Migration Tradition." *Journal of Ethnic and Migration Studies* 38 (6): 933–952.

———. 2012b. "The 'Successful' Return: Caribbean Narratives of Migration, Family and Gender." *Journal of the Royal Anthropological Institute* (N.S.) 18: 828–845.

———. 2007. *Caribbean Journeys: An Ethnography of Migration and Home in Three Family Networks*. Durham, NC: Duke University Press.

———. 2005. "Narratives of Home: Visions of 'Betterment' and Belonging in a Dispersed Caribbean Family." In *Caribbean Narratives of Belonging: Fields of Relations, Sites of Identity*, edited by Jean Besson and Karen Fog Olwig, 189–205. Oxford: Macmillan Education.

———. 2002. "A Wedding in the Family: Home Making in a Global Kin Network." *Global Networks* 2 (3): 205–218.

———. 1999. "Narratives of the Children Left Behind: Home and Identity in Globalised Caribbean Families." *Journal of Ethnic and Migration Studies* 25 (2): 267–284.

———. 1993. *Global Culture, Island Identity: Continuity and Change in the Afro-Caribbean Community of Nevis*. Reading: Harwood Academic Publishers.

———. 1985. *Cultural Adaptation and Resistance on St. John: Three Centuries of Afro-Caribbean Life*. Gainesville: University of Florida Press.

Øien, Cecilie. 2006. "Transnational Networks of Care: Angolan Children in Fosterage in Portugal." *Ethnic and Racial Studies* 29 (6): 1104–1117.

ONS. 2011. *Polish People in the UK*. 25 August 2011.

Oppong, Christine. 2006. "Demographic Innovation and Nutritional Catastrophe: Change, Lack of Change and Difference in Ghanaian Family Systems." In *African Families in a Global Context*" (Research Report No. 131), edited by Göran Therborn, 49–78. Göteborg: Elanders Infologistics Väst AB.

Orellana, Marjorie F., Barrie Thorne, Anna Chee, and Wan Shun Eva Lam. 2001. "Transnational Childhoods: The Participation of Children in Processes of Family Migration." *Social Problems* 48 (4): 572–591.

Oso, Laura. 1998. *La Migración hacia España de Mujeres Jefas de Hogar*. Madrid: Ministerio del Trabajo y Asuntos Sociales, Instituto de la Mujer.

Ostergaard-Nielsen, Eva. Ed. 2003. *International Migration and Sending Countries: Perceptions, Policies and Transnational Relations*. London: Palgrave Macmillan.

Palmer, Robert. 1977. "The Italians: Patterns of Migration in London." In *Between Two Cultures. Migrants and Minorities in Britain*, edited by James L. Watson, 242–268. Oxford: Basil Blackwell.

Papastergiadis, Nikos. 2000. *The Turbulence of Migration: Globalization, Deterritorialization and Hybridity*. Cambridge: Polity Press.

Parreñas, Rhacel S. 2010. "Transnational Mothering: A Source of Gender Conflicts in the Family." *North Carolina Law Review* 88: 1825–1856.

———. 2008. "Transnational Fathering: Gendered Conflicts, Distant Disciplining and Emotional Gaps." *Journal of Ethnic and Migration Studies* 34: 1057–1072.

———. 2005a. *Children of Global Migration: Transnational Families and Gendered Woes*. Stanford, CA: Stanford University Press.

———. 2005b. "Long Distance Intimacy: Class, Gender and Intergenerational Relations Between Mothers and Children in Filipino Transnational Families." *Global Networks* 5 (4): 317–336.

———. 2003. The Care Crisis in the Philippines: Children and Transnational Families in the New Global Economy." In *Global Women: Nannies, Maids, and Sex Workers in the New Economy*, edited by Barbara Ehrenreich and Arlie R. Hochschild, 39–54. London: Granta Books.

———. 2001a. "Mothering From a Distance: Emotions, Gender, and Intergenerational Relations in Filipino Transnational Families." *Feminist Studies* 27 (2): 361–390.

———. 2001b. *Servants of Globalization. Women, Migration and Domestic Work*. Stanford, CA: Stanford University Press.

Passel, Jeffrey, and D'Vera Cohn. 2008. "Trends in Unauthorized Immigration: Undocumented Inflow Now Trails Legal Inflow." Washington, DC: Pew

Hispanic Center, October. Accessed 30 April 2013, http://pewhispanic.org/files/reports/94.pdf

Perrons, Diane, Ania Plomien, and Majella Kilkey. 2010. "Migration and Uneven Development Within an Enlarged European Union: Fathering, Gender Divisions and Male Migrant Domestic Services." *European Urban and Regional Studies* 17: 197–215.

Pe-Pua, Rogelia. 2003. "Wife, Mother, and Maid: The Triple Role of Filipino Domestic Workers in Spain and Italy." In *Wife or Worker? Asian Women and Migration*, edited by Nicola Piper and Mina Roces, 157–180. New York: Rowman and Littlefield Publishers.

Pe-Pua, Rogelia C., Colleen Mitchell, Stephen Castles, and Robyn Iredale. 1998. "Astronaut Families and Parachute Children: Hong Kong Immigrants in Australia." In *The Last Half-Century of Chinese Overseas*, edited by Elizabeth Sinn, 279–298. Hong Kong: Hong Kong University Press.

Pessar, Patricia. 2005. "Women, Gender and International Migration Across and Beyond the Americas: Inequalities and Limited Empowerment." In expert group meeting on international migration and development in Latin America and the Caribbean. Mexico City: United Nations.

Pessar, Patricia, and Sarah Mahler. 2003. "Transnational Migration: Bringing Gender in." *International Migration Review* 37 (3): 812–846.

Peterson, Jean T. 1990. "Sibling Exchanges and Complementarity in the Philippine Highlands." *Journal of Marriage and Family* 52: 441–451.

Peterson, V. Spike. 2010. "Global Householding amid Global Crises." *Politics & Gender* 6 (2): 271–281.

Pfau-Effinger, Birgit. 2000. "Conclusion: Gender Cultures, Gender Arrangements and Social Changes in the European Context." In *Gender, Economy and Culture in the European Union*, edited by Simon Duncan and Birgit Pfau-Effinger, 262–276. London and New York: Routledge.

Philpott, Stuart B. 1973. *West Indian Migration: The Montserrat Case*. London: The Athlone Press.

———.1968. "Remittance Obligations, Social Networks and Choice among Montserratian Migrants in Britain." *Man* 3 (3): 465–476.

Pilon, Marc. 2003. "Foster Care and Schooling in West Africa: The State of Knowledge" (The UNESCO 2003 EFA Monitoring Report). Institute Recherche pour le Developpement, Unité d'Enseignement and de Recherche en Démographie.

Pingol, Alicia. 2001. *Remaking Masculinities: Identity, Power, and Gender Dynamics in Families with Migrant Wives and Househusbands*. Quezon City: University of the Philippines.

Plaza, Dwaine. 2000. "Transnational Grannies: The Changing Family Responsibilities of Elderly African Caribbean-Born Women Resident in Britain." *Social Indicators Research* 51: 75–105.

Portes, Alejandro. 2001. "Introduction: The Debates and Significance of Immigrant Transnationalism." *Gobal Networks* 1: 181–193.

———. 1996. "Transnational Communities: Their Emergence and Significance in the Contemporary World-System." In *Latin America in the World-Economy*, edited by Roberto Patricio Korzeniewwicz, 151–168. London: Greenwood Press.

Portes, Alejandro, Luis E. Guarnizo, and Patricia Landolt. 1999. "The Study of Transnationalism: Pitfalls and Promise of an Emergent Research Field." *Ethnic and Racial Studies* 22 (2): 217–237.

Portes, Alejandro, and Rubén G. Rumbaut. 2001. "Defining the Situation: The Ethnic Identities of Children of Immigrants." In *Legacies: The Story of the Immigrant Second Generation*, edited by Alejandro Portes and Rubén Rumbaut, 147–191. Berkeley: University of California Press.

Pottinger, Audrey M. 2005. "Children's Experience of Loss by Parental Migration in Inner-City Jamaica." *American Journal of Orthopsychiatry* 75 (4): 485–496.

Pribilsky, Jason. 2004. " 'Aprendemos a Convivir': Conjugal Relations, Co-parenting, and Family Life Among Ecuadorian Transnational Migrants in New York City and the Ecuadorian Andes." *Global Networks* 4: 313–334.

———. 2001. "Nervios and Modern Childhood: Migration and Shifting Contexts of Child Life in the Ecuadorian Andes." *Childhood* 8 (2): 251–273.

Price, Charles Archibald. 1963. *The Method and Statistics of "Southern Europeans in Australia."* Research School of Social Sciences. Canberra: Australian National University.

Prothero, R. Mansell, and Murray Chapman. 1985. *Circulation in Third World Countries.* London: Routledge & Kegan Paul.

Putnam, Robert, Robert Leonardi, and Raffaela Nanetti. 1993. *Making Democracy Work. Civic Traditions in Modern Italy.* Princeton: Princeton University Press.

Pyle, Jean L. 2006. "Globalization and the Increase in Transnational Care Work: The Flip Side." *Globalizations* 3 (3): 297–315.

Queirolo Palmas, Luca, and Maurizio Ambrosini. 2008. "Les Leçons de l'Immigration Latino-Américaine vers l'Europe et l'Italie." In *Nouvelles Migrations Latino-Américaines en Europe. Bilans et Défis*, edited by Isabel Yépez del Castillo and Gioconda Herrera, 85–99. Barcelona and Louvain-la-Neuve: Publicacions i Editions de la Universidad de Barcelona and Presses Universitaires de Louvain.

Raijman, Rebeca, Silvina Schammah-Gesser, and Adriana Kemp. 2003. "International Migration, Domestic Work, and Care Work: Undocumented Latina Migrants in Israel." *Gender & Society* 17: 727–749.

Ramirez, Hernan, and Pierrette Hondagneu-Sotelo. 2009. "Mexican Immigrant Gardeners: Entrepreneurs or Exploited Workers?" *Social Problems* 56: 70–88.

Ratha, Dilip, Mohapatra, Sanket, and Ani Silwal. 2011. *The Migration and Remittances Factbook 2011.* Accessed August 30, 2011. http://econ.worldbank.org/WBSITE/EXTERNAL/EXTDEC/EXTDECPROSPECTS/0,,contentMDK:21352016~pagePK:64165401~piPK:64165026~theSitePK:476883,00.html

Ratha, Dilip, and Ani Silwal. 2012. "Remittance Flows in 2011—An Update." *Migration and Development Brief 18.* Accessed May 8, 2012. http://siteresources.worldbank.org/INTPROSPECTS/Resources/334934-1103150115165/MigrationandDevelopmentBrief18.pdf

Ravenstein, Ernest George. 1885. "The Laws of Migration." *Journal of the Statistical Society of London* 48: 167–227.

Razavi, Shahra. 2007. *The Political and Social Economy of Care in a Development Context: Conceptual Issues, Research Questions and Policy Options.* Vol. Programme Paper Number 3, Gender and Development: UNRISD.

Razy, Elodie, and Virginie Baby-Collin. 2011. "Special Issue: La famille transnationale dans tous ses états." *Autrepart* 57/58.

Reyes, Melanie M. 2008. "Migration and Filipino Children Left-behind: A Literature Review." Manila: Miriam College and UNICEF. Accessed August 16, 2011. http://fahnoe-domains.ph/filer/toledo-cebu/Synthesis_StudyJuly12008.pdf.

Reynolds, Tracey. 2012a. "Men's Business? Black Men Caring Within Black-led Communication Organisations." In *Critical Approaches to Care: Understanding Caring Relations, Identities and Cultures*, edited by Georgia Philip, Chrissie Rogers and Sussie Weller, 82–91. London: Routledge.

———. 2012b. "Access for BAME Elders: Exploring Personalised Care Planning." *Runnymede Trust Bulletin*, Winter edition, February 2012.

———. 2010a. "Introduction." *Ethnic and Racial Studies* 33 (5): 749–760.

———. 2010b. "Transnational Family Networks, Cultural Belonging and Social Capital among Second-Generation British-Caribbean 'Returning' Migrants." *Ethnic and Racial Studies* 33 (5): 797–815.

———. 2006. "Bonding Social Capital within the Caribbean Family and Community." *Community, Work and Family* 9 (3): 273–290.
———. 2004. "Families, Social Capital and Caribbean Young People's Diasporic Identities." Working Paper Series 11, Families & Social Capital ESRC Research Group, London South Bank University.
Reynolds, Tracey, and Elisabetta Zontini. 2006. "A Comparative Study of Care Provision Across Caribbean and Italian Transnational Families." Working Paper Series, Families and Social Capital ESRC Research Group, London South Bank University.
———. 2007. "Assessing Social Capital and Care Provision in Minority Ethnic Communities: A Comparative Study of Caribbean and Italian Families." In *Assessing Social Capital: Concept, Policy and Practice*, edited by Rosalind Edwards, Jane Franklin and Janet Holland, 217–233. Cambridge: Cambridge Scholars Press.
Robeyns, Ingrid. 2003. "Sen's Capability Approach and Gender Inequality: Selecting Relevant Capabilities." *Feminist Economics* 9 (2–3): 61–92.
Roseneil, Sasha, and Shelley Budgeon. 2004. "Cultures of Intimacy and Care beyond 'the Family': Personal Life and Social Change in the Early 21st Century." *Current Sociology* 52 (2): 135–159.
Rossi, Alice S., and Peter Henry Rossi. 1990. *Of Human Bonding: Parent–Child Relations Across the Life Course.* New York: Aldine de Gruyter.
Rossi, Giovanna, and Donatella Bramanti. Eds. 2012. *La Famiglia Come Intreccio di Relazioni. La Prospettiva Sociologica.* Milano: Vita e Pensiero.
Rossi, Giovanna, Roberta Bonini, and Stefania Meda. 2010. "Rethinking Family, Gender and Generations in the Light of the Migration Process. A Qualitative Study on the Experience of Two Generations of Moroccan, Egyptian and Pakistani Women in Northern Italy." In ESA RN13 Interim meeting "Geographical Mobility and Family Life: How to (Re-)Think Family in a Mobile World?" Wiesbaden, Germany.
Rouse, Roger. 1991. "Mexican Migration and the Social Space of Postmodernism." *Diaspora* 1 (1): 8–23.
Rubenstein, Hymie. 1987. *Coping with Poverty. Adaptive Strategies in a Caribbean Village.* Boulder: Westview Press.
Rubery, Jill, Mark Smith, and Colette Fagan. 1998. "National Working-Time Regimes and Equal Opportunities." *Feminist Economics* 4 (1): 71–101.
Ruddick, Sara. 1989. *Maternal Thinking. Towards a Politics of Peace.* Boston: Beacon Press.
Rumbaut, Rubén G. 2002. "Severed or Sustained Attachments? Language, Identity, and Imagined Communities in the Post-Immigrant Generation." In *The Changing Face of Home: The Transnational Lives of the Second Generation*, edited by Peggy Levitt and Mary C. Waters, 43–95. New York: Russell Sage Foundation.
Rutherford, Jonathan. 1990. *Identity: Community, Culture, Difference.* London: Lawrence & Wishart.
Ryan, Louise. 2011 "Transnational Relations: Family Migration Among Recent Polish Migrants in London." *International Migration* 49: 80–103.
———. 2007. "Migrant Women, Social Networks and Motherhood: The Experiences of Irish Nurses in Britain." *Sociology* 41 (2): 295–312.
———. 2004. "Family Matters: (E)migration, Familial Networks and Irish Women in Britain." *The Sociological Review* 52 (3): 351–370.
Ryan, Louise, Rosemary Sales, Mary Tilki, and Bernadetta Siara. 2009. "Family Strategies and Transnational Migration: Recent Polish Migrants in London." *Journal of Ethnic and Migration Studies* 35: 61–77.
———. 2008. "Social Networks, Social Support and Social Capital: Polish Migrants in London." *Sociology* 42 (4): 672–690.

Safri, Maliha, and Julie Graham. 2010. "The Global Household: Toward a Feminist Postcapitalist International Political Economy." *Signs* 36 (1): 99–125.
Sahlins, Marshall. 1972. *Stone Age Economics*. Chicago: Aldine.
———. 1965. "On the Sociology of Primitive Exchange." In *The Relevance of Models in Social Anthropology*, edited by Michael Branton, 139–236. London: Tavistock.
Sánchez-Carretero, Cristina. 2005. "Motherhood from Afar: Channels of Communication among Dominican Women in Madrid." *European Journal of International Migration and Ethnic Relations* 43: 145–164.
San Martín, Carolina. 2006. "El Acceso de los Extranjeros al Mercado de Trabajo: Régimen General y Contingente." *Revista del Ministerio de Trabajo y Asuntos Sociales* 63: 139–173.
Santos, Beatriz. 2006. *From El Salvador to Australia: A 20th Century Exodus to a Promised land*. PhD diss., Australian Catholic University.
Saraceno, Chiara. 2010. "Social Inequalities in Facing Old-Age Dependency: A Bi-generational Perspective." *Journal of European Social Policy* 20(1): 32–44.
Sarausa, Carmen. 2001. "Leaving Home to Help the Family: Male and Female Temporary Migrants in 18th Century Spain." In *Women, Gender and Labour Migration: Historical and Global Perspectives*, edited by Pamela Sharpe, 29–59. London and New York: Routledge.
Save the Children. 2006. *Left Behind, Left Out: The Impact on Children and Families of Mothers Migrating for Work Abroad*. Colombo: Save the Children, Sri Lanka.
Saxenian, AnnaLee. 2005. "From Brain Drain to Brain Circulation: Transnational Communities and Regional Upgrading in India and China." *Studies in Comparative International Development* 40 (2): 35–36.
Scalabrini Migration Center. 2004. *Hearts Apart: Migration in the Eyes of Filipino Children*. Episcopal Commission for the Pastoral Care of Migrants and Itinerant People-CBCP/Apostleship of the Sea-Manila.
Schmalzbauer, Leah. 2008. "Family Divided: The Class Formation of Honduran Transnational Families." *Global Networks* 8: 329–346.
———. 2004. "Searching for Wages and Mothering from Afar: The Case of Honduran Transnational Families." *Journal of Marriage and Family* 66: 1317–1331.
Schneider, David M. 1984. *A Critique of the Study of Kinship*. Ann Arbor: University of Michigan Press.
Scott, Sam. 2006. "The Social Morphology of Skilled Migration: The Case of the British Middle Class in Paris." *Journal of Ethnic and Migration Studies* 32 (7): 1105–1129.
Segal, Aaron (1996) 'Locating the Swallows: Caribbean Recycling Migration'. Paper presented at the Caribbean Studies Association conference, San Juan, Puerto Rico, 27-31 May 1996.
Sevenhuijsen, Se. 2000. "Caring in the Third Way: The Reflection Between Obligation, Responsibility and Care in the Third Way Discourse." *Critical Social Policy* 20 (1): 5–37.
———. 1998. *Citizenship and the Ethics of Care: Feminist Considerations on Justice, Morality and Politics*. London: Routledge.
Shain, Yossi. 2007. *Kinship and Diasporas in International Affairs*. Ann Arbor: University of Michigan Press.
Sharpe, Pamela. 2001. *Women, Gender and Labour Migration: Historical and Global Perspectives*. London and New York: Routledge.
Sheller, Mimi, and John Urry. 2006. "The New Mobilities Paradigm." *Environment and Planning A* 38 (2): 207–226.
Shimoda, Yukimi. 2012. *From the Porous Spaces on the Bubble: The Life and Work of Japanese Expatriate Employees in Indonesia and Their Relations with the Host Society*. Unpublished PhD thesis, The University of Western Australia, Perth.

Shinozaki, Kyoko. 2012. "In the Absence of Mothers: Fathers' On-site Parenting in the Global Care Chains and Their Dependent Migration from the Philippines to Germany." Paper presented at the international conference Transforming Gender Orders. Intersections of Care, Family and Migration, Frankfurt, Germany, January 18–20.

Silva, Elizabeth B., and Carol Smart. 1999. *The New Family?* London: Sage Publications Ltd.

Singh, Supriya. 2011a. "Indian Students in Melbourne: Challenges to Multiculturalism." *Journal of Intercultural Studies* 32 (6): 673–689.

———. 2011b. "Transnational Community and Money in the Indian Diaspora in Melbourne." Paper presented at the City, Community and Globalisation Roundtable.

———. 2006. "Towards a Sociology of Money and Family in the Indian Diaspora." *Contributions to Indian Sociology* 40 (3): 375–398.

———. 1997. *Marriage Money: The Social Shaping of Money in Marriage and Banking.* St. Leonards, NSW: Allen and Unwin.

Singh, Supriya, and Mala Bhandari. 2012. "Money Management and Control in the Indian Joint Family Across Generations." *The Sociological Review* 60 (1): 46–67.

Singh, Supriya, and Anuja Cabraal. 2010. "Indian Student Migrants in Australia: Issues of Community Sustainability." *People and Place* 18 (1): 19–30.

Smart, Carol, and Bren Neale. 1999. *Family Fragments?* Cambridge: Polity Press.

Smith, Andrea, Richard Lalonde N., and Simone Johnson. 2004. "Serial Migration and Its Implications for the Parent–Child Relationship: A Retrospective Analysis of the Experiences of the Children of Caribbean Immigrant." *Cultural Diversity and Ethnic Minority Psychology* 10 (2): 107–122.

Smith, Michael Peter. 2001. *Transnational Urbanism.* Routledge: London.

Smith, Raymond T. 1996. *The Matrifocal Family. Power, Pluralism and Politics.* New York: Routledge.

Soehl, Thomas, and Roger Waldinger. 2010. "Making the Connection: Latino Immigrants and Their Cross Border Ties." *Ethnic and Racial Studies* 33 (9): 1489–1510.

Solé, Carlota, and Sonia Parella. 2003. "The Labour Market and Racial Discrimination in Spain." *Journal of Ethnic and Migration Studies* 29 (1): 121–140.

Solimano, Andrés. 2009. *Migration and Democracy: Issues for Latin America and Europe at a Time of Global Recession.* International IDEA, Sweden.

Sørensen, Ninna N. 2004a. "The Development Dimension of Migrant Remittances." IOM Working Paper Series. Geneva: International Organization for Migration.

———. 2004b. "Narratives of Longing, Belonging and Caring in the Dominican Diaspora." In *Caribbean Narratives*, edited by Jean Besson and Karen F. Olwig, 222–243. London: Macmillan.

Sørensen, Ninna Nyberg, and Luis Guarnizo. 2007. "Transnational Family Life Across the Atlantic: The Experience of Colombian and Dominican Migrants in Europe." In *Living Across Worlds: Diaspora, Development and Transnational Engagement*, edited by Ninna Nyberg Sørensen, 151–176. Geneva: International Organization for Migration.

Sori, Ercole. 1979. *L'Emigrazione Italiana dall'Unità alla Seconda Guerra Mondiale.* Bologna: Il Mulino.

SPF Affaires étrangères. 2011. "Family Reunion." Accessed 14 March 2011, http://diplomatie.belgium.be/en/services/travel_to_belgium/visa_for_belgium/long_stay/family/family_reunion/with_child_or_grandchild/.

Stacey, J. 1998. *Brave New Families: Stories of Domestic Upheaval in Late Twentieth Century America.* New York: Basic Books.

Stenning, Alison, and Stuart Dawley. 2009. "Poles to Newcastle: Grounding New Migration Flows in Peripheral Regions." *European Urban and Regional Studies* 16: 273–294.

Storey, Keith. 2001. "Fly-in/Fly-Out and Fly-Over: Mining and Regional Development in Western Australia." *Australian Geographer* 32 (2): 133–148.

Suárez-Orozco, Carola, Irina L. G. Todorova, and Josephine Louie. 2002. "Making up for Lost Time: The Experience of Separation and Reunification Among Immigrant Families." *Family Process* 41 (4): 625–643.

Sutton, Constance R. 2004. "Celebrating Ourselves: The Family Reunion Rituals of African-Caribbean Transnational Families." *Global Networks* 4 (3): 243–257.

Svašek, Maruska. Ed. 2008. "Transnational Families and Emotions." *Journal of Intercultural Studies* 29 (3): 247–266.

Svašek, Maruška, and Zlatko Skrbiš. 2007a. "Passion and Powers: Emotions and Globalisation." *Identities* 14 (4): 367–383.

———. Eds. 2007b. Special Issue: "Emotions and Globalisation." *Identities: Global Studies in Culture and Power* 14 (4).

Swing, William L. 2010. *The Director General's Report to the Council*. Geneva: International Organization for Migration.

Taylor, Jill C., and Janet G. Simmonds. 2009. "Family Stress and Coping in the Fly-in Fly-out Workforce." *The Australian Community Psychologist* 21 (2): 23–35.

Thai, Hung Cam. 2012. "The Dual Roles of Transnational Daughters and Transnational Wives: Monetary Intentions, Expectations and Dilemmas." *Global Networks* 12 (2): 216–232.

Therborn, Göran. 2004. *Between Sex and Power: Family in the World 1900–2000*. London: Routledge.

Thomas, William I., and Florian Znaniecki [1918–1927]. 1974. *The Polish Peasant in Europe and America* (Vols. 1–2). New York: Octagon Books.

Thomas-Hope, Elizabeth. 2002 . "Skilled Labor Migration from Developing Countries: Study on the Caribbean Region." *International Migration Paper No. 50*. Geneva: International Labor Organization.

Thompson, Paul, and Elaine Bauer. 2000. "Jamaican Transnational Families: Points of Pain and Sources of Resilience." *Wadapagi: A Journal of the Caribbean and Its Diaspora* 3 (2): 1–36.

Thompson, S. L.. 1980. *Australia Through Italian Eyes: A Study of Settlers Returning from Australia to Italy*. Melbourne: Oxford University Press.

Thorne, Barrie, and Marilyn Yalom. 1982. *Rethinking the Family. Some Feminist Questions*. Boston: Northeastern University Press.

Tilly, Charles. 2007. "Trust Networks in Transnational Migration." *Sociological Forum* 22 (2): 3–24.

Tolstokorova, Alissa V. 2010. "'Where Have All the Mothers Gone? The Gendered Effect of Labour Migration and Transnationalism on the Institution of Parenthood in Ukraine." *Anthropology of East Europe Review* 28 (1): 184–214.

Toro-Morn, Maura I. 1995. "Gender, Class, Family, and Migration: Puerto Rican Women in Chicago." *Gender & Society* 9: 712–726.

Trajano, Wilson Filho. 2009. "The Conservative Aspects of a Centripetal Diaspora: The Case of the Cape Verdean Tabancas." *Africa* 79 (4): 520–542.

Tronto, Joan. 1993. *Moral Boundaries: A Political Argument for an Ethic of Care*. London: Routledge.

Trost, Jan. 1998. "LAT Relationships Now and in the f+Future." In *The Family: Contemporary Perspectives and Challenges*; Festschrift in honor of Wilfried Dumon, edited by Koen Matthijs, 209–220. Leuven: Leuven University Press.

TUC. 2008. "Hard Work, Hidden Lives. The Full Report of the Commission on Vulnerable Employment." Accessed June 27, 2009. http://www.vulnerableworkers.org.uk/cove-report/full-report/.

Tung, Rosalie. 2008. "Brain Circulation, Diaspora, and International Competitiveness." *European Management Journal* 26: 298–304.

Twigg, Julia. Ed. 2000. *Bathing—The Body and Community Care.* London: Routledge.

Twum-Dansoo, Afua. 2009. "Reciprocity, Respect and Responsibility: The 3Rs Underlying Parent–Child Relationships in Ghana and the Implications for Children's Rights." *The International Journal of Children's Rights* 17 (3): 415–432.

Tymczuk, Alexander, and Esben Leifsen. 2012. "Care at a Distance: Ukrainian and Ecuadorian Transnational Parenthood from Spain." *Journal of Ethnic and Migration Studies* 38 (2): 219–236.

UK Border Agency. 2009. "Accession Monitoring Report May 2004–March 2009." Accessed August 24, 2011. http://www.ukba.homeoffice.gov.uk/sitecontent/documents/aboutus/reports/accession_monitoring_report/

Urry, John. 2003. "Social Networks, Travel and Talk." *British Journal of Sociology* 54 (2): 155–175.

———. 2002. "Mobility and Proximity." *Sociology* 36 (2): 255–274.

———. 2000. *Sociology Beyond Societies: Mobilities for the Twenty-First Century.* London: Routledge.

———. 1990. *The Tourist Gaze.* London: Sage.

Vaiou, Dina. 1996. "Women's Work and Everyday Life in Southern Europe in the Context of European Integration." In *Women of the European Union. The Politics of Work and Daily Life*, edited by Maria Dolors García-Ramon and Janice Monk, 61–73. London: Routledge.

Van Dijk, Rijk. 2002. "Religion, Reciprocity and Restructuring Family Responsibility in the Ghanaian Pentecostal Diaspora." In *The Transnational Family. New European Frontiers and Global Networks*, edited by Deborah Fahy Bryceson and Ulla Vuorella. Oxford: Berg.

Vatz Laaroussi, Michèle, and Claudio Bolzman. 2010. "Familles Immigrantes et Réseaux Transnationaux: Des Articulations Théoriques aux Stratégies Politiques." *Lien Social et Politiques* 64 : 7–25.

Vertovec, Steven. 2009. *Transnationalism.* London: Routledge.

———. 2004. "Cheap Calls: The Social Glue of Migrant Transnationalism." *Global Networks* 4 (2): 219–224.

———. 2001. "Transnationalism and Identity." *Journal of Ethnic and Migration Studies* 27 (4): 573–582.

———. 1999. "Conceiving and Researching Transnationalism." *Ethnic and Racial Studies* 22 (2): 447–462.

Viruell-Fuentes, Edna A. 2006. " 'My Heart Is Always There': The Transnational Practices of First-Generation Mexican Immigrant and Second-Generation Mexican American Women." *Identities: Global Studies in Culture and Power* 13 (3): 335–362.

Voigt-Graf, Carmen. 2003. "Indians at Home in the Antipodes: Migrating with Ph.D.s, Bytes or Kava in Their Bags." In *Culture and Economy in the Indian Diaspora*, edited by Bhikhu Parekh, Gurharpal Singh and Steven Vertovec, 142–164. London: Routledge.

Waerness, Kari. 1984. "The Rationality of Caring." *Economic and Industrial Democracy* 5: 185–211.

Wall, Karin. 2007. "Immigrant Families." In *Blackwell Encyclopedia of Sociology*, edited by George Ritzer, 2252–2255. Oxford: Blackwell Publishing.

Wall, Karin, and José São José. 2004. "Managing Work and Care: A Difficult Challenge for Immigrant Families." *Social Policy and Administration* 6: 591–621.

Wall, Karin, and Cátia Nunes. 2010. "Immigration, Welfare and Care in Portugal: Mapping the New Plurality of Female Migration Trajectories." *Social Policy and Society* 9 (3): 1–12.

Walsh, Katie. 2008. "Travelling Together? Work, Intimacy, and Home amongst British Expatriate Couples in Dubai." In *Gender and Family Among Transnational Professionals*, edited by Anne Coles and Anne-Meike Fechter, 63–84. New York and London: Routledge.

———. 2006. "British Expatriate Belongings: Mobile Homes and Transnational Homing." *Home Cultures* 3 (2): 123–144.

Waring, Marilyn. 1999. *Counting for Nothing: What Men Value and What Women Are Worth*. Toronto: University of Toronto Press.

Wasem, Ruth Ellen. 2005. "US: Immigration Policy on Permanent Admissions." Congressional Research Service, the Library of Congress. Accessed October 27, 2005. http://www.ilw.com.

Waslin, Michel. 2009. "Immigration Policy and the Latino Community Since 9/11." In *Immigration Policy and Security. U.S., European, and Commonwealth Perspectives*, edited by Terri Givens, Gary P. Freeman and David L. Leal, 39–51. New York and London: Routledge.

Waters, Johanna. 2002. "Flexible Families? 'Astronaut' Households and the Experiences of Lone Mothers in Vancouver, British Columbia." *Social and Cultural Geography* 3 (2):117–134.

Weeks, Jeffrey, Brian Heaphy, and Catherine Donovan. 2001. *Same Sex Intimacies: Families of Choice and Other Life Experiments*. London: Routledge.

Weenink, Don. 2008. "Cosmopolitanism as a Form of Capital: Parents Preparing Their Children for a Globalized World." *Sociology* 46 (2): 1089–1106.

Weine, Stevan, Norma Ware, and Alma Klebic. 2004. "Converting Cultural Capital among Teen Refugees and Their Families from Bosnia-Herzegovina." *Psychiatric Services* 55 (8): 923–927.

Wellman, Barry. 1988. "Structural Analysis: From Method and Metaphor to Theory and Substance." In *Social Structures: A Network Approach*, edited by Barry Wellman and Stephen D. Berkowitz, 19–61. Cambridge: Cambridge University Press.

Werbner, Pnina. 1999. "Global Pathways. Working Class Cosmopolitans and the Creation of Transnational Ethnic Worlds." *Social Anthropology* 7 (1): 17–35.

White, Anne. 2011. *Polish Families and Migration Since EU Accession*. Bristol: The Policy Press.

Whitehead, Ann, and Iman Hashim. 2005. "Children and Migration." Background paper for DFID migration team. Accessed January 4, 2011. http://www.childtrafficking.com/Docs/dfid_05_child_mig_bac_0408.pdf.

Whitehouse, Bruce. 2009. "Transnational Childrearing and the Preservation of Transnational Identity in Brazzaville, Congo." *Global Networks* 9 (1): 82–99.

Widmer, Eric D. 2010. *Family Configurations. A Structural Approach to Family Diversity*. Farnham: Ashgate.

Widmer, Eric D., and Riitta Jallinoja. 2008. *Beyond the Nuclear Family. Families in a Configurational Perspective*. Bern: Peter Lang.

Widmer, Eric, Anna-Maija Castrén, Riitta Jallinoja, and Kaisa Ketokivi. 2008. "Introduction." In *Beyond the Nuclear Family: Families in a Configurational Perspective*, edited by Eric Widmer and Riitta Jallinoja, 1–11. Bern: Peter Lang.

Wilding, Raelene. 2006. " 'Virtual' Intimacies? Families' Communication Across Transnational Contexts." *Global Networks* 6: 125–142.

Wilding, Raelene, and Loretta Baldassar. 2009. "Transnational Family-Work Balance: Experiences of Australian Migrants Caring for Ageing Parents and Young Children Across Distance and Borders." *Journal of Family Studies* 15: 177–187.

Williams, Allan M., Russell King, Anthony Warnes, and Guy Patterson. 2000. "Tourism and International Retirement Migration: New Forms of an Old Relationship in Southern Europe"" *Tourism Geographies* 2 (1): 28–49.

Williams, Allan. 2007. "Listen to Me, Learn with Me: International Migration and Knowledge Transfer." *British Journal of Industrial Relations* 45(2): 361–382.

Williams, Fiona. 2010. "Migration and Care: Themes, Concepts and Challenges." *Social Policy and Society* 9 (3): 385–396.

———. 2004. *Rethinking Families*. London: Calouste Gulbenkian Foundation.

Williams, Fiona, and Anna Gavanas. 2008. "The Intersection of Child Care Regimes and Migration Regimes: A Three-Country Study." In *Migration and Domestic Work: A European Perspective on a Global Theme*, edited by Helma Lutz, 13–28. Ayeburry: Ashgate.

Wilson, Peter J. 1973. *Crab Antics: The Social Anthropology of English-Speaking Negro Societies of the Caribbean*. New Haven, CT: Yale University Press.

Wimmer, Andreas, and Nina Glick Schiller. 2002. "Methodological Nationalism and Beyond: Nation–State Building, Migration and the Social Sciences." *Global Networks* 2 (4): 301–334.

Yeates, Nicola. 2012. "Global Care Chains: A State-of-the-Art Review and Future Directions in Care Transnationalization Research." *Global Networks* 12 (2): 135–154.

———. 2009. *Globalizing Care Economies and Migrant Workers: Explorations in Global Care Chains*. Basingstoke: Palgrave Macmillan.

———. 2005a. *Global Care Chains: A Critical Introduction* (No. 44). Geneva: Global Commission on International Migration.

———. 2005b. "Global Care Chain: A Critical Introduction." *Global Migration Perspectives* 4: 1–19.

———. 2005c. "A Global Political Economy of Care." *Social Policy & Society* 4 (2): 227–234.

———. 2004. "Global Care Chains." *International Feminist Journal of Politics* 6 (3): 369–391.

Yeoh, Brenda S. A., Shirlena Huang, and Theodora Lam. 2005. "Transnationalizing the 'Asian' Family: Imaginaries, Intimacies and Strategic Intents." *Global Networks* 5 (4): 307–315.

Zechner, Minna. 2008. "Care of Older Persons in Transnational Settings." *Journal of Aging Studies* 22: 32–44.

Zelizer, Viviana A. 2005a. *The Purchase of Intimacy*. Princeton: Princeton University Press.

———. 2005b. "Circuits within Capitalism." In *The Economic Sociology of Capitalism*, edited by Victor Nee and Richard Swedberg, 289–322. Princeton: Princeton University Press.

———. 1989. "The Social Meaning of Money: 'Special Monies.' " *The American Journal of Sociology* 95: 342–377.

Zentgraf, Kristine M., and Norma Stoltz Chinchilla. 2012. "Transnational Family Separation: A Framework for Analysis." *Journal of Ethnic and Migration Studies* 38 (2): 345–366.

Zontini, Elisabetta. Forthcoming. 'Growing Old in a Transnational Social Field: Mobility, Identity and Belonging among Italian Migrants', *Ethnic and Racial Studies*.

———. 2012. "Care Arrangements of Elderly Transnational Migrants: Between Family, Community and the State." In *Critical Approaches to Care: Understanding Caring Relations, Identities and Cultures,* edited by Georgia Philip, Chrissie Rogers and Susie Weller, 171–182. London: Routledge.

———. 2010. "Enabling and Constraining Aspects of Social Capital in Migrant Families: Ethnicity, Gender and Generation. *Ethnic and Racial Studies* 33 (5): 816–831.

———. 2007. "Transnational Families." In *Sloan Network Encyclopedia*. Sloan Work and Family Research Network.

———. 2006. "Italian Families and Social Capital: Care Provision in a Transnational World." *Community, Work and Family* 9 (3): 325–345.

———. 2004a. "Immigrant Women in Barcelona: Coping With the Consequences of Transnational Lives." *Journal of Ethnic and Migration Studies* 30: 1113–1144.

———. 2004b. "Italian Families and Social Capital: Rituals and the Provision of Care in British-Italian Transnational Families." Working Paper Series 6, Families and Social Capital ESRC Research Group, London South Bank University.

Zontini, Elisabetta, and Tracey Reynolds. 2007. "Ethnicity, Families and Social Capital: Caring Relationships Across Italian and Caribbean Transnational Families." *International Review of Sociology/ Revue Internationale de Sociologie* 17 (2): 257–277.

# Contributors

**Marina Ariza** is Professor at the Instituto de Investigaciones Sociales, Universidad Autónoma de México. Her main areas of research expertise include female migration, family, gender, urban labor markets, demographic processes and methodological reflection. Marina's main publications refer to Dominican (*Ya no soy la que dejé atrás. . . . Mujeres migrantes en República Dominicana*, UNAM–IIS/ Plaza y Valdés, 2000) and Mexican international migration (*El País Transnacional: Migración mexicana y cambio social a través de la frontera*, UNAM–IIS, 2007, reprinted in 2010, coedited with Alejandro Portes); family sociodemographic transformations (*Imágenes de la familia en el cambio de siglo*, UNAM–IIS, 2004, coedited with Orlandina de Oliveira); and, more recently, methodological issues in migration research (*Métodos cualitativos y su aplicación empírica. Por los caminos de la investigación sobre migración internacional*, UNAM–COLEF, 2012, coedited with Laura Velasco). Her current research project involves a comparative analysis of female labour markets and family dynamics between Dominican and Mexican immigrants living in Madrid and New York. During 2012, she was awarded the *Sor Juan Inés de la Cruz* distinction for her academic achievements.

**Loretta Baldassar** is Professor in the Department of Anthropology and Sociology at the University of Western Australia and Adjunct Principal Research Fellow, School of Political and Social Inquiry, Monash University. Loretta has published extensively on transnational migrants, families and caregiving, including *Families Caring Across Borders* (with Baldock and Wilding, Palgrave, 2007) and *Intimacy and Italian Migration* (edited with Gabaccia, Fordham University Press, 2011), as well as more than 20 journal articles and book chapters on this subject. She has extensively researched and written about Italian migration to Australia, including the award-winning books *Visits Home* (Melbourne University Press, 2001) and *From Paesani to Global Italians* (with Pesman, University Western Australia Publishing, 2005). Loretta served a term as Director at the Monash Centre in Prato, Italy, from 2009 to 2011, where she began new research projects on second-generation migrants in Italy and student study abroad and internationalisation in the academy. She is currently working on three volumes: *China in the World: Migration, Integration, Diaspora Formations and Transnational Linkages* (with Kee, McGill Queen's Press, Forthcoming), *Conflicting Identities: Refugee Protection and the Role of Law* (with Kneebone and Stevens, Routledge, Forthcoming) and *Chinese Migrants in Prato* (with Johanson, McAuliffe and Bressan).

**Paolo Boccagni** is Lecturer at the Department of Sociology and Social Research, University of Trento. His main areas of work are migration studies, social welfare, transnationalism and qualitative research. His recent fieldwork experiences have involved migrants' patterns of integration and transnational participation, as well as issues related to migration and well-being, ethnocultural diversity and social remittances. He has published extensively on transnational family life, care migration, political transnationalism and the migration-development nexus. His publications include articles in *Journal of Ethnic and Migration Studies, International Journal of Social Welfare, European Journal of Social Theory, Qualitative Research* and *Global Networks*.

**Claudio Bolzman** is Professor at the Graduate School of Social Work, University of Applied Sciences Western Switzerland (HES-SO), and at the Department of Sociology, University of Geneva. He leads the Research Centre on Cultural Diversity and Citizenship (CEDIC) at the HES-SO. From 2002 to 2007, he was the General Secretary of the International Association for Intercultural Research (ARIC). His main research areas are migrations, migrations policies, transnational families, life course and intergenerational relations. He is the author or coauthor of fourteen books and more than eighty papers in collective books and peer-reviewed journals about these issues. His recent publications include articles in *International Migration*, *European Journal of Social Work* and *Retraite et société* (*Retirement and Society*).

**Paola Bonizzoni** is Lecturer at the Department of Social and Political Sciences of the University of Milan. She completed a PhD in sociology with a thesis on Latin American family reunification and transnational family life. She has taken part in several international research projects on female migration, family reunification and domestic work, and she has recently coordinated research on second-generation and reunified immigrant youth's integration pathways. She has published in national and international journals with a specific focus on transnationalism and family reunification.

**Anuja Cabraal** is Research Fellow at RMIT University. Her main areas of research are social exclusion, financial exclusion, microfinance, migration and mobility and the Indian diaspora in Australia. She has done extensive work in the area of social and financial exclusion in Australia examined through the lens of microfinance and capabilities. Anuja also has an interest in research methods and provides training and advice to other academics on research methods and qualitative analysis.

**Karen Fog Olwig** is Professor at the Department of Anthropology, University of Copenhagen. She has published extensively on Caribbean migration with a particular focus on the significance of family networks in migration processes. Her particular interests have been generational relations, the mobility of children and social practices of relatedness within the context of migration. Recent publications include *Caribbean Journeys: An Ethnography of Migration and Home in Three Family Networks* (Durham, NC: Duke University Press, 2007), and *"Integration"—Migrants and Refugees between Scandinavian Welfare Societies and Family Relations*, special issue of *Journal of Ethnic and Migration Studies*, 2011, edited with B. R. Larsen and M. Rytter.

**Asuncion Fresnoza-Flot** is FNRS Postdoctoral Researcher at the Interdisciplinary Research Center on Families and Sexualities (CIRFASE) at the Catholic University of Louvain, Belgium. She is also affiliated with the Unité de Recherches "Migrations et Société" (URMIS) at the University Paris Diderot–Paris 7 (France). Her research interests mainly focus on transnational families and childhood in the migration context. Her most recent articles are published in *Global Networks* (2009), the *Asia Pacific Journal of Anthropology* (2010), *Cahiers du Genre* (2011) and *Migrations Santé* (2012). She also published two book chapters in *Diasporic Journeys, Ritual, and Normativity among Asian Migrant Women* (Eds. P. Werbner and M. Johnson, Routledge, 2011) and *Human Security: Securing East Asia's Future* (Ed. B. T. C. Guan, Springer, 2012).

**Majella Kilkey** is Senior Lecturer in the Department of Sociological Studies at the University of Sheffield, UK. She researches in the field of family social policy, particularly from a comparative cross-national perspective, and making strong disciplinary links to sociology. Her current research interrogates family policies and practices through the lens of migration. Recent publications include *Gender, Migration and Domestic Work: Masculinities, Male Labour and Fathering in the UK and USA* (with Diane Perrons, Ania Plomien, Pierrette Hondagneu-Sotelo and Hernan Ramirez, Palgrave 2013), and articles in *Global Networks*, *International Migration*, *Men and Masculinities*, *Social Policy and Society*, *Time and Society*, *Feminist Economics*, *Community, Work and Families* and *European Urban and Regional Studies*. With Helma Lutz and Ewa Palenga-Möllenbeck, she edited the 2010 special issue *Domestic and Care Work at the Intersection of Welfare, Gender and Migration Regimes: European Experiences* (*Social Policy and Society*, 9:3).

**Valentina Mazzucato** is Professor of Globalization and Development at Maastricht University, the Netherlands. She heads several international research projects on transnational families with specific reference to caregiving arrangements (www.tcra.nl) financed by the Netherlands Organization for Scientific Research (NWO) and NORFACE. Some of her latest publications appear in *Journal of Marriage and Family* (73, 4, 2011), *Population Space and Place* (2010; 10, 2004), *Global Networks* (9, 2, 2009), *World Development* (2009), and book chapters in *The Encyclopedia of Global Human Migration* (Blackwell, 2012), *Multi-sited Ethnography: Theory, Praxis and Locality in Contemporary Social Research* (Ashgate, 2009), *Migration and Development Within and Across Borders* (IOM, 2009) and *Globalization and Development: Themes and Concepts in Current Research* (Kluwer Academic Publishers, 2004). Professor Mazzucato is regularly invited to speak in public fora on the effects of transnational lives for development in Africa and migrant integration in Europe. She has lived in and conducted research on numerous African countries in the past twenty years.

**Laura Merla** is Sociologist and Deputy Director of the Interdisciplinary Research Centre on Families and Sexualities (CIRFASE) at the Catholic University of Louvain, Belgium. She studied political sciences at the Université libre de Bruxelles (Belgium) and completed a PhD in sociology at the Université catholique de Louvain (Belgium, 2006). Over the last five years, she has conducted research on Latin American transnational families in Europe and Australia funded by the European Commission, the Belgian National Funds for Research and the Belgian Science Policy. Her current research project examines the interplay between intrafamilial dynamics and the exchange of care between adult Latin American migrants and their parents. Laura is an active member of several international networks, such as the International Sociological Association, the Imiscoe Research Network and the Transnational Lives, Mobilities and Gender Network. Laura's recent publications on transnational families include a special issue of the journal *Recherches sociologiques et anthropologiques* Vol. 41(1) (coedited with Loretta Baldassar), two papers published in the journals *Autrepart* Vol. 57–58 and *International Migration* (published online), three forthcoming papers in *Global Networks* and *Cahiers Genre et Développement*, and a forthcoming book, *Transnational Family Solidarity in Local Contexts,* published by Routledge.

**Miranda Poeze** is a PhD candidate at the Maastricht University. Her current research focuses on Ghanaian transnational families in the context of parental migration. Through qualitative research in both Ghana and the Netherlands, she assesses how caregiving relationships and parenthood configurations adapt to the migration context and how this is experienced by both the migrant parents as well as the left-behind children.

In addition, she focuses on the role of gender and migration policies in shaping these relationships. This research is embedded in the 'Transnational Child-Raising Arrangements (TCRA)' research project, which applies a multi-sited and mixed-method approach in order to assess the impact of international migration on different actors in the transnational caregiving arrangement.

**Tracey Reynolds** is Reader in Social and Policy Research in the Weeks Centre for Social and Policy Research, London South Bank University, UK. Tracey's research interests include Caribbean families and kinship networks; youth and transnational identities; parenting and child rearing and women in the labour market and have led to several publications in these areas. Journal articles include 'Exploring the Absent/Present Dilemma: Black Fathers, Family Relationships and Social Capital in Britain', *The Annals of the American Academy of Political and Social Science* (2009); 'Caribbean Second Generation Return Migration: Identities, Transnational Family Relationships and "Left Behind" Kin in Britain', *Mobilities* (2011); and '"Them and Us": "Black Neighbourhoods" as a Social Capital Resource among Black Youths Living in Inner-City London, U.K', *Urban Studies* (2013). She is also the author of *Caribbean Mothers: Identity and Experience in the UK* (Tufnell Press, 2005). Her most recent publication is a coauthored book, *Transational Families: Ethnicities, Identities and Social Capital*, with Harry Goulbourne, John Solomos and Elisabetta Zontini, (published by Routledge, 2010).

**Supriya Singh** is Professor, Sociology of Communications, RMIT University. Her research interests are in the social shaping of money and banking, the Indian diaspora in Australia, the user-centred design of information and communication technologies and qualitative research. She is currently a senior project leader with the Smart Services Cooperative Research Centre and Program Leader for the Community, Migration and Development Program of the Global Cities Research Institute at RMIT University. Her books include *Migration, Belonging and the Nation State* (Cambridge Scholars Publishing, 2010, with Alperhan Babacan as first editor); *Marriage Money: The Social Shaping of Money and Banking* (Allen & Unwin, 1997); *The Bankers; Australia's Leading Bankers Talk about Banking Today (*Allen & Unwin, 1991); *Bank Negara Malaysia: The First 25 Years, 1959–1984* (Bank Negara Malaysia, 1984); and *On the Sulu Sea* (Angsana Publications, 1984). Her forthcoming book with Rowman & Littlefield is *Globalization and Money: A Global South Perspective.*

**Karin Wall** is Director of Research and Professor of Sociology of Families at the Institute for Social Sciences at the University of Lisbon (ICS-UL). She coordinates the Observatory on Families and Family Policies at

ICS and has worked since 1995 as an expert on family policies for the European Commission and the Council of Europe. Her research focuses on family and care policies in Europe, family forms and interactions, family and the life course, immigrant families, gender and the conjugal divisions of paid and unpaid work. She is currently working on a cross-national study of family trajectories and social networks across three generations, involving both quantitative and qualitative methods. She is also conducting comparative research on parental leave policies, men's changing roles and identities in family life, migrant families and the policies and practices of care for young children and elderly persons. Previous publications on families and migration include: 'Immigration, Welfare and Care in Portugal: Mapping the New Plurality of Female Migration Trajectories', *Social Policy and Society* (2010); 'Immigrant families', *Blackwell Encyclopedia of Sociology* (2007); and 'Managing Work and Care: A Difficult Challenge for Immigrant Families', *Social policy and Administration* (2004).

**Raelene Wilding** is Senior Lecturer in Sociology at La Trobe University, Melbourne. Her research uses qualitative methods to investigate identities and relationships in a mobile world, with specific attention to the roles new communication technologies play in transforming intimate relations. Her most recent project examines the potential for digital media artforms and practices to create local and global sites of belonging for young people from refugee backgrounds in Australia. Her books include *Families Caring Across Borders* (with Loretta Baldassar and Cora Baldock, Palgrave 2007) and *Race and Ethnic Relations* (with Farida Fozdar and Mary Hawkins, Oxford University Press, 2009), and she has also published in numerous journals, including *Global Networks, Journal of Sociology, Journal of Ethnic and Migration Studies* and *Continuum.*

**Elisabetta Zontini** is Associate Professor in Sociology in the School of Sociology and Social Policy at the University of Nottingham. Previously, she was a Visiting Fellow at the International Gender Studies Centre at Oxford University and Research Fellow in the Families and Social Capital ESRC Research Group at London South Bank University. She has conducted ethnographic research in the areas of gender and migration and transnational families in Italy, Spain and the United Kingdom, and she has published extensively in these areas. She is the author of *Transnational Families, Migration and Gender: Moroccan and Filipino Women in Bologna and Barcelona* (Berghahn Books) and *Transnational Families: Ethnicities, Identities and Social Capital* (with Harry Goulbourne, John Solomos and Tracey Reynolds, Routledge). She is currently working on the experiences of ageing of transnational migrants and the issues of identity and belonging of transnational and diasporic youth (with Tracey Reynolds).

# Index